Medical Records In Health Information

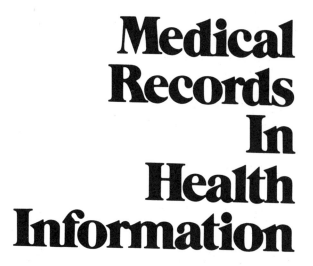

Kathleen A. Waters, RRA, M.Ed.
Associate Professor
Health Information Services
Seattle University

Gretchen Frederick Murphy, RRA, M.Ed.
Assistant Professor
Health Information Services
Seattle University

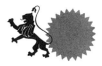

ASPEN SYSTEMS CORPORATION
Germantown, Maryland
London, England

1979

Library of Congress Cataloging in Publication Data

Waters, Kathleen A.
Medical records in health information.

Includes bibliographies and index.

1. Medical Records.   I. Murphy, Gretchen Frederick,
joint author.   II. Title.
R864.W37   651.5   79-18793
ISBN 0-89443-157-9

Copyright © 1979 by Aspen Systems Corporation

Library of Congress Catalog Card Number: 79-18793
ISBN: 0-89443-157-9

Printed in the United States of America

1 2 3 4 5

With respect, gratitude, and
active commitment to continue
the development of students in
the medical record profession
this book is dedicated to
Sister Marie Blanche Comeau, S.P.

Table of Contents

Preface

Health information in its many aspects is a subject that concerns every individual sometime during life. We recognize this from our own health experiences and more importantly from our professional work and teaching experience. We find teaching this fascinating and challenging subject to students of medical record administration a renewed source of interest as well as continued learning. Years of work and teaching experience have not tarnished our interest. In fact, we are continually encouraged to recognize and respond to the ever dynamic nature of health information—its technology, theory, and practice—so that our students and others will continue to develop this vehicle for its many uses and users.

The twentieth century has been a time of major changes in the conquest of disease, development of new technology for medical care, methods of preventing illness and disability, and in many other major discoveries and developments that have contributed enormously to better health. For some, the development of health or medical data into a useful record through completion of seemingly routine and dull methods seems vastly removed from the more publicly acclaimed medical discoveries and innovations of this century. At the record development stage, some providers and users of health care actually consider many tasks simply a matter of annoying compliance with a rule or regulation imposed by some known but unseen agency or regulatory commission.

For others, those of us who have participated firsthand in patient care through use of documented data, the development of the medical record is a stimulating and singularly rewarding experience. Daily, we are reminded of the direct link between development of data at all stages, and the life-preserving discoveries in diagnostic and therapeutic medicine.

We are afforded this continuous, firsthand reminder because of our opportunities to make complete, accurate, and useful records available in circumstances that may include the following critical situations:

- an emergency room physician treating an unknown, unconscious patient whose previous record outlines critical drug and allergy data

- a list of patients' names, addresses, and dates of primary care for the past ten months, for use by an epidemiologist studying a new, undiagnosed and serious disease outbreak

- a bar chart that points out an alarming outbreak of nosocomial infections over a three-month period for four physically separate care units in an acute care teaching hospital.

The opportunity to experience the indisputable link between development of the medical record and the continuing development of new and outstanding care methods is also available to medical records professionals who, for example, may work in such nontraditional sites as ambulatory care facilities, health planning agencies, health insurance companies, and medical record consulting firms in mental health, drug and alcohol, prison, and private practice areas. For all medical record practitioners there is inevitable assurance that our professional endeavors are integral to the full cycle that represents successful patient care and research.

It is our intent that this book be used by all those who are interested in learning about medical records and health information. All students of the allied health professions, consumers, medical and other professionals currently employed, users and providers of health care data—potential patients all—are those we hope will find a useful source of information in this book. The content follows a sequence of questions that answer such queries as what, when, where, how, and who. Answers are the people, events, methods, sites, reasons, and needs for developing and retrieving health information in its many formats. Each chapter has a list of objectives that identify what will be covered. References are available at the end of the chapters for related material on the subjects covered, and a glossary of terms is provided at the end of the book.

Acknowledgments

We are grateful to our former students who patiently helped in the development of this book. We sincerely express our appreciation to our current students, Kathy Brosnan, Tony Pizzuto, Brigitte Predel, and Joyce Rowe, who assisted in the preparation of the final manuscript. Robert Ellis, of the Lemieux Library, cheerfully provided research material and gave us excellent assistance. Sue Potter was the mainstay of all stages of manuscript development. The following medical record professionals contributed material and graciously assisted when asked: Ardis Alfrey, RRA; Joan Andenes, RRA; Emma Andersen, RRA; Harold Brown, RRA; Candace Dillman, RRA; Bill French, RRA; Mary Alice Hanken, RRA; Elaine Patrikas, RRA; Susan Stubbs, RRA; and Linda Weiland, RRA. Three reviewers who assisted immensely in refining the original manuscript are Shirley Anderson, RRA, Carole C. Johnson, ART, and Joyce E. Gormley, RRA.

Marsha Steele, RRA, is especially acknowledged for her creative illustrations throughout and for her contribution to the management resources in Chapter 8.

Chapter 1

Focusing on Medical Records in Health Care

CHAPTER OBJECTIVES

1. Identify the components of the health care delivery system
2. Recognize that patient information is inseparable from the patient
3. Relate the elements of confidentiality and continuity of recorded information to satisfactory health care
4. Relate the roles of patients, medical and allied health professionals, and organizations to the functions of recording and using health information
5. Cite various uses of recorded health information
6. Identify various job opportunities in medical record administration

THE ENVIRONMENT OF HEALTH CARE

Concepts of Health Care

How do you take care of yourself? There are as many answers to that question as there are readers of this text. Well, then, let's make the question clearer. What has been done for you or what have you done for yourself that contributes to your personal health care? Probably you brush your teeth every day. Maybe you avoid eating fatty foods. Chances are that you can remember at least one time in your life when you needed some medical or health-related attention. It may have been as simple as a vaccination in grade school or a sling applied to a broken arm in the local hospital emergency room. In each of these cases, there was a record made of what took place. You probably did not hear about that. It's almost 100 percent sure that you did not see the record or any activity involved in its development.

Because this book is about medical records, the introduction on health care will not discuss completely all facets of health care delivery. This section can be considered a framework on which we will build a thorough body of information about our major topic—medical records.

The World Health Organization (WHO) defines *health* as "the state of complete physical, mental and social well-being and not merely the absence of disease or infirmity." Other definitions of the word *health* include Webster's, which is "the condition of being sound in body, mind, or soul; especially: freedom from physical disease or pain." During the inevitable human experience of absence of health, new words appear. How many can you think of? Does your list include sick, down and out, disease, illness, pain, tension, a trip, high, paralyzed, terminal? Your list probably includes many not mentioned here.

To relieve, restore, preserve, comfort, heal—all of these words and many others are variously used to describe the act of providing health care. There are other technical terms that are used by professional health care providers, but the concept conveyed by health care is the act of healing.

This concept is as old as mankind. Ancient civilizations in all parts of the world and ancient tribes, too, were actively involved in health care. Today, computers and microfilm as well as paper are used to record the many components of health care. Recording is not new either.

The details of health care given to one individual were recorded and preserved by early man. Hieroglyphs and drawings on caves provide modern man with a detailed record of early health care. Papyrus and other early precursors of paper are also available to point out the importance early health care providers gave to recording what they knew and did about disease and patient care.

Historically as well as currently, then, documentation of health care is an essential function in the provision of that care. It provides a current record of what is done for an individual patient. Future use of the recorded information is equally important. As a memory device for those who will treat the patient in the future, the record has no equal. As a focus for research, individual or collective medical records can provide selected information that is not available from any other source.

Healing and recording, then, are two components of health care. There are many books and articles describing the other components and complexities of health care, but we will limit this discussion to the facets that most directly relate to medical records.

There are basically two kinds of health care: self-administered care and care provided at the direction of or by someone else. Most of us do not call a doctor when we have a headache. Some of us never call a doctor no matter what the pain might be. Others call the doctor as soon as they feel a mere twinge of pain or nervousness. Health care, as most of us know it, is self-directed. We seek care when we decide to. You may already know this. However, there is another concept related to this one that possibly you've not thought or heard.

Our ability to seek care when and where we choose leads to fragmented health care. Information about our care and treatment becomes scattered and separated. The surgeon has information about my appendectomy and the physician at the ski resort clinic knows all about my broken ankle. Neither the surgeon nor the ski resort clinic knows that I've been treated for an allergy by the physician who cares for the employees of the company where I work. Such a gap in the flow of information causes delays in care, creates danger for the patient, and increases the cost of health care.

This example is relatively straightforward compared with other examples of health care problems. Providing health care is complex because it involves people interacting with other people under an extraordinary number of circumstances during times of physical and emotional stress. Providers, those who treat patients or those indirectly involved in the treatment of patients, must maintain high ethical and professional standards and meet patients under numerous trying circumstances due to the very nature of illness and its physical and emotional aspects. Users, those who need professional health care and treatment, are similarly encumbered in their encounters with the providers. People, institutions, directions, medications, money, transportation, information, pain, adjustment, stamina, patience—all are part of the interaction of persons involved in health care.

The evolution of health care in this country was, for the most part, a natural, undirected process. Early in our country's history, the most familiar medical practitioner was the family doctor. In urban or rural settings, the family doctor practiced medicine out of his little black bag, and hospitals were generally thought of as the first step on the way to the cemetery. To many people, hospitals were the place their relatives went to die. Data were not available to determine public health needs and disease trends, to plan health care facilities by geographic location and population, or to study the causes of disease and promotion of health. Physicians and hospitals were the major providers and did the best they could with the available data, facilities, and educational programs.

In the early years of our country, many people never moved from the area of their birth. In fact, many lived and died in the town where they were born. Others, though they moved sometime during their life, did so infrequently. The physicians who treated this relatively stable population did so with a heavy emphasis on first-hand knowledge of their patients. Oftentimes the physician and patient were neighbors or at least inhabitants of a town or area that was not so large that it had many strangers living there. Physicians were able to treat their patients from a first-hand knowledge of the person's habits and past illnesses, along with information gathered by means of the usual human grapevine. Needless to say, a physician who at any minute might have to jump in a buggy and visit a patient hardly had time to be fully concerned with recording pertinent information. The original office records of doctors were skimpy and limited to those that were of value to the physician or to someone else who might need them in the physician's absence. Dictating machines were not available, standard formats had not been developed for keeping handwritten records, and the physician depended largely on memory for patient information. Patients were not being taught to involve themselves actively in their own health care. They relied almost completely on the advice of the physician or in some cases on the use of family remedies or folk medicine.

Twentieth-Century Direction in Health Care

During the twentieth century, health care underwent many major changes. Two changes are pertinent to our discussion: hospitals became far more active in the provision of care, and physicians became more cognizant of the need for documenting patient care. As hospitals became increasingly responsive to the needs of patients, other elements came into existence—elements related to identifying and determining standards for acceptable patient care.

The American College of Surgeons was formed in 1913, and one of its objectives was to improve standards for surgery. As one basis for training its surgeons, the college determined that work being carried out by surgeons must be evaluated. They required that candidates for fellowship in the college must submit 50 complete copies and 50 abstracts of case records of patients who had undergone major surgical procedures performed by the candidate. However, it was soon discovered that the records kept by the surgeons in their offices and the records made in the course of business by the hospitals did not contain enough information to fulfill the college's case record requirement. During the first on-site inspection of over 1,000 hospital beds in 1918, the college found only 89 of a total of 700 hospitals met the minimum standards established by the college. Recognizing a need for improvement in such areas as adequate patient care, proof of care, and medical research, a minimum requirement for hospital standardization was determined to be "that accurate and complete case records be written for all patients and filed in an accessible manner in the hospital." Hospital standardization, then, was also a development fostered by the American College of Surgeons. These two objectives—improved documentation of surgical care as a measure of the quality of that care and standardization of hospitals for the purpose of establishing a baseline guide to minimum performance—were two of the most significant indicators of what would come in American health care during the remainder of the twentieth century. They were forerunners of certification, utilization review, medical audit, health care review, professional standards review, reimbursement, continuing education, and accreditation, to name a few.

Because of the scope of the standardization program and the growth of professional organizations capable of and responsible for quality hospital programs, in 1952 the Joint Commission on Accreditation of Hospitals (JCAH) was organized. It took over the enormously effective and far-reaching standardization movement started by the American College of Surgeons. The commission is composed of 20 members appointed by the following four organizations: American Medical Association (seven members), American Hospital Association (seven members), American College of Surgeons (three members), and American College of Physicians (three members). The JCAH is incorporated in the State of Illinois as a not-for-profit corporation. A wide variety of services provided to patients in hospitals is demonstrated by the representatives of the organizations that make up the joint commission. The original purpose of this organization was to accredit hospitals as one proof that they met optimal standards established by the commission. Such accreditation is sought voluntarily by hospitals. Accreditation can assure patients that they will receive care in a facility that has met standards established by the organizations that comprise the commission. Hospitals that are accredited usually display a certificate verifying this status in a conspicuous place. Informed patient-consumers now seek such notification when looking for a hospital in which to receive treatment.

In 1969 the JCAH began to develop accreditation councils for other types of services, including: mentally retarded and other developmentally disabled persons, 1969; psychiatric facilities, 1970; and long-term care facilities, 1971. The purpose of the ambulatory health care program established in 1975 is to develop standards and survey procedures for ambulatory health care and to administer an accreditation program for qualified settings that voluntarily seek to be accredited. Original charter member organizations working with ambulatory health care were American Group Practice Association, American Hospital Association, American Medical Association, Group Health Association of America, and Medical Group Management Association. In 1978 the JCAH reorganized and retained the accreditation services under the title of programs while dissolving the companion councils. The councils were replaced with professional and technical advisory committees on standards and accreditation processes. The committees are comprised of individuals and organizations having specialized knowledge in each area of accreditation, as well as organizations or agencies that express an interest in joining the committees and that qualify for membership.

Currently, approximately 7,300 facilities, services, and programs hold JCAH accreditation. This is impressive when one considers that the accreditation programs of the joint commission survey over 4,500 facilities, services, and programs each year.

The JCAH publishes a manual for hospitals that request accreditation. This document outlines current requirements and is published annually in August. Initiated in 1978, the manual replaces other JCAH standards publications and helps facilities prepare for JCAH surveys. It is updated each year to provide the most current standards and requirements.

A major influence on the delivery of health care in our country is the federal government. This is particularly true in its many legislated programs. Exhibit 1-1 lists those federal agencies that are best known and most highly visible among health care professionals.

COMPONENTS OF HEALTH CARE DELIVERY

Health Care Delivery System

Basically, but not simply, health care is organized by a cooperative and sometimes coordinated effort of people, institutions, agencies, and organizations. Because of this, the word *system* is a euphemism when applied to the description of health care delivery. *System* has been defined as related elements interacting to form a unit or unified whole. Health care delivery today is a set of separate, related, but essentially nonunified activities that do not all work toward a single purpose. There is a decided lack of coordination and direction in health care delivery. This lack of system is, of course, not intentional. On the contrary, almost every individual or organization participating in the delivery of care has a serious commitment to work for a more unified structure so that a true system of health care can be realized. This effort will take considerable time and must begin with the planners who represent the providers and users. The planning must be a coordinated provider-user project, and objectives must be jointly established. Obviously, in our free enterprise system, with its traditional attitudes about medicine, belief in freedom of choice, and the existence of well-established health care institutions, facilities, and organizations, such a planning effort would be a monumental undertaking. Without retrenching and regrouping, however, we may never see the establishment of a true system of health care delivery. A system that is person- and family-centered, carried out by professional, technical, and vocational personnel using facilities and equipment that are physically and functionally related, delivering effective service at a cost economically compatible with individual, family, community, and national resources, seems utopian. Unless such a goal is kept before us, we will never make an effort to achieve it.

In this section we will describe in some detail those components of health care delivery that are most closely related to medical recordkeeping. There are other components, too. Perhaps the following list will serve as a reference for related readings on health care delivery:

1. Population characteristics and users
2. Technology
3. Disease trends
4. Government programs and regulations
5. Manpower
6. Finances
7. Licensing and accreditation

You may have noticed that no information component is listed. This is not an oversight, but a reflection of reality and fact. The information component of health care, while not developed as a separate entity, is an essential element of all other components of delivery. For instance, information is most easily identified in the form of patient care documentation. It can also be seen in the form of reporting used in such diverse federal programs as Medicare and the Professional Standards Review Organization (PSRO). Again, these two forms of information processing lack the characteristics of a system—not directed, not coordinated, not part of a unified whole—and only partially fit the definition of information, which is the communication of knowledge or intelligence. Another definition of information that is more appropriate for our purposes is facts, or data. A health information system will be discussed in detail in Chapter 8. If we had an information component that fit the definition of a system and satisfied the definition of information, too, what do you think it would be? Could such a component be developed? Your answer to the first question probably indicates the realistic possibility of developing such a component, if your definition includes elements such as computerization, linked data, limited access, information management, and confidentiality. The bulk of this book will be devoted, of course, to information as patient care documentation. As such, many elements in your definition of an information component of

Exhibit 1-1 Major Organizational Statutory Programs in the United States

Organizational Entity	Method	Legal Authorization
Hill-Burton State Hospital Planning Agencies	Planning and coordination; hospital services; statewide; voluntary	Federal Public Health Service Act, Amendments for Hospital Survey and Construction, 1946 (1949, 1954, 1961, 1964, 1967, 1970)
Regional Medical Programs (RMP)	Planning and coordination; primary and specialized services; regional institutional and noninstitutional providers; voluntary	Public Health Service Act, Heart Disease, Cancer, and Stroke Amendments of 1965 (1968, 1970)
Area Health Education Activities (AHEA)	Planning and coordination; areawide training; voluntary	Public Health Service Act amendments as above
Area Health Education Centers (AHEC)	As above	Public Health Service Act, Comprehensive Health Manpower Training Act of 1971
Experimental Health Services Delivery Systems (EHSDS)	Planning and coordination; areawide services delivery; all provider types; voluntary	Public Health Service Act, Partnership for Health Amendments of 1967 (establishing National Center for Health Services Research and Development)
Experimental Medical Care Review Organization (EMCRO)	Evaluation of quality of services; areawide; all provider types	As above
Comprehensive Health Planning Agencies; state (A agencies), areawide (B agencies)	Planning and coordination; state and areawide; primarily institutional services, authorized to plan for services, facilities, personnel; voluntary	Public Health Service Act, Comprehensive Health Planning Amendments of 1966 (1967, 1970)

with certification of need authority as Designated Plan Agencies (DPA)	Capital expenditures control over institutional facilities for changes above a given dollar amount; mandatory Capital expenditures control over providers receiving federal financing for Medicare, Medicaid, or maternal and child health services over program revisions of $100,000 or more for facilities/equipment; mandatory	State certification of need laws in 20 states Federal Social Security Act, Amendments of 1972, Sec. 1122
Utilization Review (UR)	Peer review; institutional services of providers receiving federal financing for Medicare and Medicaid services; mandatory	Social Security Amendments of 1965 (Medicare); 1967
State agency sample-resurvey of JCAH-approved hospital	Certification review of Medicare-approved hospitals; mandatory	Social Security Amendments of 1972
Professional Standards Review Organizations (PSRO)	Claims review; institutional and noninstitutional services of providers under Medicare, Medicaid, maternal and child health services financing; mandatory	Social Security Amendments of 1972

Sources: *Compilation of Selected Public Health Laws*, vol. 1 (Washington, D.C.: Government Printing Office, 1971). Comptroller General of the United States, *Study of Health Facilities Construction Costs* (Washington, D.C.: Government Printing Office, 1972). W. Curran, *National Survey and Analysis of Certificate-of-Need Laws, 1972* (Chicago: American Hospital Association, 1973). National Center for Health Law, *Health Planning Memorandum* (Washington, D.C.: U.S. Department of Health, Education, and Welfare, February 1973).

health care delivery will be thoroughly explored as we move through other chapters.

Patient Information Is Inseparable from the Patient

Before we dig into the various parts of health care delivery, let's take a special look at the patient and the record. Some questions should help put these into perspective. How do you differ from information about you? Are the facts that describe your individual characteristics distinct from you and those characteristics? Let's be more specific. Is the information that your blood type is A, that you were treated for pneumonia at the age of 13, and that you are currently under the care of an ear, nose, and throat specialist for upper respiratory infection and severe allergies, separate and distinct from you—your mind and body—in other words, separate from yourself? It is difficult, under the best of circumstances, to distinguish the patient from the information necessary to the care and treatment of that patient. We can describe a patient in many ways, according to many needs, according to many characteristics, yet in so doing we will inevitably compile a set of information inseparable from a particular individual. We can also compile a set of facts that, when applied to a particular patient, will describe the condition and care or treatment of that patient at a specific time. From our point of view, it is impossible to separate the patient from the patient's medical record. There is, of course, the obvious physical separateness of the two, but this is of small importance when one considers the overwhelming significance of the unity of the patient and the recorded information that describes exclusively the health care of that patient.

Relationship of Those Who Compile Patient Information to the Information Itself

Related to this concept of the unity of the patient and the record is the relationship between those who compile the patient's information and the information itself. An amazing number of people and organizations directly transmit information that is part of a patient's record.

Figure 1-1 depicts some persons who have direct and indirect contact with the patient and the patient's record.

Continuity and Confidentiality

With so many people interacting in the compilation of information about individual patients, there is a tendency for providers to overlook that unique and singular relationship of patient to information. For medical record

Figure 1-1 Direct and Indirect Impacts on the Patient Record

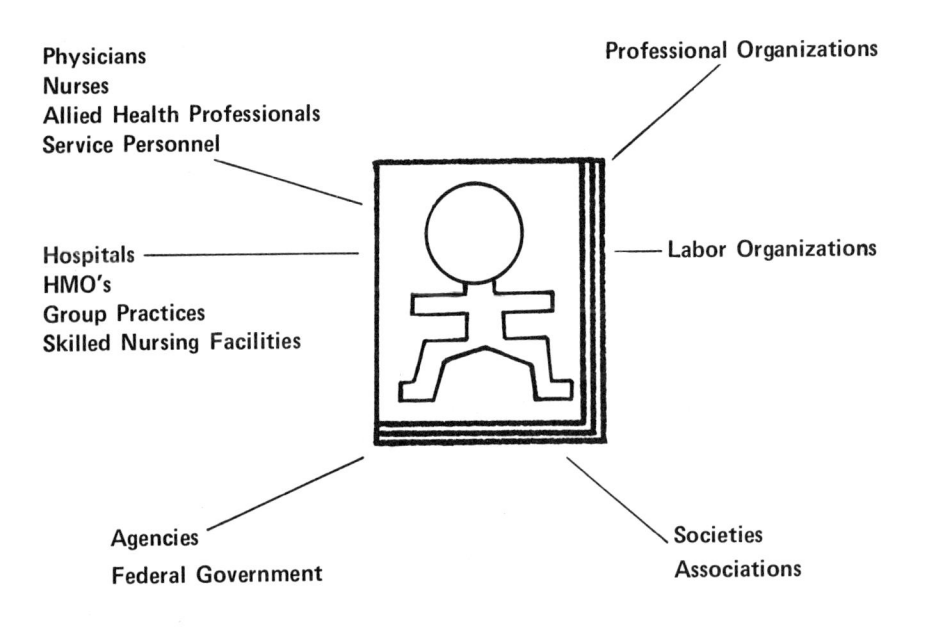

Physicians
Nurses
Allied Health Professionals
Service Personnel

Professional Organizations

Hospitals
HMO's
Group Practices
Skilled Nursing Facilities

Labor Organizations

Agencies
Federal Government

Societies
Associations

professionals, it is imperative that they develop a sense of prime responsibility for the information that identifies and describes a particular patient. Such a concern must be demonstrated in the course of developing or managing a health information system. Continuity and confidentiality of data are two essential elements of recorded information. Uniqueness of the record is centered in its unity with the patient. Continuity of events, physical characteristics, and identifying psychosocial characteristics are indistinguishable from the patient in whose record they are described, and when properly ordered, these data represent an individual as vividly as a photograph. Privacy, too, is an inherent right of a patient. One cannot separate the privacy of information from the privacy of the person to whom it relates. Because of their unique characteristics, continuity and confidentiality (privacy) share equal billing with the recording of all patient information as inseparable, unique patient extenders. Recording information about a patient brings into being an extension of that patient. Once the information is recorded, another source of information exists apart from the patient.

Figure 1-2 Patient and Information Are Inseparable

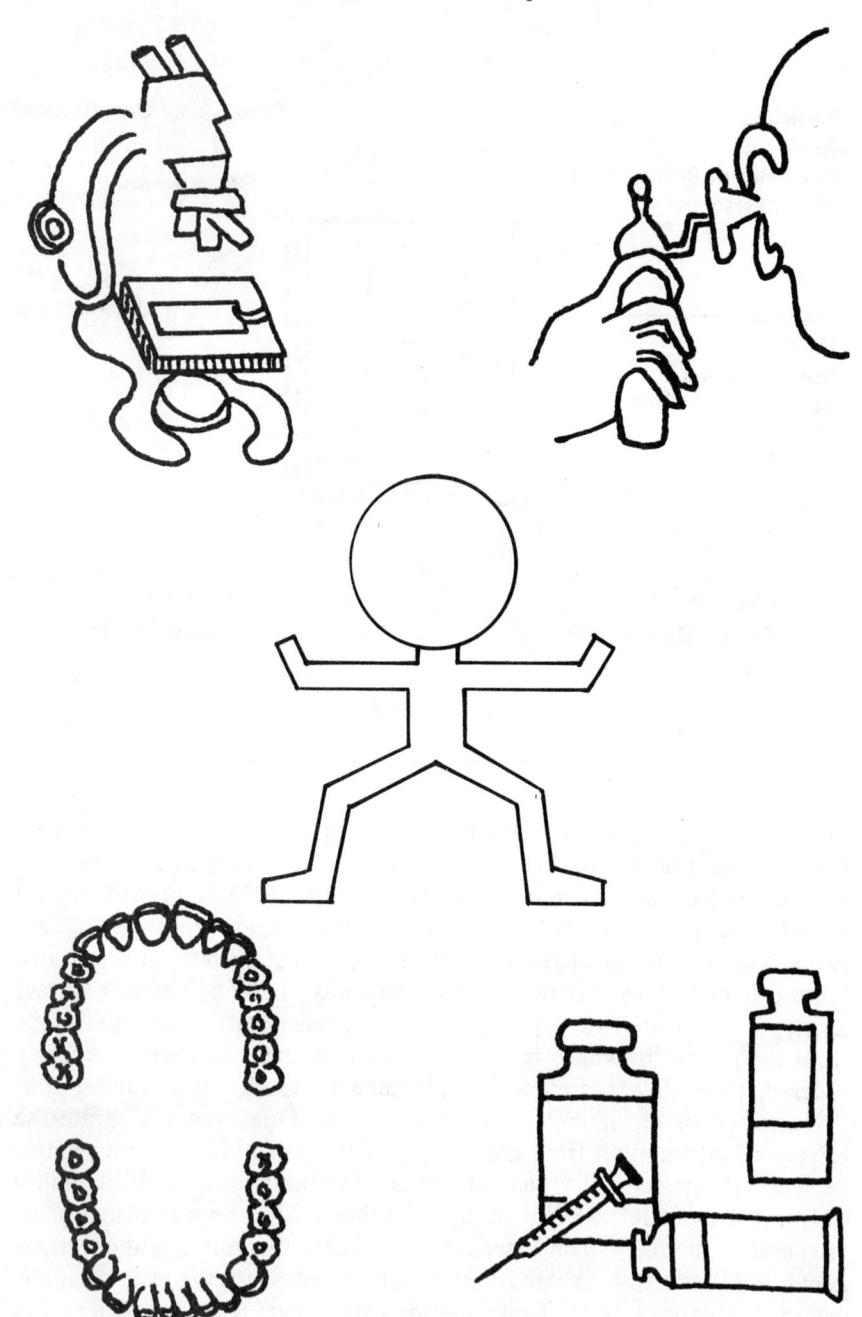

PEOPLE AND ORGANIZATIONS THAT ARE INTEGRAL TO HEALTH CARE

Let us continue to build a framework for development of the medical record. Our first consideration is people. Table 1-1 will give you a fair idea of how many people enter into health care delivery.

We will limit the list of health care personnel to seven groups:

1. Patient-consumers
2. Medical professionals (including dental professionals)
3. Nursing professionals
4. Allied health professionals
5. Service personnel
6. Professional organizations
7. Labor organizations

Patient-Consumers

Earlier we mentioned that most health care is initiated by the individual. How is this unique to American medicine? In a way, the person who seeks health care is a consumer. Perhaps you've never thought of health care as a buying-selling activity, but it is. In a free enterprise system, people can elect to receive or not to receive care. The consumer approach to health gives rise to problems of availability and cost, as well as problems of choice.

- People can wait to seek care until they are in poor health.
- Ignorance about disease and the necessity for good hygiene can delay individuals from seeking care until they are in poor health.
- Financial and cultural incapacity prevents individuals from seeking and receiving care.
- In some geographic areas health services may not be available for residents.

If patients can be made aware of their part in the delivery of care, then some discrepancies between choice and circumstance can be ironed out. Getting people to see themselves as consumers can be achieved by educating them. Education can hasten attainment of care, development of better attitudes toward care of oneself, and awareness of the importance of self-involvement in health care. For instance, examining one's own breast, not smoking, exercising regularly, eating a proper diet, and maintaining a healthy weight are all simple examples of what an average, educated consumer can do to help direct and monitor individual, personal health.

Table 1-1 Estimated Health Personnel Active Professionally in 1971

	Number	% of Personal Health Services Personnel
Total health personnel	4,250,000	
Environmental/food and drug protective services	268,000	
Personal health services	3,992,000	100.0
Fields focusing on:		
Diagnosis and treatment		
Physician, M.D.	332,000	4.0
Physician, D.O.	12,000	0.3
Physician assistant	450	0.01
Medical assistant	250,000	6.2
Ophthalmic assistant	17,500	0.4
Optometrist and optician	35,200	0.9
Podiatrist	7,100	0.1
Dentist	103,750	2.6
Dental hygienist	16,800	0.4
Dental assistant	114,000	2.8
Pharmacy	140,750	3.5
Occupational therapist	13,500	0.3
Physical therapist	24,000	0.6
Care of the dishabilitated		51.9
Midwife	4,950	0.1
Registered nurse	748,000	18.7
Practical nurse	427,000	10.7
Nursing aide, orderly, attendant	875,000	21.9
Home health aide	22,500	0.5
Counseling and education		3.2
Social worker	29,800	0.7
Psychologist	27,000	0.6
Health education/information and communication/library	41,500	1.0
Dietetic and nutritional services	37,000	0.9
Environmental health/food and drug protective services[b]	268,000	c
Machine-related technologies		6.9
Biomedical engineers and scientists	62,000	1.5
Clinical laboratory worker	150,500	3.8
EKG technician	9,500	0.2
Dental laboratory technician	31,150	0.8
Surgical and other aides	23,400	0.6

Table 1-1 continued

	Number	% of Personal Health Services Personnel
Organizational components and interrelations		10.1
Administration	48,400	1.2
Social science analysts	2,000	0.04
Medical records	54,500	1.4
Automatic data processing	2,500	0.04
Secretarial and office services	297,500	7.4
Total	3,848,800	94.4
All others	401,200	5.6
Grand total	4,250,000	100.0

[a]Categories are mutually exclusive.
[b]Does not include air and water pollution control personnel.
[c]Not included in personal health services.

Source: National Center for Health Statistics, *Health Resources Statistics 1971* (Washington, D.C.: U.S. Department of Health, Education, and Welfare, 1972).

Personal, patient-carried records are another way individuals can become more directly involved in their own care. This means people keep track of the written information about their health care and actually are responsible for physically storing and transporting their own written record.

Patient-carried records are of particular importance to the medical record professional. One mark of professional persons is that they provide a personal service. Another mark of professionalism is education of others in the professional's area of expertise. The medical record professional can serve patients most directly by educating them about the existence, content, importance, and uses of the medical record. By playing the role of patient advocate and educator, the medical record professional helps the patient understand and use the information in the record.

In recent years there has been extensive development of new technology, new practitioners, and new health professionals. It is becoming increasingly apparent that the sophisticated technical ability of contemporary health personnel must be matched by the education and involvement of patients and clients if there is to be mutually effective delivery of health care. The medical record professional can help patients prepare and communicate their own personal health information.

Patients can be involved with personal, patient-carried health records in three specific ways. First, patients could carry a card or brief summary of all their health care. This could include the names of problems, diagnoses, or surgical procedures that have been undertaken and the dates of those events. This listing could be carried on the person and made available to any health care provider. A second type of personal, patient-carried health record would be a written problem list or other detailed summary of specific medications, allergies, immunizations, dates of health care encounters, and names and addresses of physicians and other health care providers who have assisted the patient in the past. Third, patients could carry summaries of their complete medical record, including all office and hospital encounters. While this might become bulky, all data compiled in the events and treatment of illness would be centrally located and available for communication to those who needed them.

The concept of a personal, patient-carried health record has been debated in current literature. Much of the debate centers around the suppositions that patients may not want to know all the information relating to their medical care, may not be able to understand the terminology used in the medical record, and may be frightened by what they read there, thereby increasing their chance for illness. Those who believe patients must become involved in their own health care propose that the personal patient-carried health record is mandatory if patients are to follow providers' instructions and carry out their own health care when they are at home, at work, or otherwise separated from their health care providers. Advocates contend that patients must understand the effects of diet, work, exercise, life-style, drugs, alcohol, smoking, environment, stress, and related elements on health if patients are to carry out the regimen recommended by physicians and other health care providers for returning to health and maintaining health.

The debate over personal, patient-carried health records will probably go on for some time. However, many health care facilities and patient care providers are currently giving patients copies of their health records. In the studies to date, there is overwhelming evidence that patients benefit from familiarity with and responsibility for their own personal health and health records.

Collectively, educated consumers can be a mighty voice in the revision of health care delivery. The ballot box is one avenue to equitable health care that, to date, most of us have overlooked. Consumers may not be able to decide intelligently between two surgical procedures, but they can avail themselves of public information and cast an intelligent vote on health care legislation. Patient-consumer groups can actively communicate their needs to financing and planning groups in the community, work to establish acceptable fee rates for the community, develop community transportation systems for those with health-related handicaps, and participate in many other developments in the delivery of health care.

Medical Professionals

Just as the patient is the object of health care, the physician is historically the driving force behind delivery of health care. Because of the medical profession's unique role in the provision of care, its influence has permeated almost every area of the health care delivery system. Physicians have been instrumental in the design of facilities, in the education of allied health professionals, in the establishment of criteria for accrediting and licensing agencies, and even in the formation of the financial structure for the delivery of health care.

With an individual patient, the physician assumes responsibility for diagnosis, care, and treatment. This individual responsibility places the physician in a unique position to direct patients to the treatment they need. Physicians, then, must be able to furnish patients with complete diagnostic and therapeutic services within their own professional practice or suggest options where patients may obtain these services. Because the physician prescribes what will be needed for patient care, the physician comes into focus as a team leader or the one who will direct other medical professionals or allied health professionals in continued treatment. The physician is responsible not only for individual professional skills, but also for familiarity with services provided by other health professionals.

Technological developments and the information explosion have affected every segment of our society, including the medical profession. As a result, specialty medicine has evolved. There are medical and allied health specialties today that were unheard of in the 1950s. There are specialty physicians for almost every system of the body, and then some. This specialty evolution has narrowed the role of the old-time family physician and altered the concept of physician-as-healer. Still at the center of medical care, physicians now play a more specific part. They are highly educated and usually trained to treat specific categories of patients or illnesses. Physicians may practice medicine alone, in a group, in a clinic, or as a partner with a dentist, or any combination of these. For instance, a specialty physician may establish a practice with an allied health professional; an orthopedic surgeon may have as a partner a physical therapist or a rehabilitation therapist. The possibilities for cooperative professional practice are extensive because of the many specialties in medicine and allied health. Collectively, physicians have been a strong voice in American politics for many years. There is nothing to indicate that this will not continue. Some of their influence in the legislative area has included licensing laws for health care facilities, federal insurance programs for certain segments of the population such as the aged, and national health insurance.

Physicians were the first people to document health care given to patients. Their concern to record exactly what took place in their treatment of patients has greatly influenced the development of the medical record profession. In fact, it was a physician, Dr. Malcolm T. MacEachern, who originally worked with Grace Whiting Myers in the formation of the Association of Record Librarians of North America, known today as the American Medical Record Association. Not all physicians have been or are so eager as Dr. MacEachern in their relationships with medical record-keepers, and the successful medical record professional must continually be aware of new technology to help medical professionals document patient care.

Nursing Professionals

One of the oldest professions in the delivery of health care is the nursing profession. Today, nursing is represented by many skilled people. Some nurse practitioners fulfill in part the role once played by the old country doctor or the family physician. Other nurses, such as coronary care practitioners, assist heart disease patients through the use of highly modern technology that was not available prior to the 1960s. Nursing, then, has kept up to date in health care delivery by expanding the categories of practitioners and providing educational programs to meet the needs of changing technology.

In an individual role, the nurse is still the person who spends more time than anyone else with the patient in an acute, chronic, or long-term care facility. In the absence of physicians or other allied health professionals, the nursing staff offers good judgment, comfort, and care to sick patients. Nurses can be found in many job locations besides hospitals, including public health departments, community agencies, nursing homes, schools, and private physicians' offices.

Documentation of patient care is a major responsibility of nursing personnel. Nurses' recorded notes have traditionally described the sequence of events taking place during a patient's hospital stay. Activities related to an individual patient are recorded at regular intervals and include a standard set of data, such as vital signs—temperature, pulse, respiration. A more detailed description of patient documentation by nurses is provided in

Chapter 2. However, it must be mentioned here that in institutional care settings, nurses are always on duty, ready to note and record patient care events. Unlike the physician or other health care providers, they are constantly available to patients. Because of this permanency in their role, they provide unique data in patient care documentation.

Allied Health and Administrative Professionals

Occupational and physical therapists, dietitians, sanitarians, medical technologists, medical record technicians, and administrators—these and others represent the allied and administrative professions.

The functions of the allied health professionals vary from direct patient contact to no patient contact. Allied health and administrative professionals may enter the picture of patient care at any one of several points. Administrative personnel in hospitals and extended care facilities seldom interact with patients. Other administrative personnel, such as those who work with billing and other financial aspects of care, frequently interact with patients before, during, or after care has been provided.

Some allied health professionals practice individually. Included in this category are occupational therapists, physical therapists, respiration therapists, opticians, and pharmacists. Collectively, the allied health professions have influenced the delivery of health care through the performance of skills that in the past lay exclusively in the domain of medical professionals.

Some allied health professionals, such as x-ray technicians, laboratory technicians, and nuclear medical technologists, are directly involved in diagnostic patient care. Others participate in patient care only during therapy, while still others, such as medical record professionals, provide a service seldom seen by the patient. This service does not usually bring the record professional into contact with the patient, and contact between these two ordinarily is confined to a record clerk obtaining the patient's signature on various legal forms such as permits to authorize the release of information from the patient's record or consent for care.

All allied health and administrative professionals have a part in the documentation of patient care. Many of them actually participate in patient care documentation, and those who do not must utilize written patient care data for several important reasons. The hospital administrator, for instance, knows that patient records reflect the quality of patient care provided in the facility. The comptroller or financial officer of a health care facility knows that there must be sufficient, legible, and verifiable information to justify the bills that patients receive. The allied health professionals who treat or interact with patients directly are involved in recording all patient transactions so that they have communication with each other on all work shifts, 24 hours a day.

Service Personnel

While service personnel usually are not organized into formal specialty groups or educated with the allied health, administrative, or medical personnel, they play an equally important role in providing health care. The individuals in this category provide all the support needed to make patient care available. Service personnel include maintenance workers, cleaning people (housekeepers, in hospital jargon), cooks and those who deliver meals, cleanup crews, laundry workers, business clerks who perform office and clerical tasks, and groundskeepers. Organizationally they usually work in the following departments: dietary, housekeeping, maintenance or engineering, admitting, medical records, business office, computer center, and nursing. Obviously health care facilities could not operate without this group. Many service employees do come in direct contact with patients. Like all those who interact with patients, these service providers must be aware of ethical and professional aspects of their work and concerned about the confidentiality of patient data.

Personnel most directly involved in patient care documentation in the service category are in medical records, nursing, and business. They regularly use patient data in the course of their daily work. Their duties involve the use and manipulation of data instead of the creation of data. The time spent working with records and their singular concern with data entries gives them a responsibility that is oftentimes greater than that of persons who create the data entries. Data and its use are the prime concern of the record professional. Others, especially those who make original data entries, are primarily concerned with patient care and only secondarily interested in recording that care. Medical record professionals, then, are the only ones whose entire professional focus is the development, processing, retention, and retrieval of health and medical information.

Professional Organizations

Professional organizations (e.g., American Society of Allied Health Professions (ASAHP), American Hospital Association (AHA), American Medical Association (AMA), American Public Health Association (APHA)) are in many ways modern cousins of early century guilds. They provide an opportunity for individuals to pool ideas and resources. They serve to inform the group about the current state of the art in the profession of their interest and education. Through their role in the development of curriculum for schools and their voice in accrediting their members, they are a powerful entity in the total health care industry.

Labor Organizations

A strong voice in the development and delivery of industrial goods in the United States since the nineteenth century, labor organizations, more commonly called unions, now represent an increasing number of workers in health-related occupations and many health professionals. Physicians, too, have found collective bargaining an avenue of acceptable negotiation. The slow-changing role of the hospital and the people who work there is probably one reason that health workers see unions as acceptable and useful organizations.

The term *profession* enters into this discussion, too. Historically, hospitals were charitable institutions, operated by groups or individuals at their own expense to provide care for others. People who gave of themselves to do this work formed groups, started schools to teach others how to perform their skills, and eventually joined together in professional organizations. Health professionals were persons who went above and beyond the call of duty, so to speak. They could not cease to treat a patient when the clock struck 4:30, but for obvious reasons had to complete the task. Even today, professionals are expected to keep up to date in their field, share information, and maintain high ethical and moral principles. However, with the increasing availability of trained personnel, modern technology, better methods of management, and the development of specialty institutions for groups of individuals who need the same kind of health care, those who deliver health care have come to expect more equitable work hours, salaries, and benefits, and greater participation in management. Unions have offered to assist workers who aspire to equal treatment with those employed outside the health care system.

Most patients enter the health care system at their own choosing under nonemergency conditions in a physician's office. We will not discuss this health care facility thoroughly, but only mention it because it is the most frequently used health care site in our country. In fact, recent estimates indicate that only about 0.5 percent of Americans seek health services at neighborhood centers, about 11 percent use hospital outpatient facilities, about 11 percent have no regular source of care, and about 5 percent use no services at all. Thus, more Americans (65 percent) go to private physicians, and another 8 percent go to physicians in group practice. Institutions that provide facilities, equipment, and personnel for health care vary in size, scope of services, level of care, and type of care.

Type of care required influences the type of facilities and personnel required. Some institutions are designed to provide care specifically for psychiatric patients, or pediatric patients, or crippled patients, or patients with heart and lung disorders. Other institutions treat patients with acute illnesses, while still others treat patients in need of long-term care.

Level of care refers to the degree of services and care required. For example, among those who need long-term care, some may need more help than others to participate in such activities as eating, bathing, taking medications, and walking. Differences in levels of care can be seen in the differences between the services offered in intensive care units and routine care units. Intensive care is for patients who need constant surveillance because they are temporarily unable to function even at a life-support level without the help of special equipment, medicines, and personnel.

Hospitals

Hospitals are designed to play a comprehensive role in the delivery of health care. The gamut of services available in the acute care hospital closely resembles all of the services available in a home, plus a vast number of specific services related to diagnosis and treatment of disease. Comfortable surroundings, food and warmth, newspapers and television, and bathing facilities are all part of the atmosphere of the hospital. Acute care hospitals are specifically designed to treat short-term illnesses and provide emergency care. The more common medical facilities available include an x-ray department, a coronary care unit, an intensive care unit, a surgery, a laboratory, and, of course, various other care units where patients stay while being treated. Extended care hospitals treat patients with chronic illnesses or patients whose acute illness has changed to a degree that requires less extensive care than that offered in the acute care hospital.

As institutions or corporations, hospitals have all of the characteristic financial and organizational responsibilities of businesses. Hospitals are financed and chartered for operation. They may be profit or nonprofit, owned and operated through a community charter, financed through local taxes, franchised through a religious or lay organization, or federally funded and operated. Some hospitals are affiliated with universities and serve as primary teaching laboratories for students in the allied and administrative professions and nursing, health, and medical professions. Many nonuniversity-affiliated hospitals also serve as teaching hospitals.

As an indication of quality of care provided, hospitals may elect to be accredited. Accreditation rests on evaluation of the physical, medical, and administrative, as well as social and rehabilitative, services provided. For the patient-consumer, accreditation is a sign that the hospital has met optimal standards of patient care. The group responsible for voluntary accreditation is the JCAH.

Traditionally, hospitals have been the greatest source of patient records. To date, more emphasis has been given to the completeness, accuracy, and use of the hospital patient record than to the quality of records developed in any other type of health care facility.

Health Maintenance Organizations (HMOs)

As the name implies, the health maintenance institution focuses on preventive as well as acute care and treatment. Designed to utilize collectively all fiscal as well as physical resources, HMOs include outpatient or clinic facilities as well as hospital beds. Prepayment for medical care is the characteristic that makes HMOs different from other types of health care facilities. Kaiser-Permanente is perhaps the best known HMO, although Group Health Cooperative of Puget Sound also has achieved national recognition. The Puget Sound group provides satellite clinic facilities as well as centrally located hospital units. These two HMOs are especially well known because of their early development and continued success.

The philosophy that nurtured the development of HMOs was that of medicine without crisis. The contention is that if patients can make regular prepayments of fixed amounts for their health care needs, when the time comes for treatment, they will unhesitatingly seek care and not worry unnecessarily about the cost of that care. Equally important, patients will seek care before they are acutely ill. If practiced this way, there are several benefits. Two will be mentioned here. More patients receive care through an HMO facility, and the records reflect more emphasis on health care than traditional medical records usually reflect. From the organization's point of view, a regular and reliable source of payment assures easier budget projection, greater cost control, and smoother service. Exhibit 1-2 lists the characteristics of HMOs.

A recent three-year study showed that hospital admissions for HMOs as a whole were 22 percent lower than for a control group and 33 percent lower among pediatric patients. This lower level of hospitalization for the study group was attributed to the HMO's emphasis on ambulatory, diagnostic, and therapeutic medical services. There was a substantial increase in the cost of ambulatory services, but this was offset by the reduction in hospitalization costs. Wider use of ambulatory services, including preventive care, without increase in total cost is considered a better use of health care money. In this same study a periodic followup review indicates a high level of enrollee satisfaction.

Exhibit 1-2 Characteristics of Health Maintenance Organizations (HMOs)

Sponsor	Any for-profit or not-for-profit organization (including Foundation for Medical Care, labor union, hospital, medical center, community group, government, insurance company, bank, or other corporation)
Patient Population	Voluntarily enrolled, as on a defined geographic (or other) basis
Services	
Type	Comprehensive (including M.D., laboratory, x-ray, nursing, drugs, ambulatory, and in-hospital)
Place	Group practice facility (free-standing or attached to hospital, community center, and so on)
Equipment, Records	Shared
Financing	Fixed premium
Out-of-pocket cost	Relatively low
Payment basis:	
To system	Capitation
To M.D.	Salary, capitation
M.D. Personnel	Closed panel (hired by system)
Cost Control	
Prospective budget	Yes
Claims and other types	
of peer review	Yes
M.D. liability	Shares percentage of risk

Sources: Comptroller General of the United States, *Study of Health Facilities Construction Costs* (Washington, D.C.: Government Printing Office, 1972).
R. Egdahl, "Foundations for Medical Care," *N. Engl. J. Med.* 288:491-99 (March 8, 1973).

From February to August 1977 a national HMO census survey was conducted under the combined auspices of the Group Health Association of America, Incorporated, the American Association of Foundations for Medical Care, the Blue Cross Association, the Health Insurance Association of America, and the National Association of Blue Shield Plans. About 93 percent of all known plans responded to this survey. The number of operational HMOs had increased by nearly 15 percent between 1976 and 1977. This census survey showed that the larger and older HMOs accounted for 71 percent of the total membership in all HMO-type plans, which was

6,330,676 during this period. Members of HMOs under age 65 used an average of only *488* hospital days per one thousand enrollees as compared with the general population of the United States under 65, who used an average of *908* hospital days per one thousand. The degree to which HMOs have met their philosophical and operational intentions is seen in some of these studies. A great deal has been written about HMOs, and they are likely to continue to be a major development in the U.S. health care delivery system.

An interesting aspect of the HMO structure for the health record professional is the opportunity to develop an almost ideal health information system. Because of broad-ranging HMO care and prepaid scheduling, individuals and families could use only the HMO for patient care and not shop around as so many consumers do. This gives a health information professional the opportunity to develop a complete record on all family members in one source file.

Group Practice

Group practice is care provided by several physicians who usually represent a fairly broad spectrum of medical specialties. Group practice benefits the patient because it brings together the physicians and allied health professionals who can collaborate in patient care and treatment, often while the patient is in the office. Physical therapy, podiatric services, or provision of optometric aids can be scheduled before the patient goes home. Delays, phone calls, extra trips, and other patient inconveniences are lessened in group practice. Perhaps the most important benefit of group practice is the personalization that it affords. The patient receives the care and advice of everyone in a centralized, personalized setting. Physicians who specialize in family practice often offer their services through a group.

Ambulatory Care Facilities and Clinics

Ambulatory care facilities started receiving noticeable attention in the early 1970s. Federal construction funds shifted from acute care to ambulatory care facilities in 1972. This came about with the recognition that low-income states had at least as many or more hospital beds in relation to population as high-income states. This called attention to a need for alternatives to high-cost hospital care. Rural communities had long received a preponderance of inpatient facilities funds, and their ambulatory projects and services were carried out mostly in public health centers rather than outpatient facilities. By early 1972, half of the federally supported facilities projects and almost 45 percent of the funds involved ambulatory care.

Ambulatory care, however, remains rather fragmented or segmented. Many ambulatory care facilities have not integrated their service approach and still emphasize particular diseases, health problems, forms of treatment, or age or sex groups. Child care, mental health, and family planning are some examples of ambulatory care services.

Clinics are organized to serve patients through the cooperative efforts of several physicians or groups practicing together. That is, a clinic is often simply a physical site that provides office space for several physicians. They may also share the laboratory and x-ray facilities but do not necessarily collaborate in providing patient care. Some clinics feature prepayment or other types of membership similar to that of HMOs. Clinics do offer collaborative medical treatment from physicians located there and provide ready referral service when specialists or special services are needed. Lower costs of shared facilities and equipment can be an incentive for physicians to practice in a clinic. Speedy transmittal of patient information between the practitioners can also be established, making patient data immediately available to those who need it.

Long-Term Care Facilities

After acute care, or sometimes apart from acute care, patients may need continued or custodial care. Facilities that provide continuing care are generally called skilled nursing facilities or intermediate care facilities. Through skilled nursing and rehabilitative services, continued care completes the program initiated in the hospital. Custodial care maintains the best quality of living when ongoing medical and nursing support is required. Prevention and intervention activities are adapted as a component of long-term care. Patients in long-term care facilities need professional monitoring of their progress, skilled nursing, and daily health maintenance through proper hygiene, nutrition, and exercise. In addition to all the physical care, patients require facilities and activities, such as an entertainment center for group and individual social activities, and beauty and barber shops, that promote the health of the whole person. Off-site programs are often utilized, too, in long-term care; patients visit cultural or sporting events, or go sightseeing.

Health records for long-term patients are maintained in the facility. They are subject to federal certification requirements in Standards of Participation for Skilled Nursing Facilities (SNFs) and Intermediate Care Facilities (ICFs) when the patients are beneficiaries of Medicare or Medicaid funds. Specialized long-term care settings for the mentally retarded are subject to Federal Standards for Participation in Institutions for the Mentally Retarded (IMRs). Content, organization, and documentation standards are defined for all of these applications.

Agencies, Associations, and Societies

Extensions of the individuals who participate in the delivery of health care are the organized groups and agencies that collectively provide a variety of health-related services, such as obtaining health aids, equipment, and funding for patients, lobbying for health care legislation, and filling the scholarly, research, and educational needs of medical specialist members.

Agencies are usually funded through the cooperative efforts of government at its various levels. Some agencies are backed by foundations or philanthropists, but the most common agency, the community agency, usually gets its funds through a local drive or good neighbor campaign, along with federal matching funds. The primary role of the agency is to coordinate activities and provide information that is not specifically offered anywhere else in the health care system. The need for agency service is an example of one omission in our health care delivery system.

Patients who are ill, handicapped, elderly, poor, or unfamiliar with sources for funds, services, drugs, or health aids, often need direction when they leave the physician's office. This is the role of the agencies—to provide someone who will find out what is available and how it can be obtained. This may be one part of an agency's role. An agency can also provide the aids, equipment, and funding that a patient may need.

With more federal money being spent in the delivery of health care, agencies were a natural outcome in the expenditure of federally budgeted funds on broader health care services for an increasing population of patients.

Allied health professionals, nurses, and medical professionals are all represented by collective groups known as associations. The American Medical Record Association (AMRA), for example, represents those who practice the medical record profession at its several levels. Associations serve their membership by providing programs for continuing education of members, journals with up-to-date research and information, accreditation or licensing standards, curriculum direction to professional schools, and so on. Some associations have legislative interests and spend money on lobbying at various levels of government for or against legislation that can affect their profession in some way.

Societies are a branch of the medical professions for the most part. They share with academies the role of academic, scholarly, research, and other educational functions and are usually organized as components of particular medical specialties. Medical societies also serve a broader purpose than those previously mentioned by publishing the names of members as a service to patient-consumers. Such societies usually do not limit membership to one specialty group, but are composed of physicians of all specialties from a certain geographic area, for instance. Some societies also are formed to provide medical care for members, much as medical insurance groups do.

Federal and Local Government

It is impossible to talk about health care delivery in the United States without recognizing the various roles played by agencies, branches, bureaus, and legislative arms of our government. It is equally impossible to describe that vast and complex governmental involvement in health care in one small section of a book devoted to medical record administration alone. However, we will at least describe some of the major programs, some of the major agency roles, and the impact of the government role on the consumer and health professional levels.

The Department of Health, Education, and Welfare (HEW) encompasses the largest number of health care agencies and includes, among many others, the National Library of Medicine, the Center for Disease Control, the National Center for Health Statistics, and the National Heart, Lung, and Blood Institute. The scope of HEW can be seen in Figure 1-3. Legislative influence is demonstrated through such programs as the Professional Standards Review Organization (PSRO), Medicare and Medicaid, and the American College of Surgeons (ACS) Commission on Cancer Tumor Registry Program. The Cooperative Health Statistics System is an example of a federally initiated program that relies on the private sector for full development and implementation, as reflected by its title. Many federal programs have this characteristic. Local or state money is pledged along with federal money to a program developed with federal staff and federal funds.

Built into some of the federal health care programs are controls or mandates that require compliance from those who use the funds and programs. Compliance with rules and regulations is a way of life for many who rely on federal money to do their jobs or receive reimbursement for services rendered. The Medicare program, first funded in 1967, is the result of what is perhaps the most impressive health care legislation to date. Designed for patients over 65 years of age, Medicare made a significant mark on the delivery of care for several reasons. To be eligible for reimbursement for treating those who are legitimate users of the Medicare program, physicians, clinics, and all other providers of care must document exactly what was done for the patient, the date of the event, the cost of the care, and any other pertinent information. Thus, the Medicare program heralded an increase in the amount of health care documentation. Furthermore, because of the huge population that Medicare serves, documentation tripled and, in many cases, quadrupled on its way to the nation's capitol where all such

Figure 1-3 Health Care Agencies in the U.S. Department of Health, Education, and Welfare (HEW)

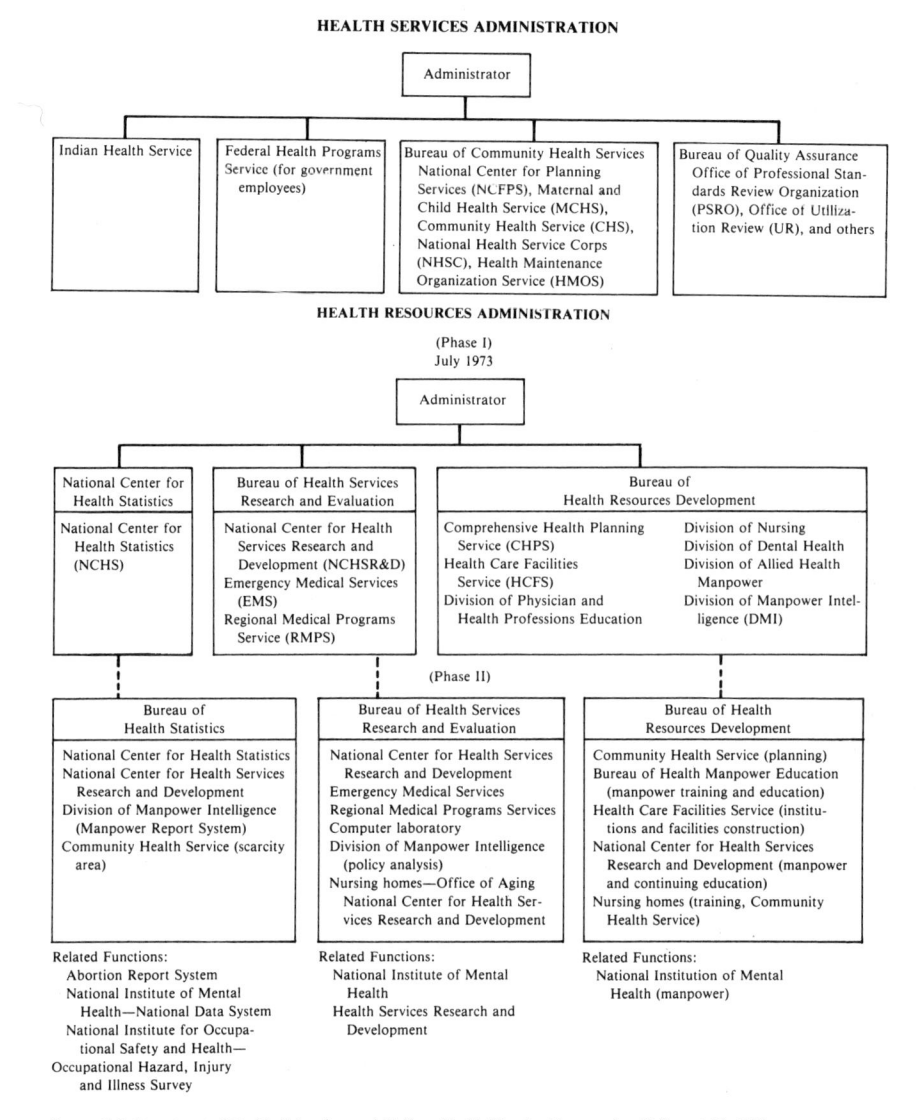

HEALTH SERVICES ADMINISTRATION

Administrator

| Indian Health Service | Federal Health Programs Service (for government employees) | Bureau of Community Health Services National Center for Planning Services (NCFPS), Maternal and Child Health Service (MCHS), Community Health Service (CHS), National Health Service Corps (NHSC), Health Maintenance Organization Service (HMOS) | Bureau of Quality Assurance Office of Professional Standards Review Organization (PSRO), Office of Utilization Review (UR), and others |

HEALTH RESOURCES ADMINISTRATION

(Phase I)
July 1973

Administrator

National Center for Health Statistics	Bureau of Health Services Research and Evaluation	Bureau of Health Resources Development	
National Center for Health Statistics (NCHS)	National Center for Health Services Research and Development (NCHSR&D) Emergency Medical Services (EMS) Regional Medical Programs Service (RMPS)	Comprehensive Health Planning Service (CHPS) Health Care Facilities Service (HCFS) Division of Physician and Health Professions Education	Division of Nursing Division of Dental Health Division of Allied Health Manpower Division of Manpower Intelligence (DMI)

(Phase II)

Bureau of Health Statistics	Bureau of Health Services Research and Evaluation	Bureau of Health Resources Development
National Center for Health Statistics National Center for Health Services Research and Development Division of Manpower Intelligence (Manpower Report System) Community Health Service (scarcity area)	National Center for Health Services Research and Development Emergency Medical Services Regional Medical Programs Services Computer laboratory Division of Manpower Intelligence (policy analysis) Nursing homes—Office of Aging National Center for Health Services Research and Development	Community Health Service (planning) Bureau of Health Manpower Education (manpower training and education) Health Care Facilities Service (institutions and facilities construction) National Center for Health Services Research and Development (manpower and continuing education) Nursing homes (training, Community Health Service)

Related Functions:
Abortion Report System
National Institute of Mental
Health—National Data System
National Institute for Occupational Safety and Health—
Occupational Hazard, Injury
and Illness Survey

Related Functions:
National Institute of Mental
Health
Health Services Research and
Development

Related Functions:
National Institution of Mental
Health (manpower)

Source: U.S. Department of Health, Education, and Welfare, *Health Planning Memorandum* 48 (August 16, 1973).

documents eventually go. Medicaid, the other large federal health service program, added to the documentation load. Exhibit 1-3 describes the scope of the two programs.

Although the Medicare program functions with an intermediary, that is, a regional insurance company or health care organization, the rules and regulations are federally mandated. Paper documentation in the form of tapes or printouts is utilized to satisfy administrators who must determine if legislative intent is being carried out at the local level in health care delivery.

Exhibit 1-3 Federal Medicare and Medicaid Programs

	Medicare	Medicaid
Eligible beneficiaries	1. Social Security retirees and other aged 2. Chronically disabled; certain others	1. Recipients of categorical aid programs (e.g., Aid to Families with Dependent Children) 2. Medically indigent, determined by each state: 23 states limit their programs to (1); 28 states cover both (1) and (2)
Coverage Basic services	*Part A:* Hospital care; skilled nursing facility care; home health services (with time limits)	*Mandatory:* States must provide physician services, inpatient and outpatient hospital services, skilled nursing facilities, and home health care; family planning
Supplementary	*Part B:* Physician, home care; physical therapy, and outpatient hospital services	*Optional:* State may provide drug, dental, and eye services
Financing	Social Security, plus 1. individual premiums (Part B) 2. deductible (Parts A and B) 3. copayments (Parts A and B)	Government revenues (federal and state) matched by 1. monthly premiums from medically indigent 2. copayments imposed by states
Proportion of personal health care covered for eligible groups	42 percent	26 percent

Sources: Social Security Amendments of 1972 (P.L. 92-603)
    Perspective (1972),
    Health Law Newsletter, 25 (May 1972), from the book *The Care of Health Communities,* by Nancy Milio. Reprinted with permission of Macmillan Publishing Co.

Other federal health care programs may be implemented through grants. Grants have played a major role in providing buildings, equipment, research monies, salaries, travel expenses, supplies, and consultative services for ongoing and new health care programs of all types. Such grant support has been used by universities, organizations, private companies, individual medical researchers, and allied health professionals. Curriculum revision, development of new health professions, medical discovery through research, additional buildings for hospitals and research centers, and education of the public about high health risks such as cigarette smoking and high blood pressure are all examples of activities that were funded through federal appropriations approved by the U.S. Congress and provided through the direction of federal agencies and programs.

Local government plays a similar health care role. By local we mean state, city, county, borough, or any other nonfederal regional or sectional government body. State agencies and state health care programs are frequently subsidized by the federal government, but may also be directly funded by the state. Licensing of facilities and personnel are two functions commonly performed by state agencies. Mortality and morbidity studies are also frequently carried out by the state. State or local agencies often are involved in determining the need for expenditures for equipment, buildings, or additions to existing buildings. Comprehensive planning functions are also performed locally to coordinate and control health care provision and prevent duplication of costly facilities and equipment.

PATIENT-CONSUMER PARTICIPATION IN HEALTH CARE

Paying for Care

The most infrequently used method of payment for health care in our country is self-payment. At one time almost all patients paid for their own care, but that is no longer financially feasible for even the average working person. The high costs of care, whether in the physician's office, a hospital, or an extended care facility, and of drugs and other health necessities make it impossible for most people to rely on personal income and savings for health care payments.

Most Americans rely on third-party payment plans, that is, they spend a regular part of their income or work benefits on insurance and, in turn, receive full or partial payment for their health care.

Payroll deduction allows many employed patient-consumers to budget for health care on a regular basis. Most health insurance plans include benefits for families or dependents of the employee. For those of us interested in the documentation of health care, insurance companies that offer health care plans have access to some of the largest accumulations of health data anywhere in the world. This is particularly true of those companies that specialize in health insurance, such as Blue Cross or Blue Shield. Another important source of health data is the Medical Information Bureau, a private firm that services more than 700 life and health insurance companies and preserves patient care information submitted by providers. It is estimated that the bureau currently has data on file for some 12 million individuals.

Prepaid insurance offers the patient-consumer the opportunity to pay for care on a regular basis and receive care at no charge when or after treatment is received. Prepayment alleviates the need for having cash on the spot when an expensive treatment is needed or the period of illness is extensive. Kaiser-Permanente is one example of a large, prepaid medical program.

One implication of prepaid medicine for record professionals is the opportunity it offers them to compile records before care is initiated. Basic identification information and records on individual patients can be ready and waiting when treatment commences.

Selecting Care

Choosing where to go for health care and scheduling an appointment are two major decisions that a prospective patient faces. Because of increased emphasis on medical specialization, it is sometimes difficult for a patient to identify what particular physician to contact. This is especially true for those who do not have a regular physician, who have needed only occasional care in the past, or who have been treated previously only by a specialist. When a new symptom occurs, these individuals are hard put to know what physician to consult. Calling some known physician for a suggestion is one way to identify the right person for the current condition. The local medical society also can identify qualified medical practitioners.

Visiting a physician is not always the quickest or most appropriate way to receive medical attention. In some instances, initial care is provided through outpatient facilities in hospitals, neighborhood clinics, specialty community services such as mental health centers and mobile cardiac care units, among others. Such contacts are usually unscheduled, and care is provided on the spot as quickly as modern transportation will allow. In some areas, scheduling can be frustrating for the patient entering the system. Low physician-patient ratios preclude speedy scheduling, and an individual with painful or otherwise worrisome symptoms can become agitated if it is not possible to find someone to start treatment immediately. Once a visit to the physician has been accomplished, another scheduling problem can arise if adequate facilities for carrying out diagnostic tests are not available. Timing, again, can be either satisfactory or a source of increased annoyance.

Entering the system, then, can be voluntary or it can be imposed, if emergency medical needs arise. One does not need to worry about scheduling if one arrives at the health care facility in an emergency vehicle. Entry and scheduling, then, are the concern of those with nonemergency conditions. When a physician or other professional source of care—a dentist, psychologist, nurse practitioner, or physician's assistant, for example—has been identified, the prospective patient is then ready to select a particular provider.

During the initial appointment with the health professional, the patient will make judgments, possibly express doubts, raise questions, and undoubtedly seek answers, explanations, and predictions. Very often, patient and health professional relationships are built on communication compatibilities and mutual trust and respect. But it always remains the prerogative of patients to select those who will treat them. Because of this and the need to seek care from specialists, patients must develop a method for selecting care from particular professionals.

Patient-consumer selection of a professional can be based on information provided by friends, colleagues, family, other health professionals, medical and professional society bulletins, or licensing and accrediting qualifications of health professionals and facilities. Type of payment expected, costs of care, and availability of the professional and of diagnostic and therapeutic facilities also enter into consideration.

HEALTH INFORMATION: HUB OF HEALTH CARE

At the very heart of all health care is the information that describes or symbolically represents that care. Whether it is written in English or machine-readable computer language, the information about the activities, judgments, plans, problems, facts, values, and other elements of patient care is the core of that care. Health information can be defined as any data pertaining to the physical, mental, or social well-being of an individual or group of individuals. Figure 1-4 summarizes the sources of the data being fed into the sole source of health information—the patient-client record.

Throughout this book we will discuss health information in its many different formats. Because there is such a proliferation of health information, we will not confine ourselves to strict definitions, but rather will approach health information as it is known in contemporary society. Health information has various names, depending on the situation in which it is used and who is using it. Throughout the book, then, we will use many different words for health information interchangeably, including health data, medical records, health records, and many other descriptive terms that are synonymous in some way with health information in its many variations.

Figure 1-4 Health Information: The Hub of Health Care

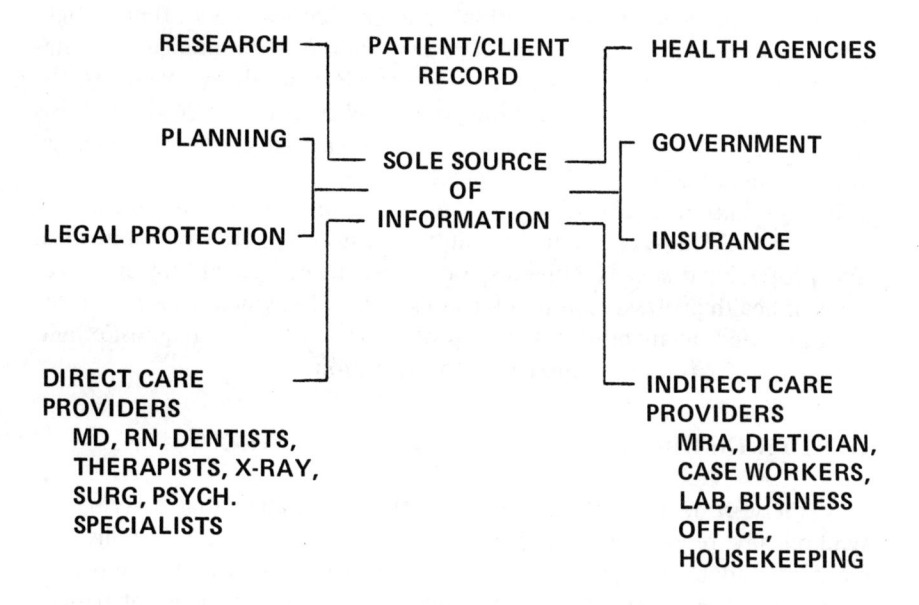

RESEARCH — PATIENT/CLIENT   HEALTH AGENCIES
RECORD

PLANNING — SOLE SOURCE — GOVERNMENT
OF

LEGAL PROTECTION — INFORMATION — INSURANCE

DIRECT CARE
PROVIDERS
  MD, RN, DENTISTS,
  THERAPISTS, X-RAY,
  SURG, PSYCH.
  SPECIALISTS

INDIRECT CARE
PROVIDERS
  MRA, DIETICIAN,
  CASE WORKERS,
  LAB, BUSINESS
  OFFICE,
  HOUSEKEEPING

Many users and providers of health information have specialty names for data. These names are often assigned to categories of data and help identify the data in particular applications. The principles applied to managing and developing data, however, are similar in most applications.

Whether health information is retained by an insurance company or developed and retained in a physician's office, the basic data and the documentation of those data remain the same. For instance, there will always be identification data—a body of information describing what has taken place in a particular encounter and identifying the providers and/or users of the data. Other elements similar for all types of health information are the confidentiality of the information, the decisions and policies regarding who can have access to the data, and retention and retrieval policies and procedures for the data.

The principles and methods used in the development, retention, and use of hospital medical records also apply to collections of health data in their many forms. Health information for evaluation is gathered by federal agencies, licensing or accrediting agencies, school health record systems, home health agencies, and others. All health information is confidential, and its retention and retrieval are controlled by policies regarding who can have copies of the information, how copies will be provided, and how data flow will be maintained so that the information is available to serve the purposes of the organization.

Health information is found in many places and in a wide variety of formats. For example, dental records, mental health records, public health records, health planning agency records, vital statistic reports, health insurance company records of patient care, school health records, and company physical examination reports are all documents of health information. These documents can originate in planning agencies, state, local, county, or federal health departments, volunteer and specialty health organizations such as the American Red Cross, the Planned Parenthood organization, and alcohol and drug treatment centers. The records that these agencies develop as they routinely collect patient data are examples of health records. Health records can be defined as documentation of health care services rendered by direct or indirect patient-provider interaction.

In the health records developed and utilized by some facilities mentioned above, little attention has been given to standardization, control, development, and regulated use of records. The records kept by these facilities are used for a single purpose, or what is defined as a single purpose at the outset. The records meet the particular needs of specialty agencies, facilities, and institutions. Among other purposes, these agencies or facilities keep records (1) as permanent documents that describe what the agency did in relation to the patient, (2) as fiscal evidence of health care events, or (3) as resources for future planning and evaluation. These reasons are analogous to the reasons medical records are created and retained in the first place. We must reiterate that the terms *health records* and *medical records* will be used interchangeably in this text because there is such a close relationship between the various types of records and the principles of recordkeeping in all health service settings. Medical records are essentially the same, whether they are kept in acute care facilities, extended nursing care facilities, dentists' offices, or institutions that provide indirect care.

Medical record professionals have a unique role in the processing of health information. This is the only professional group that has an educational background directed solely at the development, processing, retention, and retrieval of health information. Medical record professionals establish policies and develop procedures for the adequate use of medical information. But medical record professionals must work with others in the development and use of health information. In most facilities, institutions, agencies, and other health care locations, medical record professionals must educate others and continually make them aware of the importance of adequate health information systems. The medical record professional is sought out as a source of information by other health professionals in making decisions about health information policies and procedures.

With increasing emphasis on the use of information, many medical record administrators and technicians have expanded their influence beyond the hospital medical record department. The same is true of record administrators and technicians in other facilities, too. For instance, many administrators are coordinating record activities in departments outside the medical record department. Two functions they perform are the coordination of medical record information developed in admitting departments, outpatient facilities, or emergency rooms and medical care evaluation. These functions may be carried out under the auspices of an organizational unit known as the Department of Information Services. This department is a recent organizational development in many health care facilities, particularly those utilizing teleprocessing procedures. In some health care facilities the information services department is responsible for coordinating all health information and making it available to users. (See Figure 1-5.)

Medical record professionals traditionally have directed their efforts toward hospital medical records. Other types of health records deserve the profession's attention and in recent years have started to receive it. Many record professionals are now employed in nonhospital positions where they develop information systems to provide accurate, complete, and useful health records.

Figure 1-5 Department of Patient Information and Appropriate
Management Areas for an Integrated System

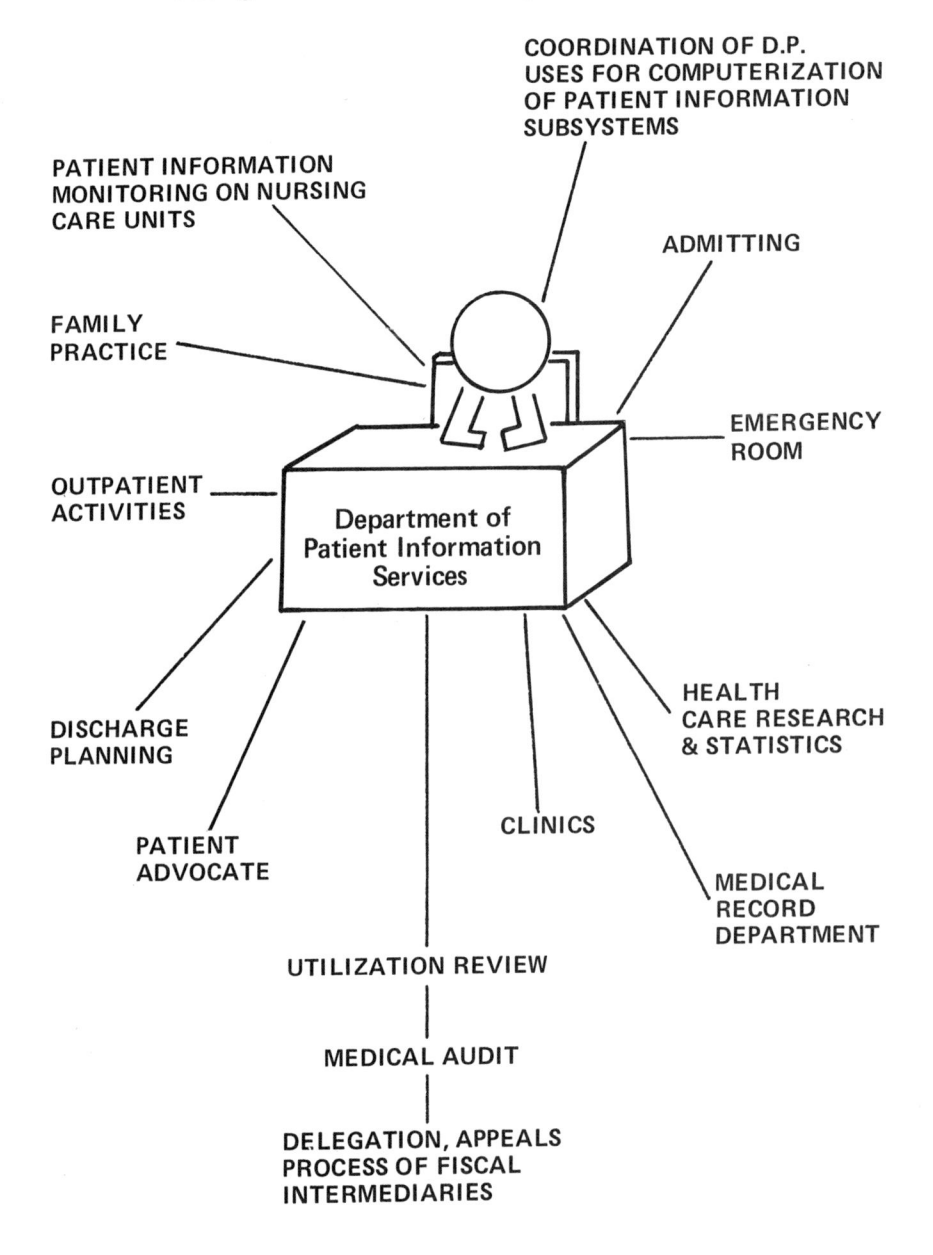

REFERENCES

Health, United States, 1978, Department of Health, Education and Welfare's annual report to Congress, March 1979.

Huffman, Edna K. *Medical Record Management*. Berwyn, Ill.: Physicians' Record Co., 1972.

Joint Commission on Accreditation of Hospitals. *Perspectives*. Chicago, Ill.

Jonas, Steven. *Health Care Delivery in the United States*. New York: Springer, 1977.

Milio, Nancy. *The Care of Health in Communities: Access for Outcasts*. New York: Macmillan Publishing Co., 1975.

Describing the Medical Record

CHAPTER OBJECTIVES

1. Identify the four major types of data entries
2. Understand the characteristics of data entries
3. Differentiate between direct and indirect patient data
4. Recognize the importance of accuracy, completeness, and usefulness of data entries
5. Identify computer compatible components of data entries
6. Relate the quality of data entries to the functions of a health information system

DATA ENTRIES AS ESSENTIAL RECORD COMPONENTS

We now know that all health records are made up of items of information or data entries. Just what does this mean? Data entries are all the bits of information that are entered into a health record. That is, they are any fact, any piece of information that a health care provider needs to know to treat a patient or client.

Consider health records in various environments. What do they look like? They are usually paper records. Many are kept in file folders. Some appear on cathode-ray terminal (CRT) screens when someone pushes a button. There is a lot of detailed information in some records. Others appear to be summarized and succinct. Record systems can be complex and expensive or simple and inexpensive. With the impact that health services have on our pocketbooks and our person, examining the record that reflects these services becomes a clear priority. The first step in this examination is to secure an adequate and informative description of medical and health records.

Data entries are of four major types:

1. Identification
2. Financial
3. Social
4. Medical/Treatment

When specialized health services are provided in such places as alcohol treatment centers, family planning clinics, and mental health clinics, unique kinds of data entries are built into the record. To define a particular health record, it is necessary to determine the circumstances in which it developed. We have defined health record as documentation of health care services rendered by direct or indirect patient-provider interaction. For our more detailed study of records in this chapter we will add to that definition a dimension that includes the setting for the development and use of those records. The expanded definition is documentation of direct or indirect health care services to patients-clients by providers and users of that data in any health-related institution.

A health record is no longer limited to traditional medical institutions or medical personnel. It is no longer limited to a written document. The concept of health records encompasses a wide range of patient problems, including those that are social and psychological. The record is the sum total of all four kinds of data entries in a given health care delivery experience. Accordingly, managers of health and medical data need to consider five major premises.

1. As a record is constructed, individual data entries that are compiled in an organized format comprise an information component.
2. All data entries are communicators that relate a message about the individual. They may be results of direct or indirect communication with the patient.
3. To provide patient information that is effective, all data entries must be accurate, complete, and useful.
4. Data entries have attributes or characteristics that determine the form in which they are presented. Data entries may be
   • Dynamic or permanent
   • Singular or cumulative
   • Measurable against a norm
   • Alphabetic, numerical, or plotted image.
5. The functions and activities of a health information system are determined by the specific characteristics and measurable qualities of data entries.

This chapter will examine these premises in greater detail and help the reader formulate images of medical and health records as they currently exist in various settings.

CONSTRUCTING THE RECORD

Let's examine the first premise in detail and explore its implications. Each data entry on your medical record represents a fact about yourself. Combined with other data entries, it becomes an individual dimension and communicates for you about you. It directs your current and future health care. It critiques your life-style. Each time you receive a health service, that experience is recorded. Sometimes the information is recorded in a complete and appropriate manner. Sometimes it isn't. If all data entries about an individual were assembled from all records that documented health services in a lifetime, they would appear as pieces of a jigsaw puzzle. Each entry is a piece of the puzzle—the more entries, the more complete the picture.

Identification Data Entries

Stop now and identify data about yourself that might appear in your family doctor's record. An example is an entry about a strained leg muscle received in a tennis game. If we turned from your family doctor's record to the community hospital record, we would expect the data on the two records to look different. Generally, data entries in a hospital medical record reflect information about the hospitalization. If the strained leg muscle was a complex fracture instead, you would probably see that condition cited in the hospital records as a reason for admission.

If you were an elderly person who fractured your hip during a lively tennis game, you would probably be admitted to the hospital for primary care and then transferred to a skilled nursing facility (SNF) for additional nursing and physical therapy before going home. You would also have a medical record in the SNF. At the time of your discharge, you might be given a copy of the patient care plan; you would need this to maintain the therapy program at home.

A data entry about identity, for instance, could be a notation in the history that reads, "this 64-year-old Negro male, born and raised in Albany, N.Y., has been treated in the past for. . . ." Another example: "This elderly Caucasian female has a well-healed surgical incision on the right upper quadrant. . . ." Data entries in the identification classification are not always as standard as they might appear when we first see them on an inpatient admission record such as the one shown in Exhibit 2-1.

Exhibit 2-1 Sample Admission Record with Identification Data Entries

| Last Name | First | Middle | Nickname | Number |

| Sex | Race | Age on Adm. | Religion | Social Security Number | Admitted from | Adm. Date | Time |

| Burial Plan | Birthdate | Birthplace | State | County | City | Marital Status | Citizenship: what country? |

| Residence prior to Institutionalization | State | County | City, Town, or Location | Street & Number | Inside City Limits? |

| Father's Last Name | First | Middle | Birthplace | Mother's Maiden Name | First | Middle | Birthplace |

| Legal Custody of Resident (if ward of county, give county) | Address | Telephone no. |

| Legal Guardian of Person | Address | Telephone no. |

| Notify in Case of Emergency | Address | Telephone no. |

| Also notify in Case of Emergency | Address | Telephone no. |

| Alternate in Case of Emergency | Address | Telephone no. |

| Supplemental Insurance | Number | Subscriber |

| Medicaid no. | Medicare no. | Discharge Date | Time | Discharge to |

Admitting Diagnosis:

Another item of identification data, ethnicity, needs a little explanation and, perhaps, promotion. Federal requirements and mandates aside, the exact origin of a patient must be known if that patient is to receive optimum care and treatment. It takes little thought to recognize that in a being as complex as a human there are many interrelationships that contribute to health or lack of health. A patient's genetic and cultural identification is important for those who need to diagnose and treat that individual. Because certain diseases are prevalent in certain races, nationalities, and populations that work or live in certain parts of the world, identification of patients by ethnic background becomes important. Two examples that support this concept are Cooley's anemia, which occurs only in people of Mediterranean background, and sickle cell anemia, which occurs almost exclusively in North American blacks.

The medical record administrator can serve as a patient advocate in promoting the collection of ethnicity data in a health information system. It is a useful entry and therefore should be collected, stored, and made available for current and future care and research. Continuing research is seldom thought of when identification information is collected, but when it is considered, it is usually based on what is currently accepted as proven. Some information elements, while still not thoroughly understood or proven, should be included for those future researchers who elect to study disease linkages not currently recognized or totally proven. For example, it took a lot of research and a vast number of records to determine the ethnic similarity of those who are diagnosed as having Cooley's anemia or sickle cell anemia.

When a health problem arises, the patient seeks help. It can be said that identification entries are usually the first entries noted on medical records. Depending on the nature of the problem and the type of provider, patients may be interviewed by a variety of people. Sometimes it seems that the interviewer wants to know more about the socioeconomic side than about the medical problems. This is not the case. Who you are, how old you are, your occupation and marital status are some of the items that identify you as an individual.

Your name or even birthdate and name are not enough. Hospitals and health care providers at all levels need to know enough information to adequately and with reasonable certainty identify individual patients on a continuing basis. One obvious reason is to notify next of kin should any emergency arise. All of the information listed in Exhibit 2-2 is collected by health care facilities to provide consistent and accurate identification information. This, in turn, provides statistics for the provider as well. For instance, knowing the number of people over 65 that are treated for a specific time period can affect planning for future services.

Exhibit 2-2 Typical Identification Data Entries

Name—full name: first, last, middle, and maiden for women
Address—full: house or apartment number, street, city, state, and zip code

Full name of next of kin
Parents' name
Birthdate
Birthplace
Social Security number
Occupation
Sex
Marital status
Ethnic origin

The National Center for Health Services Research and Development sponsored an international conference on hospital discharge abstract systems in June 1969 at Airlie House, Warrenton, Virginia. The purpose of this conference was to explore ways in which health information systems in the United States might be improved and coordinated.

Following the conference, the National Center for Health Services Research and Development appointed a steering committee to oversee implementation of the conference recommendations.

In late 1970, the National Center for Health Services Research and Development contracted with the Hospital Research and Educational Trust (HRET) of the American Hospital Association to design and develop areas of information that would further assist in implementation of the conference recommendations. The seven-month HRET contract, entitled Common Data Set for Hospital Management, had three major objectives:

1. To determine the present state of collection and use of the basic data set, or of most items of the set, by hospitals, including both those that subscribe to a collective reporting system and those that do not.
2. To determine the capability of hospitals to collect and use all or most of the data set items if they are not presently doing so.
3. To propose and/or devise training programs for staffs of institutions not presently collecting and using the basic data set, to bring them to a level of capability that would allow them to do so.

Five steps were taken by HRET to develop the information base required to accomplish the objectives of the contract.

1. A sample of community hospitals was surveyed by mail questionnaire to assess the capability of those hospitals to collect and use the basic data set, as well as to provide insight into their present methods of discharge data collection and use.
2. The allied hospital associations (metropolitan, state, and regional) were surveyed to determine their actual or planned involvement in new or existing discharge abstract systems.
3. The hospital discharge abstract systems that had been identified by the Health Services Foundation were requested to furnish lists of their subscribing institutions to provide a precise, quantitative measure of the number of hospitals actually participating in such programs, as well as to provide a means for studying characteristics of system-participating institutions.
4. Collected data produced by the previously described methods were analyzed to determine the characteristics of the potential audience(s) for the educational programs. Informal conferences were held with education specialists to determine methods—both innovational and traditional—for conducting such an educational program, and field visits were made to existing discharge abstract systems to determine their methods of training personnel in hospitals participating in their ongoing programs.
5. A short conference was held with selected participants from the original hospital discharge abstract conference to seek advice and recommendations concerning the development and progress of the contract tasks.

Here is the uniform hospital discharge data set that resulted from the efforts of the groups cited above.[1]

Hospital Discharge Data Set

A. *Person identification.* Each patient is to have a unique number within the hospital to distinguish that patient from all other patients. The patient's name need not be recorded.
B. *Date of birth.* The month, day, and year of birth.
C. *Sex.* Male or female.
D. *Social characteristics.*
1. Marital Status.
   a. Divorced or Separated is used for persons who no longer live together (whether or not legal action has been taken).
   b. Never Married (Single) refers to persons who have never been married or whose only marriage has been annulled.

    c. Now Married refers to married persons and persons who state they are living in a common-law marriage.

    d. Widowed includes widows or widowers.

  2. Race. White, Black, and Other.

E. *Residence.* Record zip code.

F. *Hospital identification.* Each hospital must have a unique number within the abstracting system.

G. *Admission and discharge dates.*

  1. Admission Date includes month, day, year, and hour (1–24) of admission.

  2. Discharge Date includes month, day, and year of discharge.

H. *Physician identification.* Each physician is to have a unique number within the hospital. The attending physician and operating physician are to be identified.

  1. Attending Physician. This is the physician who was primarily responsible for the care of the patient at the beginning of each hospital episode.

  2. Operating Physician. This is the physician who performed the principal procedure.

I. *Diagnoses.* All diagnoses that affect the current stay. Old diagnoses that relate to an earlier episode and have no bearing on this hospital stay are excluded.

  1. Principal Diagnosis is listed first and is defined as the condition established after study to be chiefly responsible for occasioning the admission of the patient to the hospital for care.

  2. Other Diagnoses to be listed are all conditions that coexist at the time of admission or develop subsequently and affect the treatment received and/or the length of stay.

J. *Procedures.*

  1. In addition to surgical procedures, all other significant procedures are to be recorded together with the dates. A significant procedure is one that carries an operative or anesthetic risk or requires highly trained personnel or special facilities or equipment. Some examples of such procedures are

    a. Cardiocatheterization

    b. Renal dialysis

    c. Angiography

    d. Exchange transfusion

    e. Endoscopy

    f. Encephalography

2. The principal procedure is to be listed first. If only one procedure was performed, it is considered the principal procedure.

In determining which of multiple procedures is the principal procedure, the following criteria are to be applied:

a. The principal procedure is one that was performed for definitive treatment rather than diagnostic or exploratory purposes, or a procedure that was necessary to take care of a complication.

b. The principal procedure is that procedure most related to the principal diagnosis.

K. *Service to which patient was admitted.*

Assignment to service is to be consistent with one of the following categories:

1. Medical
2. Surgical
3. Obstetrical
4. Pediatrics
5. Psychiatric

L. *Disposition of patient.*

1. Discharged to home (routine discharge)
2. Discharged or transferred to another institution
3. Discharged or transferred to an organized home care service
4. Died
5. Left against medical advice

M. *Principal source of payment.*

1. Self-pay
2. Worker's compensation
3. Medicare
4. Other government payments (including Medicaid)
5. Blue Cross
6. Insurance companies
7. No charge (free, special research, or teaching)
8. Other

N. *Charges.* Includes the total hospital charges for the episode of hospitalization without regard to payment.

After meeting in 1972 and 1973, the Consultants on Ambulatory Medical Care Records, U.S. National Committee on Vital and Health Statistics, recommended that the following items constitute the minimum basic data set that should be entered in the records of all ambulatory medical care. The recommendations were enacted in 1974.[2]

Basic Data Set for Ambulatory Medical Care

A. Items that characterize the patient
   1. Patient identification
      a. Name
         Surname, first name, middle initial
      b. Identification number
         A unique number that distinguishes the patient and his am-
         bulatory medical care record from all others
   2. Residence
      Patient's usual residence, to consist of street name and number,
      apartment number (if any), city, state, and zip code
   3. Date of birth
      Month, day, and year
   4. Sex
      Male or female
   5. Expected source of payment
      Government
      a. Workmen's compensation
      b. Medicare
      c. Medicaid
      d. Civilian Health and Medical Program of the Uniformed Ser-
         vices
      e. Other
      Insurance mechanism
      a. Blue Cross
      b. Blue Shield
      c. Insurance company
      d. Prepaid group practice or health plan
      e. Medical foundation
      Self-pay
      No charge (free, charity, special research, teaching)
      Other

B. Items that characterize the provider
   1. Provider identification
      a. Name
         Surname, first name, middle initial
      b. Identification number
         A unique number that distinguishes the provider from all other
         providers
   2. Professional address
      Street address, office number (if any), city, state, and zip code

3. Profession

The profession in which the provider is currently engaged

a. Physician

Include specialty, if any, as determined by membership in, or eligibility for, specialty board

b. Dentist

(Include specialty)

c. Nurse

d. Other (specify)

C. Items that characterize the patient-provider encounter

1. Date of encounter

Month, day, and year

2. Place of encounter

a. Private office

b. Clinic or health center (any except hospital outpatient department)

c. Hospital outpatient department

d. Hospital emergency room

e. Home

f. Other (specify)

3. Reason for encounter

The patient's principal problems, complaints, or symptoms on this encounter, in the patient's own words

4. Findings

All history, physical examination, laboratory, and other findings pertinent to the patient's reasons for visit or diagnoses, or both, and any other findings the provider deems important

5. Diagnosis and/or problem

The provider's current assessment of the patient's reasons for the encounter and all conditions requiring treatment, with the principal diagnosis and/or problem listed first. Principal diagnosis and/or problem is defined as the health problem that is most significant in terms of the procedures carried out and the care provided at this encounter

6. Services and procedures

All diagnostic, therapeutic, and preventive services and procedures (including history taking) performed during the encounter and those scheduled to be performed before the next encounter

7. Itemized charges

All charges to be made by the provider for services and procedures performed during the encounter or to be performed by him or his associates before the next encounter

8. Disposition (one or more)
   The provider's statement of the next step(s) in the care of the patient
   a. No followup planned
   b. Return, time specified
   c. Return, pro re nata
   d. Telephone followup
   e. Referred to other provider
   f. Returned to referring provider
   g. Admit to hospital
   h. Others

The Technical Consultant Panel on the Long-Term Health Care Data Set of the U.S. National Committee on Vital and Health Statistics met in 1977, and in 1978 recommended that the following 24 descriptive items and 2 procedural items constitute the minimum data set for long-term care clients and their use of services. This proposal awaits formal federal approval as this book goes to press.[3]

Minimum Data Set for Long-Term Care

Demographic items
1. Personal identification
2. Sex
3. Birth date
4. Race/Ethnicity
   a. Race
   b. Ethnicity
5. Marital status
6. Usual living arrangements
   a. Type
   b. Location
7. Court-ordered constraints
   a. Court-ordered care
   b. Court-ordered guardian
Health status items
8. Vision
9. Hearing
10. Communication
   a. Expressive communication
   b. Receptive communication

11. Basic activities of daily living
    a. Bathing or showering
    b. Dressing
    c. Using toilet
    d. Transferring in and out of bed or chair
    e. Urinary or bowel incontinence
    f. Eating
    g. Walking
12. Mobility
13. Adaptive tasks
14. Disruptive behavior
15. Orientation/Memory impairment
16. Disturbance of mood
17. Primary and other significant diagnoses
Service items
18. Provider identification
    a. Unique number
    b. Location
    c. Type
19. Last principal provider
20. Date of admission/Commencement of service
21. Direct services
22. Principal source of payment
23. Charges
24. Discharge/Termination of service
    a. Date
    b. Status/Destination
Procedural items
Date of report
Type of report

Financial Data Entries

The doctor's office and other health facilities are operated as businesses. As businesses, they are entitled to know who will pay services they are about to provide. Financial entries are concerned with employer, health insurance company, insurance identifier numbers, types of coverage, and methods of payment. Exhibit 2-3 shows typical financial data entries. Asking for this information is a reasonable request. While it sometimes seems that health care personnel are more concerned about who will pay the bill than they are about care of the patient, in reality financial information often helps expedite services. Today, many hospitals and clinics send reports directly to

Exhibit 2-3 Typical Financial Data Entries

Employer's name—full name of company and supervisor
Job title—occupation
Address of employer company
Name of insurance company
Type of insurance coverage
Insurance identification number
Type of payment

---

the insurance company. The reports include final diagnosis and numerical codes designating what services were provided. This practice saves time and money in information handling for the patient and the provider. Along with the identification entries, financial entries will be present on any medical or health record, regardless of the nature of the medical problem being treated.

The identification entries provide individual patient designation. Consumer status is verified through financial data entries.

Social Data Entries

Social data describe your position in human society. According to Webster, social science "deals with human society or its elements, as family, state or race, and with the relations and institutions involved in man's existence and well-being as a member of an organized community." Social data include race, family status, and role in the community. They include family information and information about a patient's current living situation. It may include data about jobs, interests, hobbies, general attitudes, and feelings about life-style. Exhibit 2-4 summarizes these entries.

Identification and financial entries are made by a clerk or secretary who interviews the patient at the beginning of care. However, an increasing

---

Exhibit 2-4 Typical Social Data Entries

Race
Family Status
Occupation
Hobbies and Interests
Family Information
Life-style
Attitude

Exhibit 2-5 Entries to the Medical Record

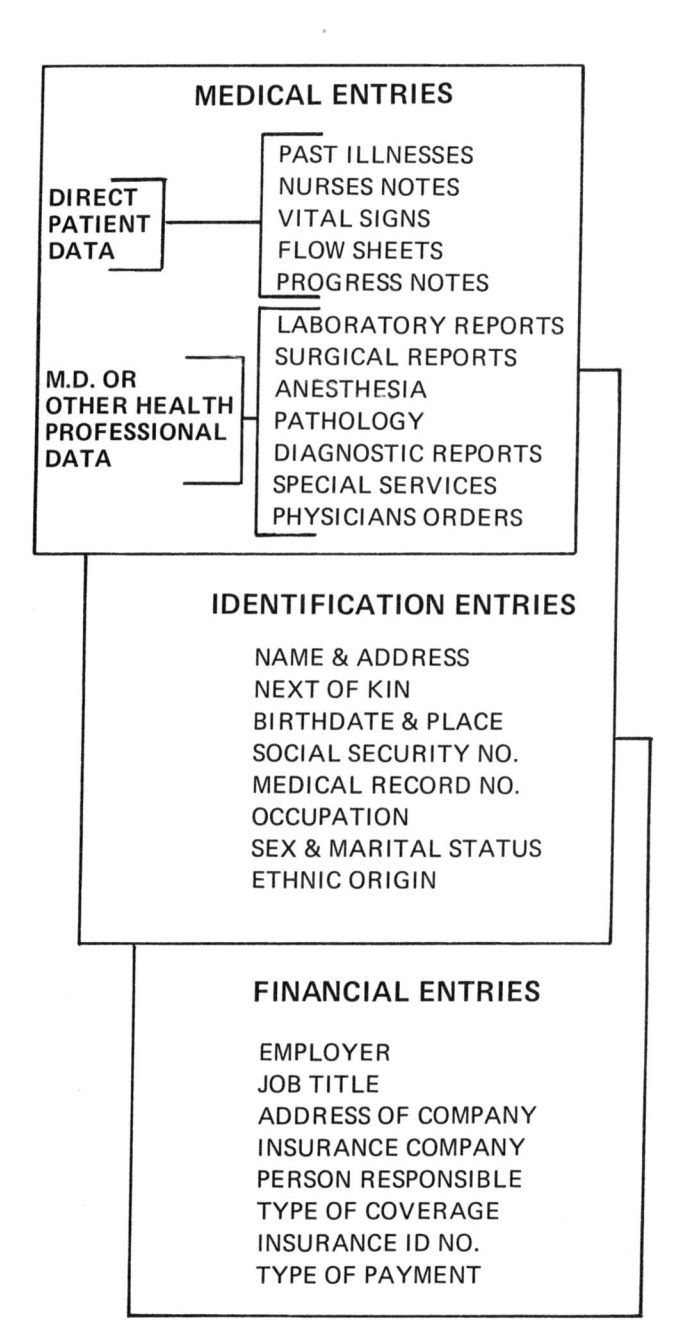

number of agencies are requesting that this information be completed directly by the patient. In some clinics, patients answer questions at a computer terminal, and the computer automatically creates a printout for the record. This printout can be read and reviewed by the patient and checked for accuracy. Having the patient record the data entries serves two purposes:

1. It requires the participation of the patient in developing an accurate medical record.
2. It frees up highly skilled health professionals for more appropriate interviewing that addresses the patient's health problems.

The advantages of computerized patient histories are itemized in Figure 2-1. A computerized patient profile is illustrated in Figure 2-2.

Medical or Treatment Data Entries

Medical data entries are made by doctors, nurses, dentists, physical and occupational therapists, psychologists, social workers, and many others who offer services to the patient. Together, they formulate a legal document that demonstrates the following:

- The patient has a need for service.
- The correct service is provided.
- The service is provided in the proper manner by the proper person.

Exhibit 2-6 Typical Medical Data Entries

Direct:
   History of past illnesses and operations
   Nurse notes
   Vital signs
   Progress notes
   EKG graphs, other direct tracings, graphs

Indirect:
   Laboratory reports
   Surgical reports, including anesthesia, post-anesthesia, and pathology
   Diagnostic and x-ray
   Physician's orders
   Graphs, flow sheets
   Specialty reports

Figure 2-1 Computerized Patient History

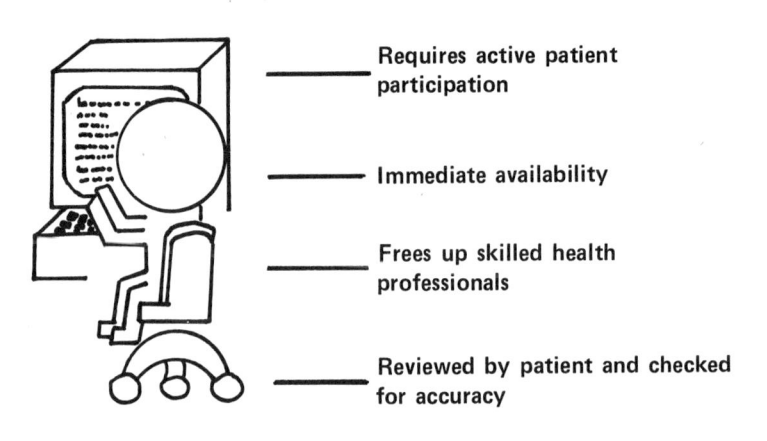

Requires active patient
participation

Immediate availability

Frees up skilled health
professionals

Reviewed by patient and checked
for accuracy

Accordingly, data entries must verify the provider's signature and the date that care was given. It must be clear who is making the written statement and when it was recorded. Therefore, all medical data entries are dated and signed by the person responsible for the service provided. Exhibit 2-7 shows a dated and signed source document for data entries. Medical entries are the largest group of data entries. They may be direct data entries by doctors, nurses, therapists, and others who write directly on the record at the time of the encounter with the patient. Or they may be indirect data entries, such as lab test results, reports of operations, computerized medication profiles, or clinical pathology reports. Data entries may record past history about the patient's medical problems or a doctor's specific plan for investigating and treating current problems. Entries should cover the patient's response to treatment as it progresses. The record may show vital signs and reflect physical parameters or descriptions of the patient's condition. The data are found on many different forms and are usually recorded in chronological sequence. They might be written on a flow sheet that records parallel information at stated intervals. Forms and formats for data entries and medical records will be discussed in more detail in Chapter 4.

Figure 2-2 Computerized Patient Profile

```
            ************
            * MEDQUEST *
            ************
```

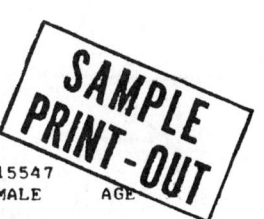

```
    DOCTOR: JONES                    CODE:    15547
                                     SEX:  FEMALE      AGE
    DATED BY PT.:  5-15-70           SS-#:
    DATE PROCESSED:  5-18-70   OCCUPATION: HOUSEWIFE
                               MARITAL STATUS: MARRIED
                               EDUCATION: TECHNICAL SCHOOL
                   ***********************
---THE PATIENT INDICATES THE FOLLOWING SYMPTOMS OR PHENOMENA MAY
HAVE BEEN NOTED (OR MAY HAVE BEEN PROGRESSIVE) DURING THE LAST YEAR:

    SEE LAST SHEET FOR CHIEF COMPLAINT.

    DYSURIA.
    UTI OR NEPHRITIS.
    URINARY FREQUENCY.
    VAGINITIS.
    DEPRESSION.

               PAST HISTORY AND REVIEW OF SYSTEMS
               **********************************

***EYES***
                              DENIES: CHANGE IN VISION,
                              DIPLOPIA, SCOTOMATA, OR
                              BLURRING OF VISION.

***EARS, NOSE, TEETH AND THROAT***
    SUSCEPTIBLE TO RECURRENT PHARYNGITIS.
                              DENIES: TINNITUS, VERTIGO,
                              DYSPHAGIA, HEARING CHANGE,
                              OR HOARSENESS.

***GASTROINTESTINAL***                                  15547
    HAS HAD HEMORRHOIDS FOR ABOUT    2 YEAR(S).
    HAS NOTED BLOOD-STREAKING OF STOOL.
                              DENIES: ABD. PAIN, MELENA,
                              DIARRHEA, CONSTIPATION,
                              HEMATEMESIS OR JAUNDICE.

***CARDIO-RESPIRATORY***                                15547
    A HEART MURMUR WAS NOTED    2 YEAR(S) AGO.

***GENITO-URINARY***
    HAS PERSISTENT DYSURIA.
    URINARY FREQUENCY: MORE THAN 10 TIMES A DAY.
    HX. OF GLYCOSURIA.
    HX. OF PROTEINURIA.
    HAS HAD UTI OR NEPHRITIS  10 TIME(S).
        LAST UTI OR NEPHRITIS WAS  1- YEAR(S) AGO.

***OBSTETRICS AND GYNECOLOGY***                         15547
    MENARCHE: BETWEEN AGES 11 AND 15.
        MENSTRUAL FLOW IS USUALLY MODERATE.
        PERIODS USUALLY LAST 3 TO 6 DAYS.
        CYCLE IS AT 3 TO 5 WEEK INTERVALS.
```

ALL DATA ENTRIES ARE COMMUNICATIONS ABOUT A PATIENT

Direct Patient Data

Facts that a patient actually provides to someone are direct data. Answering a question about one's health status, "Yes, there is diabetes in my family," is providing direct medical information. A nurse's notes made in a hospital or a long-term care facility are another example. These notes document the results of the nurse's interaction with the patient.

Vital signs such as pulse and respiration or general appearance are physical findings that can come only from the patient directly. Progress notes in medical and health records should accurately reflect the patient's condition when in direct contact with the person writing the notes. Providers of care do interpret some facts and put those facts as they perceive them into their own words, but it's still direct patient data.

Why is this important? Unlike all other data, direct patient data may be gathered straight from the source and evaluated and clarified at the outset to make sure they are accurate and complete. People can be emotionally upset when they are physically upset. Illness usually involves both. Patients may have financial worries, work pressures, or family problems over and above their illness. Consequently, they may emphasize facts that don't need emphasis and overlook facts that do. When taking direct patient data, the provider has to be skilled in communication to secure patient data that are accurate and useful. The patient may also question and correct the interviewer, if there seems to be a communication gap. It is this opportunity for corroboration of information taken directly from the patient that distinguishes direct from indirect patient data.

Indirect Patient Data

Indirect medical data from the patient are also significant, but may require interpretation before they are usable. An example would be a laboratory report. Exhibit 2-8 shows such a report. The specimen comes directly from the patient, but the analysis of it requires a technical process that doesn't directly communicate with the patient. Another example of indirect data is the information in the patient's surgical report. Patients usually do not see their surgical report. They don't know what is in the report, nor do they interact with those who are performing the surgery while it is in progress, if they are under the effects of anesthesia, as is usually the case. Surgi-

Exhibit 2-7 Data Entries Dated and Signed

DATE AND HOUR	NOTE PROGRESS OF CASE - COMPLICATIONS - CONSULTATIONS - CHANGE IN DIAGNOSIS - CONDITIONS ON DISCHARGE - INSTRUCTIONS TO PATIENT - AND FINAL SUMMARY.
MONDAY — July 6, 1980	
7 30/AM	*Afebrile — Doing well — Still has very early systolic sound, best heard in 2nd ICS -3 ICS. A soft systolic murmur is also heard. Aerating lungs well. Will get up in chair today. All tubes out.* — *Mc Glenn, MD* —

PROGRESS RECORD

cal reports may include anesthesia information and even preanesthesia information. The surgical or operative report is a narrative description of what was done to the patient in the surgical suite. While the surgery report describes in detail the procedures performed on one individual's particular anatomical tissue, it is described solely by the surgeon without the collaboration or verification of any other person present during performance of the procedure. A pathology report completes the picture and puts it all together. Pathology reports describe the tissue or specimen removed during surgery.

Data entries on diagnostic tests such as electrocardiograms and radiology reports can also be considered indirect communication from the patient. These data reflect the role of allied health professionals who are trained to provide or interpret test results in a certain area.

Physician's orders and plans are the data entries that tell what is to be done for the patient.

- Admission orders and plans specify what the patient is there for.
- Orders and plans specify investigative procedures to identify further the patient's problems. Lab work is an example.
- Orders and plans prescribe treatment, such as medication, wound dressing, and diet.
- Orders and plans specify patient education to help self-management, as in diet programs.

The physician's orders and plans are a communication link between members of the professional team to tell them what is planned for the patient. It demonstrates health care planning and rationale for treatment. The physician's orders and plans are monitored by other providers and patient data managers. Indirect medical data, then, are data the patient usually doesn't see. Somebody else takes an action as a result of looking at parts or products of the patient. It could be a blood or urine sample, an x-ray, or a scan of the patient's liver. Someone else interprets the raw data, writes or dictates a report, and transmits it to the patient record.

Exhibit 2-9 details the evolution of hospital medical records from about 1900 to the present. Note that the volume and complexity of data entries have grown as the number and types of reports have increased. We can see increasing sophistication in recordkeeping as additional health providers become available and technology is introduced.

Exhibit 2-8 Indirect Data: Laboratory Report

```
                              LABORATORY VALUES
AFOLABI, JULIUS (A39821)                                        3-30-77


URIC ACID    (MG%)

LAST VALUE      12-02-76  7.7        NORMAL: 3 - 8
MIN VALUE                 6.8
MAX VALUE                 7.8

   8.2 :
   8   H:...........................................................
   7.8 :    .             *                            *
   7.6 :                                  *
   7.4 :        *                    *
   7.2 :
   7   :      *
   6.8 :        *
   6.6 :
   6.4 :
       :++++++++++++++++++++++++++ +++++++++++++++++++++++++++++++
                    75^76                      76^77    T
*****************************************************************************

UREA NITROGEN   (MG%)

LAST VALUE      12-02-76  16         NORMAL: 8 - 20
MIN VALUE                 12
MAX VALUE                 9

   16  :      *                                        *
   15  :        *
   14  :
   13  :
   12  :      *
   11  :
   10  :
   9   :              *
   8  L:................................*......................
   7   :
       :+++ ++++++++++++++++++++++++++++++++++++++++++++++ ++++++++
                    75^76                      76^77    T
***************************************************************************

POTASSIUM   (MEQ/L)

LAST VALUE      12-02-76  3.3        NORMAL: 3.5 - 5
MIN VALUE                 3.0
MAX VALUE                 4.6

   4.8 :
   4.6 : *    *
   4.4 :
   4.2 :
   4   :      *
   3.8 :
   3.6L:......................*.........................
   3.4 :    .    *      *              *      *
   3.2 :
   3   :                              *
       :++++++++++++++++++++++++++++++++++++++++++++++++++++++++
                    75^76                      76^77    T
```

Reprinted with permission: Jenkin, M.A., M.D.,
A Manual of Computers in Medical Practice,
The Society of Computer Medicine, 1977.

Observe the increasing use of technology and consider what that means in management activities such as personnel expansion, cost increase, and control functions. To introduce typewritten reports into medical recordkeeping, managers had to add typewriters and typists to departments. Dictation equipment was required. Volume and productivity became important as more and more typed reports were added to the record. Systems were set up to establish a procedure for securing and retrieving the information. Information was dictated, reports were typed, and finished records were routed to doctors or other providers for review and signature.

In the late sixties and early seventies, computers entered the picture and brought faster processing and retrieval of information. Computers also brought new needs. Equipment costs and mutual cooperation between medical record personnel and computer personnel came into focus. Programs had to be written. Reports and formats had to be designed. Data entries moved from verbal communication and documentation to data entries transmitted on a CRT terminal. This meant data had to be read, interpreted, collapsed into computer languages, processed, stored, and retrieved. Technology and systems design had to develop and expand. The manager of patient information now had to monitor and verify developing methods. At the same time, the manager had to stay in control of the existing record development.

DATA ENTRIES MUST BE ACCURATE, COMPLETE, AND USEFUL

Consider the accuracy of data entries from two perspectives. First, accuracy originates with the patient. A patient who is not feeling well goes into a physician's office and waits 40 minutes. The patient sees the physician's nurse who asks what the problem is; the patient explains. The patient is told that the doctor will be in in a moment. After another 10 minutes the doctor enters, asks what the problem is, and again the problem is described. At this point the doctor may or may not record the information. Or the information that seems relevant in light of what the patient has said about the problem is what gets written down. In many cases the information is recorded manually on paper. In some cases a few notes may be jotted down and a fuller report later dictated for the patient's record. If a patient enters a teaching hospital, the patient provides information to a member of the house staff, that is, to an intern or resident. And that intern or resident writes down the information as the patient relates it. Later on, when the patient's personal physician comes in, some of these points may be reviewed a second time. In these examples a patient has sought health care and

Exhibit 2-9 Evolution of Data Entries on Hospital Records

Circa 1900	The patient tells doctor about illness.	The doctor may write down the information in a notebook the physician carries.
Primary care provided through community doctor		
Circa 1918	The patient tells the doctor about illness in hospital setting where standards are identified.	The handwritten paper record contains
Movement to hospital standards by the American College of Surgeons with a beginning focus on medical records		• Identification and summary of hospitalization form
		• History and physical exam
		• Progress notes
		• Reports of diagnostic tests such as x-rays
		• Reports of surgery
		• Medication records
		• Nurses' notes
		Increasing use of dictation systems. Central dictation units established in medical record departments.
Circa 1920 to 1940	The patient tells the doctor about illness. Also tells interns and residents. Some information from the doctor's office records may be available before the patient's entry into the hospital.	• Increased handwriting as procedures are established to secure complete, adequate medical records.
		• Increased variety of medical reports appear—lab tests, EKGs, EEGs, anesthesia records.

From the 1950s to early 1960s	Patients complete preadmittance questionnaires for hospital when possible. Patients tell history and facts about their illness to nurses and social service personnel. Lab and x-ray work completed prior to admission—potential for inclusion in the record.	Continued focus on streamlining and organizing the patient records. Use of central dictation units highly developed. More and more reports prepared through typing units. Forms designed to standardize record organization and structure developing. Record is becoming more and more complex. Less handwriting and more transcribing.
Mid- to late 1960s	Establishment of Medicare, requiring specified reason for hospitalization and consents from patients for transfer of records under agreements to continue hospital care in nursing facilities. Introduction of computer.	Establishment of methods to transfer information—summarize discharge status and nursing care plans. Increasing use of preadmission information to be part of patient record. Computer printouts appear.
1970s	Professional Standards Review Organization (PSRO) added to Medicare. Utilization review for length of stay and defined data items to be reported are introduced. Computerization is well accepted for function activities of medical record departments:	Records continuing to grow in complexity. Attempts made to computerize the information. Interim records emerge. Interim is printout that serves as record form between paper records and fully computerized documents: • Cumulative lab reports

Exhibit 2-9 Continued

- Discharge abstract systems
- Computer output
- Microfilm for master patient index

Computer printouts alter the paper record.

- Computerized history
- Computer-analyzed tests—EKG, EEG

Systems established that maintain the record on computer—El Camino Hospital, Mountain View, CA. Doctors and nurses form and construct the medical record through TV-like terminals on the nursing station.

Problem-oriented records evolve. Model established at PROMIS lab. Patient record on computer keyed to problem number and title—brings more structure. Data entries are constructed from words and phrases displayed on CRT screen. Physician users can gain access to particular groups of data entries as needed.

described a problem and feelings about the problem to two different people in a given time period. In both cases the information is entered by hand or dictated into a paper record system. Accurate description rests with the patient. The patient may, out of fatigue or irritation with having to repeat the information, leave out information to speed things up. When ill, the patient is especially apt to suffer from mental (memory) and physical fatigue. Or, the care provider may choose to record only those bits of the information that seem relevant.

Techniques of interviewing definitely influence data accuracy. For the most part, health providers are skilled interviewers, and errors in data accuracy will usually be the result of memory lapses or distractions caused by interruptions or inability to concentrate. Health providers also suffer from fatigue.

In a study, patients admitted to a hospital were provided with copies of their health history and physical examination records and asked to read them through and make corrections where there were errors. Many patients made additions, deletions, and actual corrections of information about their own past history or about their current health problems and feelings about their problems. One reason that the information appears inaccurate is that the patient is communicating with another human being, and this communication is facilitated or retarded by the receiver's attitude and listening skills. With the introduction of the computer in the role of information receiver, patients' willingness to communicate increased. The computer was a nonjudgmental machine with plenty of time that expressed no opinion about patients' responses to embarrassing questions and simply allowed patients to enter the information at their own speed. All studies of patient-machine interactions have shown that the histories and the patients' accounts of their problems gathered in this way are far more complete, comprehensive, and accurate than they had been in the traditional oral/manual mode. Exhibit 2-10 shows a sample printout from a computer questionnaire.

The communication model in the computerized system must be put into an automated language. This is a problem. It is expensive, and must be tailored to the clinic or hospital. It must be cost-justified in a health information system. But the benefits in accuracy and completeness of the information have been demonstrated.

Other methods that improve the accuracy and completeness of data entries generated by patients include giving questionnaires to patients with enough time for them to complete the forms and review them with an interviewer. This method also improves accuracy and completeness of data.

Exhibit 2-10 Sample Computer Printout from Questionnaire

```
DOCTOR: JONES                    CODE:   15547
                                 SEX:  FEMALE      AGE: 34
DATED BY PT.:  5-15-70           SS-#:
DATE PROCESSED:  5-18-70    OCCUPATION: HOUSEWIFE
                            MARITAL STATUS: MARRIED
                            EDUCATION: TECHNICAL SCHOOL
                   ********************
---THE PATIENT INDICATES THE FOLLOWING SYMPTOMS OR PHENOMENA MAY
HAVE BEEN NOTED (OR MAY HAVE BEEN PROGRESSIVE) DURING THE LAST YEAR:

    SEE LAST SHEET FOR CHIEF COMPLAINT.

    DYSURIA.
    UTI OR NEPHRITIS.
    URINARY FREQUENCY.
    VAGINITIS.
    DEPRESSION.

             PAST HISTORY AND REVIEW OF SYSTEMS
             **********************************

***EYES***
                                 DENIES: CHANGE IN VISION,
                                 DIPLOPIA, SCOTOMATA, OR
                                 BLURRING OF VISION.


***EARS, NOSE, TEETH AND THROAT***
    SUSCEPTIBLE TO RECURRENT PHARYNGITIS.
                                 DENIES: TINNITUS, VERTIGO,
                                 DYSPHAGIA, HEARING CHANGE,
                                 OR HOARSENESS.

***GASTROINTESTINAL***                               15547
    HAS HAD HEMORRHOIDS FOR ABOUT   2 YEAR(S).
    HAS NOTED BLOOD-STREAKING OF STOOL.
                                 DENIES: ABD. PAIN, MELENA,
                                 DIARRHEA, CONSTIPATION,
                                 HEMATEMESIS OR JAUNDICE.

***CARDIO-RESPIRATORY***                             15547
    A HEART MURMUR WAS NOTED   2 YEAR(S) AGO.

***GENITO-URINARY***
    HAS PERSISTENT DYSURIA.
    URINARY FREQUENCY: MORE THAN 10 TIMES A DAY.
    HX. OF GLYCOSURIA.
    HX. OF PROTEINURIA.
    HAS HAD UTI OR NEPHRITIS  10 TIME(S).
        LAST UTI OR NEPHRITIS WAS  1- YEAR(S) AGO.

***OBSTETRICS AND GYNECOLOGY***                      15547
    MENARCHE: BETWEEN AGES 11 AND 15.
        MENSTRUAL FLOW IS USUALLY MODERATE.
        PERIODS USUALLY LAST 3 TO 6 DAYS.
        CYCLE IS AT 3 TO 5 WEEK INTERVALS.
```

Health providers other than physicians are now involved in the collection of data, especially in the area of history and physical examinations. Physician's assistants, medexes, nurse practitioners, and other highly trained health professionals who are skilled in certain topics of medicine and interviewing are now interacting directly with patients in the gathering of this information. Data entries should improve in accuracy, completeness, and usefulness because of this. This is true because there is less of a rush involved in securing these data entries. These new practitioners are assuming several other tasks besides information gathering. As a result, overall workload is shared, and there is more time for some important activities that were rushed through in the past. Physicians have more time to devote to the judgmental aspects of patient care, and data entries that must be made by physicians should now be more thorough and complete.

Still another approach to information gathering for data entries would be a combination of an interview by a skilled health professional, use of a computerized questionnaire, patient interaction with a terminal, and a physical exam by the physician. All in all, whatever method is used, the accuracy of data entries should be verified at the outset.

Information generated by other sources must also be accurate. For example:

- There is an operative report completed after the operation with no final diagnosis.
- There are four laboratory slips with no patient identification on them.
- There is a diagnosis listed on the summary sheet that is not mentioned anywhere else in the record.
- In reviewing the nurses' notes, there is a statement that the patient received penicillin as ordered by the physician. The doctor's orders show no orders for penicillin.
- The nurses' notes state patient's appetite excellent. There is an entry on the multidisciplinary progress notes by the dietitian that says appetite poor—75 percent return on all trays for the past three days.

These examples show the inaccuracy that can happen when data entries are improperly changed, omitted, or otherwise incorrect in content, sequence, or expression. To monitor these data and reduce the number of errors, the medical record manager must assume responsibility for teaching and continuously working with those who are involved in the entry of data. If possible, the medical record administrator should assist those who enter data. By providing personnel, equipment, and a system that facilitates data entry, the accuracy level of entries can be greatly enhanced.

Those who would understand data entries must know where to look for data entries and the relationship of one entry to others. An information component is made up of several data entries. For example, all entries about diet must coincide with one another. If there is an entry by nursing regarding a patient's food intake, it should agree with statements by the physician, dietitian, and possibly the x-ray department. Entries regarding medication dosages and times should be in agreement. This means that all entries describing medication types, amounts, and times taken should agree with one another. Data entries in the pharmacy should verify what is entered on the patient's record. Prescriptions for the patient should also be in agreement with the entries in the pharmacy or the patient's clinic, hospital, or office record.

These examples help us understand the relationship of data entries and also how one could establish a monitoring system to verify accuracy and completeness. The health record professional must know what each entry should consist of and what the total information component should reflect in patient services. Only then can the professional examine records generally, and particularly for adequacy and completeness.

All entries that are made in a narrative mode must have a *date*, a *body of information*, a *signature*, and the *professional title* or designation of the person making the entry. One measure of the completeness of narrative data entries, then, is the presence of all four items in the entry. The question of completeness of information often can be resolved only in particulars, for instance, if there is a correct signature and date, or if the frequency of entries about hospitalization or clinic service seem to justify or follow along with the procedures and practices of the institution. Those who review data entries become skilled in recognizing patterns of information components because they have practice in reading and relating single entries to the totality of entries.

All records are monitored for accuracy and completeness to assure that they contain minimal information as set forth in preestablished standards or bylaws. The system will also review the content of the record to identify incomplete information about service rendered. The monitoring can also survey the level of audit done in cooperation with the medical audit program used to review the quality of medical care. Accuracy and completeness, then, are inseparable in the maintenance of an adequate information system for patients. With the use of deficiency lists, check sheets, and other monitoring devices, medical record professionals have established procedures whereby records can be circulated back to providers—physicians, nurses, and others—for correction or completion of information. The providers are ultimately responsible for completing the information and are obliged to sign their portion of the information to verify the accuracy and completeness of their own entries.

When record managers entered into health information processing, they devised a system to centralize the information on a given patient. Now, if patients enter an institution and indicate that they were treated there the previous year, information on previous treatment can be made available to the present staff. Setting up unit records to make available all fragments of information on a given patient remains an underlying task for the patient information manager. Known as a unit record system, it compiles all information and records in one document and file folder. Some large facilities treat patients with chronic or recurring diseases and accumulate many sheets in a document. Thick documents may be divided for ease of handling. However, all components of the document remain in one record and storage unit.

The computer offers a unique opportunity for verifying accuracy and completeness of records. The computer can work with an interviewee through a terminal and remind the individual that a piece of information is missing or was not entered correctly. This is accomplished through programs that are written to control what the computer receives. For example, a patient is admitted to the obstetrical ward, and her age is listed as 04. That information isn't compatible with the characteristics of an obstetrical patient, and the computer would communicate this data entry error via CRT display. This kind of monitoring can also be done when patients work with medical history questionnaires.

Another example of computer assistance in monitoring accuracy and completeness is the problem-oriented medical record system established in the PROMIS program. All data entries on the physician's plans, doctor's orders, progress notes, and so on, are keyed into a given problem number and title. If the patient enters the institution with three problems—for instance, heart failure, pulmonary edema, and cataracts—the computer will wait for the clinician's entry on the titled and numbered problem before it carries out the order. If the physician orders drug therapy for heart failure, the computer will wait to enter problem number 1, heart failure, and indicate the drug order. It will then acknowledge that it has received the information and transmit the order directly to the pharmacy. The information will appear on a CRT screen in the pharmacy and sound a small whistle to tell the staff that an order has come in. The staff in the pharmacy will usually fill the prescription immediately, acknowledge it through the terminals, and with the help of the computer, decrease their inventory for that medicine by the amount called for in the prescription. The terminal will automatically print out a label for the prescription with the specific instructions sent in by the physician and have the order available for the patient within a matter of minutes. By 1990, the whole teleprocessing system will probably work like the one illustrated in Figure 2-3.

Exhibit 2-11 is an example of the pharmacy record and medicine label. Since the computer produces gummed labels for each new medication order, the pharmacists do not have to type them. The label showing the patient's name, bed location, attending physician, and the medication ordered is affixed to the container of the patient's initial supply of medication. This supply is just enough to last until the next unit dose servicing of the patient's nursing station. The patient's medication allergies are printed alongside the label to assist the pharmacist in checking for allergy problems.

Technology obviously helps promote accuracy. The computer requires the physician to key in the prescription for the problem in question, verifies what that problem is, and sends the order to the pharmacy staff exactly as the physician entered it for the problem listed. All this and a printout of the correct prescription label are based on the single order of the physician. This is how technology has effectively enhanced the accuracy and completeness of the information network. Health information managers can expect to see computers handling more and more data entries. The medical information system created by Technicon for El Camino Hospital in Mountain View, California, is an excellent example of an on-line computer system in which data entries are made by physicians, nurses, and allied health personnel of all professions. The entries are stored on a magnetic disc while the patient is in the hospital. Entries may be called up on the screen as needed by persons who are properly identified with badges and ID numbers.

When the patient is discharged, the stored information is accumulated and combined with summary information about laboratory results, radiological tests, and medication, and selected nursing summary discharge care plans. These data are automatically printed out and sent to the medical record department, where they become part of the patient record.

An interesting feature of the system is that the physician's orders are numbered sequentially. This means that each order is given a number as it occurs, and these numbers serve as an index to determine if specific orders were carried out. Upon discharge, the medical record department then uses these numbers as an aid in analyzing the record for completeness.

Figure 2-3 Teleprocessing in 1990

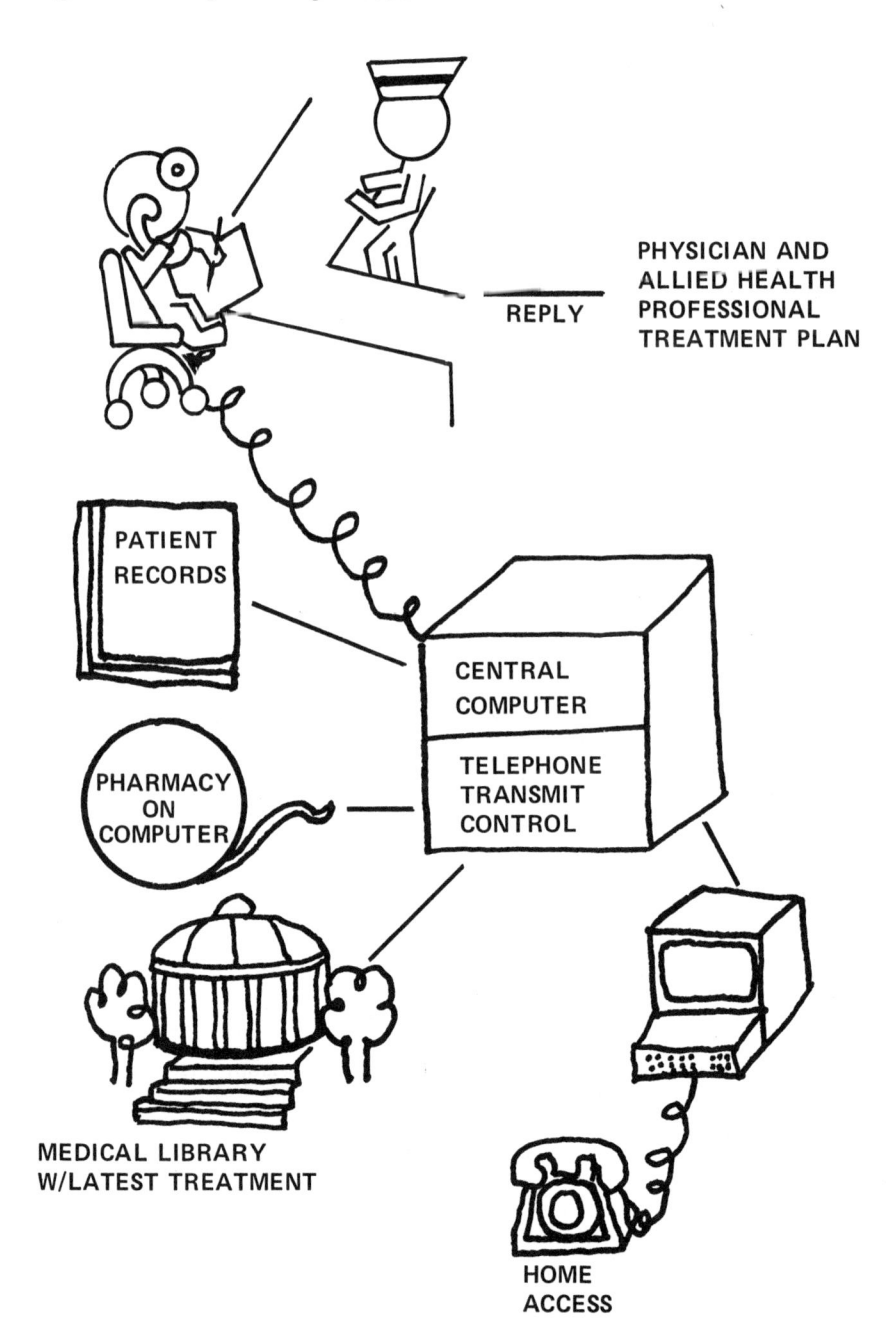

PHYSICIAN AND
ALLIED HEALTH
PROFESSIONAL
TREATMENT PLAN

REPLY

PATIENT
RECORDS

CENTRAL
COMPUTER

TELEPHONE
TRANSMIT
CONTROL

PHARMACY
ON
COMPUTER

MEDICAL LIBRARY
W/LATEST TREATMENT

HOME
ACCESS

Exhibit 2-11 Prescription Record and Medication Label

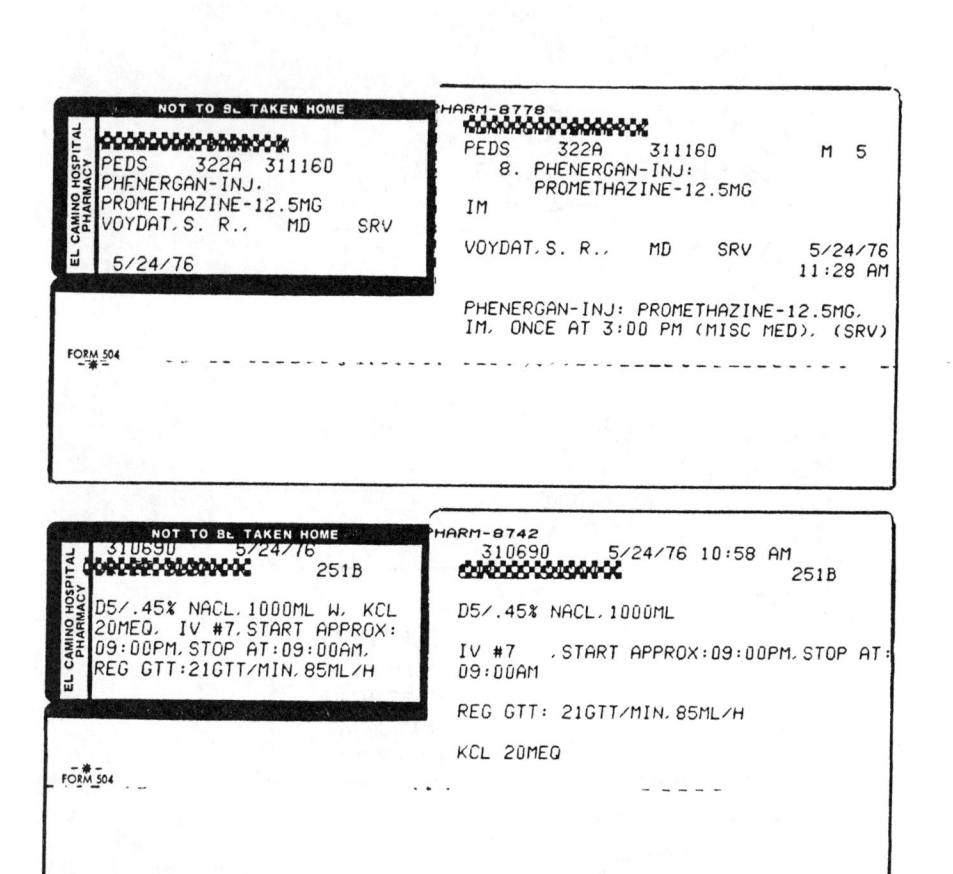

Source: Melville H. Hodge, *Medical Information Systems* (Germantown, Md.: Aspen Systems Corporation, 1977). Reprinted with permission.

Patient information managers, medical records personnel, health information analysts, and allied health professionals in all health care facilities need to understand that there must be a system, whether manual, mechanical, or computerized. The system must meet the needs of the institution in establishing the patient record through secured data entries. Data entries must be developed in an appropriate manner to verify accuracy and completeness of those entries according to standards established by the institution.

The health information manager must consider the flow of information in the institution. Information may come from the admissions office, outpatient department, hospital emergency room, patient receptionist in a specialty clinic, or social worker in a psychiatric facility. The flow of information must be coordinated to facilitate and promote the most accurate and complete collection of data from the time the patient enters the system until the patient is discharged. Following discharge, the information is transmitted via the record to the next agency or facility.

The purpose of maintaining health records in all environments is to provide maximum information to those caring for the patient. We must first consider usefulness of data entries in terms of availability for the individual patient's needs. Usefulness of data entries is the reason that the medical records professional, as a *patient advocate*, develops a system and methods to maintain records in the facility.

There are two major methods or systems of recordkeeping—the source-oriented record and the problem-oriented record. Each was designed to promote maximum use of the data entry in patient information. The source-oriented record maintains all reports and data from a given department in one section. The record is organized so that data entries are seen in chronological sequence within each section. The viewer picks up the source-oriented record and looks for an identifying tab or color border that indicates that the sheet comes from the x-ray section, the laboratory section, the progress notes, or the nurses' notes. The reader turns to the section of choice in the record and locates the specific entries desired—for example, test results on a liver function scan. The source-oriented record was a widely accepted design for medical records from the beginning of record standardization in the 1920s until the mid-1960s.

THE PROBLEM-ORIENTED MEDICAL RECORD

Lawrence L. Weed, M.D., introduced the concept of the problem-oriented medical record (POMR). The purpose of the POMR is to make patient data entries more useful by keying them to a table of contents that Dr. Weed calls a problem list. His theory is that each patient seeks help with a list of

active health problems and that the clinician establishes a plan to investigate, diagnose, treat, and educate the patient about each of these problems.
Dr. Weed perceives the traditional physician's orders as plans and keys
them to a problem number and title. He then keys the progress notes to that
number and title.

The progress notes in the POMR have four components: subjective
information from the patient and provider indicating their perception of
current conditions; objective data, which are lab reports, test results,
observations from physical examination of a wound, and so on; assessment
of the patient's condition by the physician or other providers; and the plan
for continued treatment or therapy. Dr. Weed labeled these elements of the
progress notes—subjective data, objective data, assessment, and plan
—SOAP. Organizing progress notes in this manner is known as SOAPing.

Dr. Weed's method is used by physicians and other providers and is
widely accepted by health care institutions in psychiatry, mental retardation, and other health care areas. To a large extent, Dr. Weed's documentation plan has been accepted outside the health care industry. The entire
concept of the problem-oriented record is illustrated in Figure 2-4.

Part of Dr. Weed's rationale for establishing his system was to allow a
reviewer to audit the care provided to patients. In the source-oriented
method it is difficult to determine why a given prescription was ordered. It
is difficult to find out exactly what the patient's condition was at 10 A.M.
on the previous Friday with respect to the heart problem, weight problem,
insomnia, or depression. Dr. Weed maintains that the organized method
that identifies each provider's selection of tools to treat the patient, whether
the tool is investigative or therapeutic, is the best means for promoting maximum patient care. His system requires that plans, therapy, and progress
notes be keyed to the problem in question. Exhibit 2-12 is a sample problem
list.

Exhibit 2-12 Sample Problem List

PROBLEM LIST: Example I
PATIENT NAME: 38-year-old male
  #1 Epigastric distress
  #2 History of intermittent liquid stools
  #3 Overweight (= 35%)
  #4 Smoking
  #5 Family history of lung cancer (father)
  #6 Anxiety about excessive job mobility
  #7 Inflamed asymptomatic conjunctivae
  Temporary Problem A: Abnormal chemistry

Figure 2-4 The Problem-Oriented Medical Record: Component Parts and Sequence

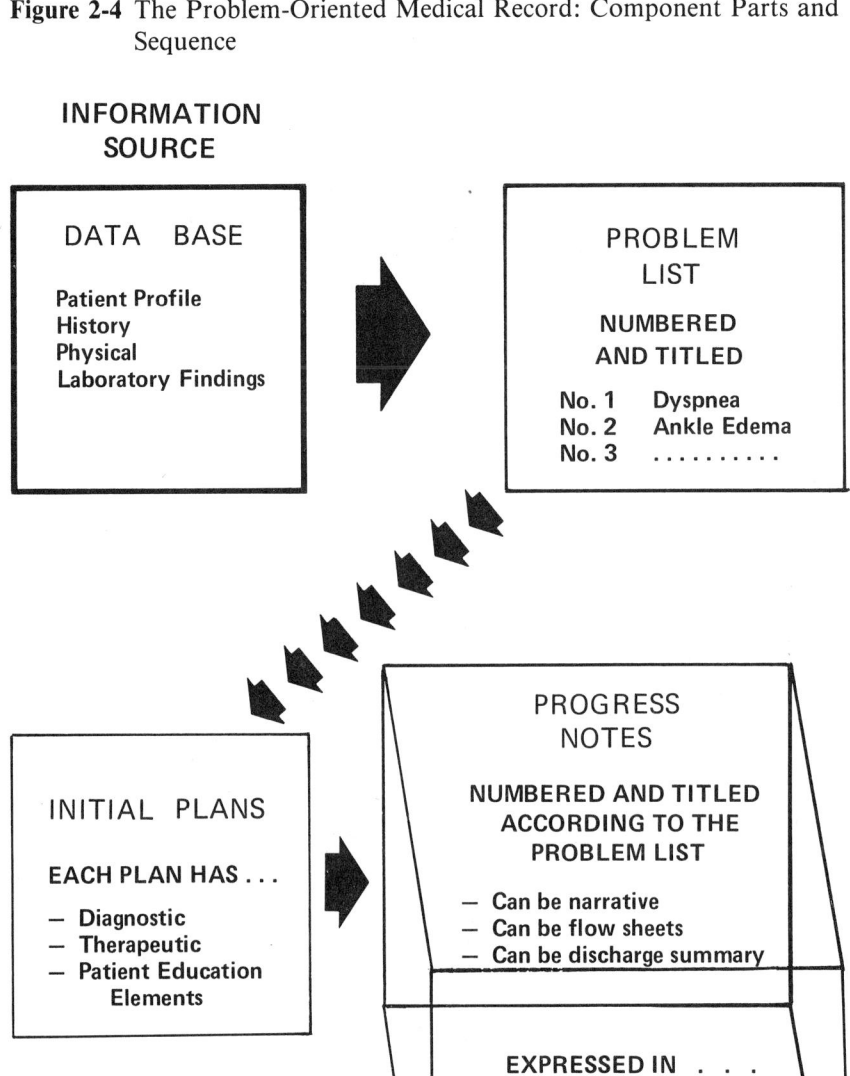

INFORMATION
SOURCE

DATA BASE

Patient Profile
History
Physical
Laboratory Findings

PROBLEM
LIST

NUMBERED
AND TITLED

No. 1   Dyspnea
No. 2   Ankle Edema
No. 3   . . . .

INITIAL PLANS

EACH PLAN HAS . . .

— Diagnostic
— Therapeutic
— Patient Education
    Elements

PROGRESS
NOTES

NUMBERED AND TITLED
ACCORDING TO THE
PROBLEM LIST

— Can be narrative
— Can be flow sheets
— Can be discharge summary

EXPRESSED IN . . .

S ubjective — patient described

O bjective — clinical observations and
                diagnostic findings

A ssessment — physician's judgment

P lan — action taken as a result of
         the assessment

The POMR is a major change in methodology for health care providers. It has had major impact on the health care industry. Its format has served as an instrument in computerizing data entries. The PROMIS reference program is based on the POMR system. If the information in the record is to be of any use to the patient, provider, or planners of health care, it must be auditable. Dr. Weed's belief is that only the problem-oriented system is auditable. One purpose of the POMR is to consider the whole patient and all of the patient's problems. POMR organizes the narrative data in records, and the problem list properly profiles a given patient's condition.[4] Health record professionals have adapted Dr. Weed's system to a variety of settings. The problem-oriented system is flexible enough to be used in alternative health care delivery systems, such as psychiatric hospitals. In this situation the staff felt that patients needed to see their problems listed, but they also needed to see their strengths listed so that the strengths were always evident and could be used for reinforcement in treatment. Assets were added to the POMR and provided a focus for motivation. Assets remained on the list even when problems were added or listed as no longer active. The result was a document that is useful to staff, germane to the individual, personalized, and holistic.

Usefulness of data entries is also considered from the point of view of statistics, epidemiology, and general health services planning, as well as individual health services planning. These perspectives on data usefulness will be covered elsewhere in the book.

THE CHARACTERISTICS OF DATA ENTRIES

Data entries may be dynamic or permanent. The status of your health may change. Your date of birth never will. Your name may change, but your parents' dates of birth or places of birth will not. Laboratory values may change with the state of your health. Those values are dynamic. Your chromosomes will always remain the same. Their record is permanent.

The difference between dynamic and permanent data entries can affect the design of forms, the review of information for completeness, and the methods used to gather and verify data. These tasks are a primary concern of the health records manager.

Data entries also may be singular or cumulative. Some data entries, such as laboratory test results or blood analyses, are recorded and compiled in a cumulative fashion. Certain laboratory values are determined by machine or by processing every ten seconds, and the data are recorded in a cumulative form. Other information is recorded as a single entry. Individual progress notes, for example, are singular entries.

Data entries are inherently sequential—some are necessarily so. A provider needs to know what drugs a patient took on a previous day before prescribing drugs for the patient today. Today's data entry is necessarily based on yesterday's entry.

Many data entry values are relative to a norm. For example, test results are usually stated in numbers and actually describe the relationship of a patient's performance on a particular test to a norm or standard range of test values. This is true of many other data entries. Descriptions of appetite, height, growth weight, urine output, blood pressure, and hematocrit are all examples of data entries that are relative to norms or standards.

Another attribute of data entries is currentness. Entries are current when they are recorded close to the time the event takes place. The time between the information gathering and the entering of the data should be as short as possible. Lack of currentness is a frequent problem in manual systems. The physician orders a lab test; the test is completed, but the information is not filed soon enough for the next clinic visit. This causes a lapse in the flow of information. It also may lead to the expense and inconvenience of another test. It certainly creates frustration and lack of continuity of care for the patient. For efficiency in communicating data entries in the problem-oriented system, Dr. Weed focuses on recording diagnostic test results in numbers and on flow sheets as much as possible. Exhibit 2-13 is a sample data sheet showing information in numerical form. The graph in Exhibit 2-14 contains information that has been translated from narrative or numerical data and listed on a computer printout. It gives the viewer information on data entries, but the form of the information is a graph or plot. Tests that use scanners are frequently printed out on plotters. The selection of the form and format of data entries, comprehension of narrative entries and their appropriateness, use of numerical entries, and implementations of a system such as the problem-oriented medical record all require decisions by the health information manager. The medical or health record system is tailored to meet the needs of the patient, the providers, and appropriate accrediting and licensing agencies in a given location.

Here again computer technology enters the picture. The many data entries that were formerly narrative descriptions of the way a patient felt, or descriptions of the way a patient looked, or statements of a problem, such as "I feel tired all the time, or have difficulty breathing," can be given numerical equivalents and stored in a computer. When a patient states a problem to the physician, the physician simply keys in a number on the terminal. The printout of that entry has been translated into a standard narrative statement, such as "I feel tired all the time." So the entry and retrieval forms that the data take are no longer limited. Even expressions of laboratory values as they deviate from the norm can be stated in percentages

Exhibit 2-13 POMR Flow Sheet—Numerical Data Entries

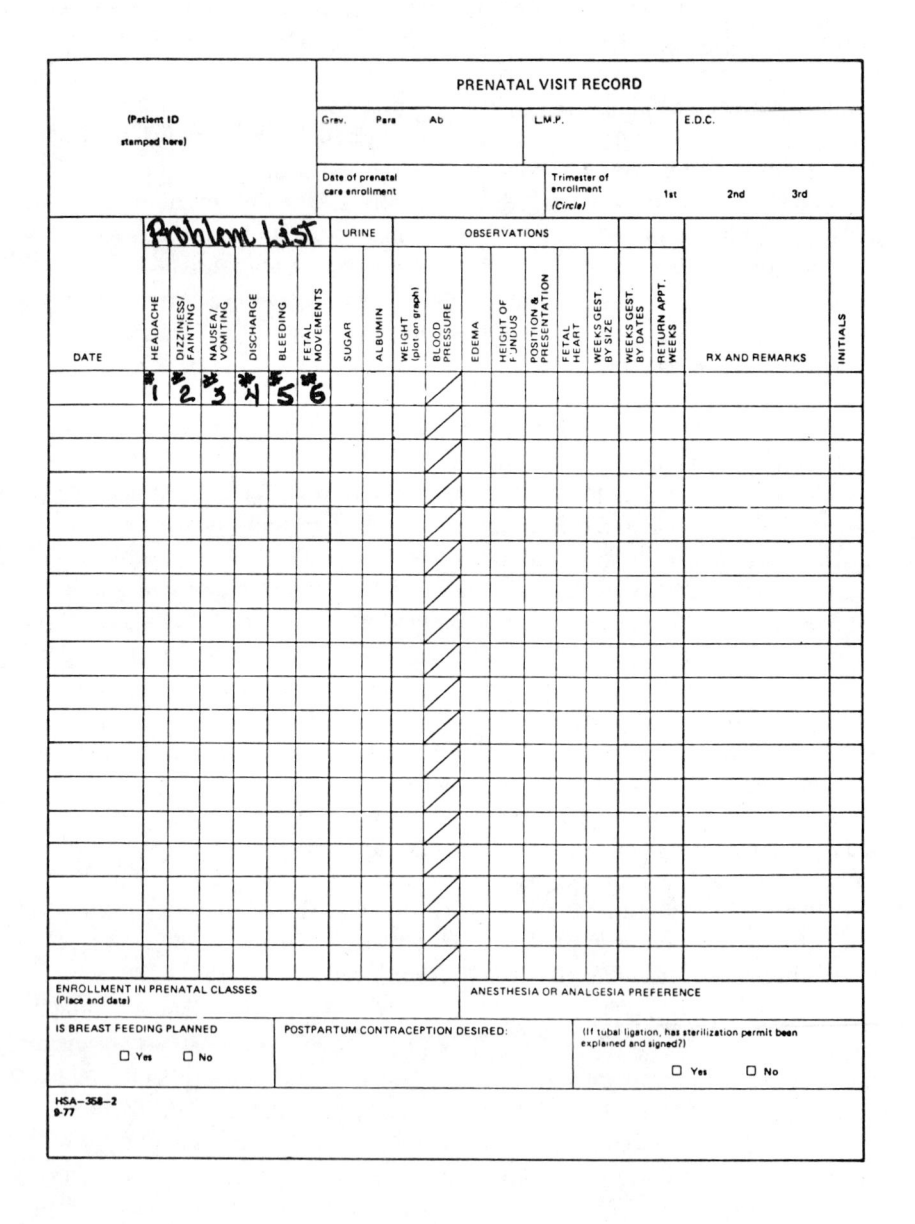

Exhibit 2-14 POMR Flow Sheet—Blood Pressure and Medication Graph

```
                    HYPERTENSION CLINIC DATA SHEET                          FORS
   A39821                                                                03-31-77
   AFOLABI, JULIUS
   T-2
      INITIAL   VISIT: 04-02-75      BP: 184/114 (137)      WGT: 145
      LAST      VISIT: 02-10-77      BP: 112/80 (90)        WGT: 140

      CURRENT MEDICATIONS                        LAST LAB VALUES
   ALDOMET          500 MG BID          URIC ACID     7.7    (12-01-76)
   DYAZIDE          1 QD                BUN          16.0    (12-01-76)
   K SUPL           1 BID               POTASSIUM     3.3    (12-01-76)
                                        HGB          14.6    (12-01-76)
                                        RENIN          .6    (04-02-75)

                        BLOOD PRESSURE/MEDICATION GRAPHS
      >200 :
       200 :
            :
       190 :
            :
       180 :S
            :
       170 :
            : S
       160 :
            :
      .150 :      S                       S
            :                             S
       140 :           S                 S
            : S  S          S        S
       130 :                    S   S        S
            :               S                  S
       120 :           S                  S      S
            :
       110 :D                                          S
            :
       100 : D                    DD
            :        D            D        D
        90 : D  D  D          D        D
            :
        80 :      D  D       D        D  D     D    D
            :           D
        70 :
       < 70 :
            :+++++++++++++++++++++++++++++++++++++++++++++++++++++
                        75^76                        76^77    T

   DIUCARDIN    +..+-...-..........+......+....0
   ALDACTONE    +..+0
   ALDOMET         +...............................................
   K SUPL          +...............................................
   DYAZIDE                     +............._.........
```

Reprinted with permission: Jenkin, M.A., M.D.,
A Manual of Computers in Medical Practice,
The Society of Computer Medicine, 1977.

instead of numerical figures or plotted visually. Whatever makes the information most readable and comprehensible to the provider of care is the form that the data entry should take. The discharge summary report in Exhibit 2-15 illustrates different attributes of data entries. Notice how various data entries are brought together in a summary of the health services provided during a particular hospitalization.

Exhibit 2-15 Sample Discharge Summary Report

Admitted: 6/29/78
Date Discharged: 7/09/78

D
I
R
E
C
T

HISTORY: This is the first University Hospital admission for this 6-year-old white female referred from St. Petersburg, Florida. The patient was noted to have a murmur at the age of 4 years and since she was asymptomatic, no surgery was advised. In December 1978 she was seen by a pediatric physician who again noted the murmur and advised cardiac catheterization. Diagnosis of atrial septal defect was made. She has been asymptomatic throughout; however, surgery was advised and the patient's family chose to come to _____

PAST MEDICAL HISTORY: Noncontributory to the present illness.

FAMILY HISTORY, REVIEW OF SYSTEMS: Noncontributory to the present illness.

D
I
R
E
C
T

PHYSICAL EXAMINATION: She is a well-developed white female child in no distress. Pulse 98 and regular.
Skin: no lesions.
HEENT: within normal limits. The patient has small tonsils without inflammation or exudation.
Neck: supple, without masses.
Chest: the lungs are clear to percussion and auscultation.
Cardiovascular: she has a regular rhythm, no cardiomegaly to percussion. There is a slight right ventricular heave, Grade II/VI soft, systolic murmur over the entire precordium, and no diastolic murmur can be heard.
Abdomen: within normal limits. The liver cannot be palpated.
Genitalia and Rectal: within normal limits.
Neurological examination: within normal limits.

Exhibit 2-15 Continued

I
N
D
I
R
E
C
T

LABORATORY DATA: Urinalysis, 0-1 white cells per high-power field, otherwise entirely normal. Hematocrit ranged from 36 on admission to 35.5 on discharge. White count 8,000 to 11,000. Urine culture showed no growth. Blood culture showed no growth. BUN preoperatively was 21 mg. %, glucose 71 mg. %. Postoperative BUN was 10 mg. %.

X-RAYS: Cardiac series: congenital heart disease, left to right shunt of large volume at the atrial level. Postoperative chest films were satisfactory.

EKG: Normal sinus rhythm, right bundle branch block, right ventricular hypertrophy, right axis deviation.

HOSPITAL COURSE: The patient was taken to the operating room on July 2, 1978, where open heart repair of the atrial septal defect was accomplished. The postoperative course was completely benign. She developed a slight pericardial friction rub, which was felt to be of little or no consequence. The patient was discharged in satisfactory condition one week postoperatively, to come back to surgery clinic for follow-up on two occasions, and then to return to Florida to the care of her private physician. Suggest electrocardiogram follow-up in one to two months to evaluate change in right ventricular hypertrophy.

FINAL DIAGNOSIS: Congenital heart disease, atrial septal defect.

THE FUNCTIONS AND ACTIVITIES OF A HEALTH INFORMATION SYSTEM

Data entries must be brought together in an organized document to be meaningful. We have seen examples of data entries throughout this chapter. They represent the range of data entries possible in a variety of health care settings. The reason for focusing on the data entry is threefold.

First, as computer technology influences recordkeeping in health care, each data element will come under careful scrutiny. This is because computers potentially can increase accessibility through faster storage and retrieval. However, planning must be specific if computer storage is to be great enough to accommodate computerized records. Decisions about the computer file design—whether to make it of a fixed length or a variable length—will become paramount. It will be vital in this planning to analyze thoroughly each data entry to determine whether to keep it and how to collapse and store it on the computer. Computer storage is expensive. The individual patient record will be evaluated for the volume of space it uses and how fast it may be read. What types of data entries should be maintained on a computer record? What types could be purged immediately after treatment is completed?

A second reason for focusing on the data entry is that specific functional operations in medical and health records departments are determined by characteristics and qualities of data entries. We will look more closely at this concept.

Recall that data entries must be verified and analyzed for completeness. Generally, verification and analysis are done by trained personnel in a records department. We call this function chart analysis. All records are verified for consistent order of assembly; the entire record is carefully reviewed. Specific areas that are incomplete are identified. Notice is given to the providers who must complete the items. As a follow-up, the health record department must provide a means by which the physician or other provider may come and rectify the deficiencies in the record.

Since the effectiveness of a medical record system can be measured by the number of complete records available for use by and for patients, record deficiencies are monitored on a regular basis. Reports on the status of incomplete records are often sent to medical staff members, administrative personnel, nursing and allied health personnel, and others who need the information.

Data entries are used to document the care rendered. This documentation, in turn, is needed to initiate payment. Someone must review the medical record to determine the reason for and the type of treatment provided and to transmit that specific information to third-party payers such as Blue Cross and Blue Shield. Records should be reviewed immediately after patient discharge in cooperation with the business office. It is the first step in securing payment for services provided.

Data entries that record the step-by-step progress of treatment are required by providers to direct continued patient care. When patients are transferred from one facility to another, an abstract or summary of the treatment and a patient care plan should accompany the patient. Such a plan would include current diagnosis, medications, nursing care activities, and physician's orders for continuing the care at the next location.

Data entries require updating. When patients reenter a health care setting, updated information is added to the record. Health record personnel review the master patient index to learn whether the patient has been treated in the past. If so, the card is pulled or the computer display is called up and the new admission data is added to the document. In some hospitals, this process also automatically creates an admission register, adds to the admission list for the day, and provides input for the calculation of the census. (The census is the daily count of patients in the facility.)

If the patient is returning for treatment at the facility, records from previous admissions are pulled and made available to the physician and other providers. If the patient is a new patient, an initial record must be prepared and a corresponding card added to the master patient index.

Data entries are used to verify that care has been provided. Particular kinds of health problems will generate particular kinds of data entries. For instance, a blood count, urinalysis, and chest x-ray might be performed on all patients. However, patients with peptic ulcers would probably have additional tests, such as an upper GI (gastrointestinal) x-ray series. Health care professionals review the care provided by evaluating patient's records. They select particular diagnoses and review the corresponding records to see if appropriate care was provided. Medical record department personnel, working with medical staff committees, pull records, review them to see if the data entries document the specific kinds of activities that should have been performed, prepare reports showing the results of such review, and direct the records back to committee for recommended action. This is an ongoing process in medical and health record departments. Data entries from patient records are used to measure the care provided and feed back the analysis of that care to physicians and other providers.

To retrieve the records of patients who have the same selected diagnosis, someone must first identify them. This is done through review of the disease and operation index, a numerical index of patient problems, diagnoses, and procedures by individual categories. For instance, hypertension might be coded in one system as 437.5. In a disease index system, there is a separate card, page, or file for Hypertension 437.5. One operation carried on in medical record departments is the coding of all patient diseases and the recording of the patient's name on the appropriate disease index card, such as Hypertension 437.5 or Cancer of the Prostate 637.3.

Review of a particular diagnosis or problem by an evaluating committee is integrally involved in coding and indexing operations. The diagnosis or problem is used to retrieve the names of patients who fall into the category under study. When someone pulls patient records from the main files, a chart out guide is prepared that records the date and name of the person removing the record and the reason for removing it. This guide is filed in the record location so that other requesters will be directed to the location of the patient record. The guide is removed when the record is refiled.

Data entries documenting diagnostic tests, medications, and special treatments are coded and indexed for access. Individual providers who wish

Figure 2-5 Functional Operations Related to Data Entries

Data Entries Target Functional Operations

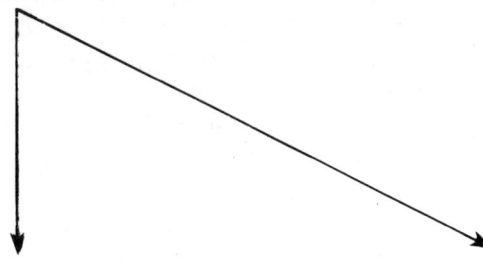

- To evaluate completeness of medical records, analysis and verification of data entries is required.
- To secure completeness of individual data entries, it is necesarry to initiate and follow-up on physician and other providers' data entires.
- Continuous assessment of patterns of documentation in patient records is achieved through monitoring adequacy of data entries.
- Reimbursement operations depend on prompt, accurate information on medical diagnosis and procedures to initiate payment.
- Information for individual patient's continuing medical care, legal assistance and health or life insurance are routinely abstracted from medical records.
- Follow-up systems for tracking cancer and other chronic health conditions are established and maintained through ongoing procedures in patient record departments.
- Effective inter-facility transfer programs and home health care programs require information from nursing entries in patient care plans.
- Facts drawn from data contained in patient records provide statistics for health agency review, assessment and planning operations.
- Patient records are used for medical staff activities that monitor and evaluate care through utilization review and medical audit functions.
- Data entries are coded and indexed by numbering systems so that research programs may be developed and sustained.
- Individual patient records are maintained in filing systems to be available for continuing care.

to study the effects of a certain medication on patients with the same diagnosis might request those particular records.

Figure 2-5 shows many functional operations carried out in a health or medical record system that relate back to characteristics and attributes of data entries. Other functional operations we have not discussed are statistics, cancer registry reports, legal requests, and pulling and filing clinic charts. These functions will be addressed in succeeding chapters.

Our third reason for focusing on the elementary unit of data entries is their role in the construction of vital, effective, action research programs to increase available health care resources for larger patient populations. Health care data, looked at collectively, are the source and measurement for meeting this need. The critical importance of having health care data that are accurately and comprehensively collected, stored, and made available for research is featured in the statement by the American Hospital Association (AHA) on the definition, need for, and use of health care data that appears in Appendix 2A. The statement was approved by the AHA House of Delegates on August 30, 1977.

In summary, data entries are the core of all information processing. The quality and usefulness of the information are directly proportionate to the accuracy and completeness of the data entries. Data entries determine the formats of medical forms, a characteristic on which Chapter 4 focuses.

NOTES

1. *Common Data Set For Hospital Management*, DHEW Pub. No. (HRA) 74-3026, U.S. Govt. Printing Office (1974).

2. *Ambulatory Medical Care Records: Uniform Minimum Basic Data Set*, U.S. Dept. of Vital & Health Statistics; Series 4, #16, National Center for Health Statistics, Rockville, Md. (Aug., 1974).

3. *Long-Term Health Care: Minimum Data Set*; USDHEW Office of Health Policy, Research and Statistics, National Center for Health Statistics, Sept. 8, 1978.

4. Lawrence L. Weed, *Your Health Care & How to Manage It* (Essex Junction, Vt.: Essex Publishing Co. Inc., 1975).

Appendix 2A

Health Care Data

This statement, S032, was developed in response to new concerns that have emerged as demands for health care have increased. The American Hospital Association's Council on Research and Development appointed a working party to revise S008, Statement on Health Data Systems, published in 1973, which stressed the need to develop useful data systems. The new statement, S032, elaborates upon the responsibilities attendant to the development of such systems.

On March 3, 1977, the Council on Research and Development approved the revised statement and recommended that the 1973 statement be rescinded. Following review and comment by various policymaking bodies within the Association, the AHA House of Delegates on August 30, 1977, approved the statement on Health Care Data (S032), which supersedes S008.

Hospitals generate *health care data* (see Glossary) to satisfy their various internal information requirements and to meet the increasing demands for data from users outside the institution. More detailed data on a broader range of subjects will be required as the decision-making process changes at all levels of the health care delivery system. As the number of potential users of the data continues to increase, hospitals will need to apply data effectively and to meet efficiently the data needs of other organizations.

The American Hospital Association for some time has recognized the importance of expanding both the content and use of health care data. This statement identifies the important issues arising from increasing demands for data and assesses the implications of these developments for hospitals and other health care institutions. Many of these issues have not yet been resolved, and hospitals therefore have both an opportunity and an obligation to contribute their experience and expertise to discussions with other concerned public and private organizations.

Source: ©1978 by the American Hospital Association, 840 North Lake Shore Drive, Chicago, Illinois 60611.
Printed in the U.S.A. All rights reserved. Catalog no. S032. 12M-3/78-6102.
Reprinted with permission.

The expectations and needs of institutions that generate and use data frequently differ from those of individuals and organizations seeking access to these data. Cooperation among data collectors and providers is therefore essential as pressures increase to provide data for a variety of public and private purposes. The Association urges its member institutions to participate in the development and operation of cooperative arrangements with other data providers and with users to establish coordinated, efficient, and effective *health care data systems* (see Glossary) at the local level. State and regional hospital associations should assist their members to develop and participate in such systems at the state and regional levels and to facilitate their integration at the national level. These arrangements should identify the types of data covered by the agreement and specify the terms and conditions under which data may be released to users by data providers, individually or collectively. These conditions will vary, depending on the data providers and users involved and on the needs for data. Hospitals and their representatives must participate in determining these conditions in order to voice their interests in controlling the use of data generated in hospitals.

The Association will guide and advise its membership on technical and policy issues related to data at the local and state levels. This guidance should include assistance during the negotiation of agreements on local and regional data systems. Integrated, coordinated data systems at these levels are especially important if national data needs are to be met by existing data systems.

Standardization

Standardization means the compilation of data from diverse sources so that data can be organized, analyzed, and fed back to users.* Standardization will occur either de facto or de jure, and the Association believes that the necessary standardization should take place without legislation. Integrated voluntary health data systems are more likely to meet diverse needs for data than a single mandatory data system, which would be less responsive to local and regional data needs and to existing data systems and data providers. Voluntary cooperative arrangements are necessary to coordinate the components of data systems and to develop specifications for data sets.

A voluntary system for the provision of health care data poses difficulties in the coordination of a large number of individual data systems, but the benefits anticipated from the success of such a system, such as greater flexibility and responsiveness to the need of both data providers and users,

---

*Familiar examples of standardization in other health care contexts include the *Chart of Accounts* and the *International Classification of Diseases, Adapted.*

compensate for these deficiencies. In the interest of cost containment, elements of data, wherever possible, should be recorded only once, and users should accept the least expensive means of reproducing these elements.

Types of Health Care Data

There are many types of health care data that are useful in a variety of applications. The incidence and type of illness and disability, life expectancy, and mortality rates are described by population-based health statistics. Environmental and social conditions and health hazards can be studied along with other determinants of health. Once the extent of illness is known, the social and economic consequences of poor health can be identified. In addition, health care resources, including the supply of manpower, facilities, and services, can be described statistically. Resource statistics may be related to utilization statistics covering ambulatory care, the types of practice providing services, and inpatient services. Finally, information on health care costs, financing, and sources of expenditures are useful in an increasing variety of analyses.

Management Applications of Health Care Data

Health care data are employed successfully in the internal operations and planning of hospitals. Hospitals and other health care institutions should continue to make effective use of data in management, and all managers should apply data to improve their operations. Data generated within an institution are used to construct profiles over a period of time for determining changes in departmental performance. Cross-sectional comparative data profiles derived from health care data systems enable health care institutions to evaluate their performance in light of the experience of similar institutions. Specific data used in this regard include comparisons of expenditures, productivity, staffing levels, utilization, and occupancy rates. Such data also are useful in providing feedback for monitoring the effects of programs directed at specific operational problems.

Patient Care Data

Patient care within hospitals can best be evaluated and managed when adequate information about large numbers of inpatients and ambulatory care patients and their treatment is available. Information about length of stay, diagnoses, therapies, tests, case outcomes, and procedures can be aggregated and analyzed to gauge the quality, effectiveness, and appropriateness of care rendered to patients in hospitals and by health care professionals. Several health care data systems specialize in the collection, analysis, and feedback of such data to member institutions.

Health Care Resources

Decisions about the allocation of health care resources require the best available data, both on the current deployment of facilities, services, and manpower, and on the expected future availability of these resources. This information can be used to identify areas suffering from shortages of resources as well as those with an overabundance and is, therefore, a prerequisite of any attempt to alter the existing resource distribution. Aside from use in such decisions at the community, regional, and national levels, these data are useful to the individual institution as it plans to meet anticipated future demands for services.

As decisions about the distribution of health care resources are increasingly made in an atmosphere of real or perceived resource constraints, accurate information is required for the evaluation of alternative uses and for selection of the most efficient resource use.

Research and Development

Health services research and development has been defined in the AHA statement *Health Services Research and Development (S026)* as the "systematic process of adding to useful knowledge, either through discovery of new knowledge (research) or through new applications for existing knowledge (development)." Research and development activities can be conducted in health care institutions or by outside researchers. In either case, the purpose of these activities is to contribute to efficiency and effectiveness in the delivery of health services, and the availability of accurate data is important in determining the validity of research. These activities are particularly concerned with the effects of organization, management, financing, public policy, and the allocation of health resources on access to services, quality and outcome of services, and efficiency of the delivery system. Many disciplines contribute to health services research and development, which complements biomedical and clinical research and epidemiology.

Minimum Uniform Basic Data Sets

Hospitals, their representatives, and other providers and users of health care data should involve themselves in the development of *minimum uniform basic data sets* (see Glossary) at the relevant geographical and political levels. Such data sets consist of a limited number of standardized data items and relevant uniform definitions to meet the needs of multiple users. The raw data in each set can be aggregated and rearranged in various ways to construct data displays and tabulations to meet the specific needs of most data users.

The items collected in minimum uniform basic data sets must be kept to a manageable number if they are to serve as an efficient method for collecting large amounts of frequently demanded data. However, endorsement of the concept of minimum uniform basic data sets should not be construed as approval of any specific form or format for the collection of such data. This endorsement does not preclude the collection of additional, optional information within the individual institution or within a particular geographic area when necessary. These additional data items will not replace the basic subset of data items.

Minimum uniform basic data sets are essential to meet the differing needs of governmental and private providers and users of data at the national, state, regional, and local levels. Data sets for different purposes, such as billing, quality control, or discharge abstracting, may be necessary. Each basic data set should include a uniform subset of data that links all data sets. Without such a uniform subset of data, it would be impossible to perform analyses requiring the linkage of data collected in different data sets. The detailed specifications of these data sets must be developed as part of the cooperative arrangements among public and private data providers and users.

Auditing

No data system can be more reliable or useful than the quality of data submitted to it. It is not necessary, however, for all data collected routinely by hospitals and other health care institutions to be transmitted to other collection sites for verification. A system for periodic data audits with certification of the data recording, record-keeping, and recovery procedures must be maintained in order to protect standards of uniformity, comparability, and quality. The data systems of institutions could then be approved if they comply with the standards or guidelines that have been enunciated by the participants. The standards for data quality should be realistic and reasonable. Comparisons among institutions could be rendered valueless by data of dubious accuracy. Therefore ensurance of data quality is essential to the integrity of the entire system.

Provisions for audit and certification of data and data systems also reduce the need for large data collections. Data contained in records or original entry in institutions, but certified by a procedure such as this, can be retained for later use, if necessary, in special surveys, samplings, and prospective and retrospective studies.

Need for Cooperation

Major federal initiatives in the area of health care data have already been undertaken. The data needs of the health care field, however, cannot be satisfied exclusively by federal efforts in data collection because jurisdiction is lacking at the state and substate levels where health care data are generated. Although there has been an increasing willingness to enlist existing health care data systems in meeting federal program needs, even greater efforts are essential if these programs are to fulfill their evaluative and regulatory intentions. Cooperation among the federal government, health care data systems, and health care institutions is essential to meet current data needs.

Private voluntary providers and users of health care data should increase their efforts to establish coordinated, effective data systems at the local level and to establish such systems at the state, regional, and national levels through the appropriate organizations. The state and federal governments should similarly strengthen their efforts to involve more of these established providers and processors of health care data in their programs.

Access to Data

Agreements regarding access to data should be negotiated by representatives of data systems, data providers, such as hospitals, and potential users. Although data providers should attempt to formalize and impartially apply standards for access and usage to the requests of all potential data users, they must always exercise their judgment in evaluating each request for data. The ultimate responsibility for determining whether or not data will be released must remain with the data provider.

Consent should be given by the data provider only when need is adequately demonstrated. Providers may legitimately impose fees to defray the costs of collecting, producing, and distributing requested data. All users of data must respect agreements regarding confidentiality and privacy in the handling and usage of data. All institutions contributing data to data systems or other aggregations must be guaranteed access to their data and to the resulting tabulations and statistical arrays.

Education

Each cooperative arrangement must include provisions for educating and guiding participants toward agreements on joint data collection and usage. The educational role should include the provision of information on effective and innovative data applications to internal operations and decision making, especially because of the growing usage of health care data. Education should also be provided on the issues of privacy, confidentiality, and security, both within the data system itself and among participating organizations. Education is especially important within a voluntary cooperative network of health care data systems because it can stimulate innovation in data applications and uses.

Privacy

Wherever possible, only aggregate data should be released. Individual data will not be released except in those instances where such data must be released. Individual patient care data must be protected to the maximum possible extent. Privacy is the right of individuals to determine what information about themselves will be disclosed to others, what will be withheld, and under what conditions. Privacy is not an absolute or overriding right, but it must be carefully weighed against other rights.

The existence of health care data that are generated by the health delivery system poses an additional problem because, although they relate to an individual's personal health matters, they are rarely under the direct control of the individual and therefore are not disclosed by him. However, because the original release of personal information does not constitute a waiver of the individual's right to privacy at subsequent stages of the data flow, this right must be respected throughout the data system. The same consideration must be accorded to personal data that are produced by the health care services system.

Confidentiality

The issue of confidentiality arises after information has been obtained originally by a data system. It arises from the need to ensure that data are released only to authorized persons having legitimate access to them. Data providers and users jointly share a responsibility to those who have disclosed and entrusted data to them, although the full extent of this responsibility has not yet been determined by law or custom.

When data are released by a data system, they should avoid unnecessary detail when possible. The principles embodied in contracts covering submission of information to a data system at the entry level must be respected at all higher levels of aggregation to maintain the integrity of the system. Negotiations may be necessary to resolve discrepancies between systems with conflicting standards of confidentiality for data release. Hospitals and other original sources of data should emphasize to employees the confidentiality of these data.

Security

Security relates to the physical protection of data in contrast to confidentiality, which deals with the conditions governing release of data to authorized persons. Hospitals and other health care institutions must assume responsibility for ensuring that only legitimate use is made of data they retain and that there is not unauthorized access to data.

Organizations receiving, processing, or handling health care data must take all necessary and reasonable precautions to prevent theft, destruction, and other forms of unsanctioned access. Employee educational programs and other measures should be undertaken to maintain confidentiality and security. Extensive use of computers to which access can be gained by telephone lines requires security precautions beyond those needed to guard against physical thefts and break-ins.

Identifiers

Identification of patients and providers is a legitimate requirement for certain reporting purposes. When identifiers are necessary because of legislative mandate or because identification is essential to the achievement of a user's purpose in requesting data, and data providers agree to release the requested information, identifiers should be expunged from the record as early as possible after the data have been utilized. Consistent with principles of privacy, confidentiality, and security, data with identification of patients and providers should be released only for the purpose specified and only to those authorized to receive such data, whether authorized by law or by consent of those identified.

Governance and Coordination

Effective governance is required for the standardization of data and for the successful operation of any data system. Private, voluntary cooperative bodies should provide sufficient governing authority for the conduct of most health care data systems, but public bodies must participate in these arrangements to ensure that their data needs are met.

Providers and users of health care data must have a voice in defining, establishing, and governing such data systems. Hospital associations, medical associations, planning agencies, state health departments, Blue Cross/Blue Shield, and other third-party payment plans and medical care foundations, are examples of organizations that would typically participate because of the health care industry's need to control the uses of the data it generates. Providers of data also should participate in considering proposals for major changes in data collection and transmission. Proposed revisions should be tested and introduced in an orderly manner, and changes in the information to be collected or the reporting format should convey sufficient benefits to warrant any added cost and/or loss of continuity in an historical perspective.

Conclusions

Hospitals and other providers and users of health care data must actively cooperate in arrangements for development of local, regional, state, and national health care data systems if these data are to be used effectively throughout the delivery system.

Hospitals have both an opportunity and an obligation to participate in the organization of voluntary health care data systems that best meet the needs of hospitals and the public. The expertise and experience of hospitals and health care institutions in generating and using data qualify them for a major role and responsibility in contributing solutions to the problems produced by increasing data usage and in protecting their patients' right of privacy to the maximum extent possible.

GLOSSARY

Health care data—Quantitative and qualitative indicators that reflect selected predefined facets of health care services. They encompass, but are not limited to, patient care data, data on professionals and institutions providing health care services, billing and financial statistics, and measures of institutional output and performance. Health care data is a category of indicators relating to health care, health resources, and health status.

Health care data system—The aggregation of operations and procedures, men and machines, united to accomplish specific objectives in the collection, processing, analysis, and/or feedback of health care data. The interaction of the components of such a system accomplishes more than could the sum of its parts because its parts work together and enhance one another. Systems consist of integrated subsystems, so that a state health care data system might be composed of several integrated local and regional systems.

Minimum uniform basic data set—An array of specified information elements and their standardized definitions developed for a specific purpose that are regularly collected by agreement among institutions and individuals providing health care services, regardless of the specific format or form on which they are reported.

Chapter 3

Uncovering the Dynamic Memory of the Medical Record

CHAPTER OBJECTIVES

1. Recognize the memory element of the record as an essential and dynamic characteristic of patient care
2. Relate the characteristic of dynamic growth of the patient record to the record's use in patient care and research
3. Identify the responsibilities of data providers in the development of memory elements and information design
4. Recognize the advantages of computer technology in the development, retention, and retrieval of memory elements
5. Relate individual memory elements to their use in describing collective care
6. Understand the role and function of statistics in health information management
7. Differentiate between descriptive and inference statistics

DYNAMIC GROWTH OF THE MEDICAL RECORD

Medical records are used individually for patient care and collectively for research and other reasons. Records are initiated before birth for patients who receive prenatal care. The information about the baby, who is one of the subjects in prenatal records, changes and grows throughout the lifetime of the living person. The documentation on records is not completed for the individual until after death with the narrative analysis of the autopsy report. Each patient record evolves and gradually forms the basis of a health profile. Beginning with genetic information, the patient record unfolds as a medical history and memory source for health care providers. In group and

97

family practice clinics where patients are followed for a long time, this record is based on a program for continual health care.

As individuals move from one area to another, change physicians, or cease to participate in group practice programs, continuity of patient information is broken. It becomes more difficult to keep track of all incidents of care. Physicians and allied health professionals usually have only one portion of an individual's health record to work with at any one time. Finding the memory elements and pulling them together with current records to expedite care is a critical issue.

- The first goal of medical recordkeeping is to uncover the memory elements for individual patients.
- The second goal of medical recordkeeping is to uncover the memory elements as they reflect collective health care. Data for evaluation, research, education, and active use of health statistics are all included in this goal.

Recognition of Memory Elements in the Patient Record

Generally, there are three categories of information recorded. Records on acute spells of illness include documentation of short-term or limited illnesses, such as measles or influenza. Information is also collected for the management of chronic conditions that require ongoing treatment. Hypertension and diabetes are well-known examples of chronic illnesses. There is also descriptive information, which includes demographic data and facts about the social, economic, psychological, and educational status of an individual. Much of the data base on the patient is descriptive. Often descriptive information is interwoven with data on acute and chronic illnesses in a patient's medical record. These come together to form a three-dimensional picture. The clinician must pull together the person with the information about the person and then provide for health services that meet that patient's unique needs.

First, the physician must identify and collect the appropriate information about the patient to establish a data base that is as accurate and comprehensive as possible.

Second, information must be sorted and selected to yield the data that is most useful at a given time in treating the patient. For instance, the information required to treat periodic bouts with allergy will not be the same as that required to treat hypertensive cardiovascular disease.

Third, health care professionals must identify, select, and adapt appropriate methods that will help them retrieve the data quickly. These methods can range from simple paper records housed in a manual file to sophisticated computer equipment in which records are stored on magnetic tape and retrieved through computer terminals. To present information to the provider of care at the time it is needed, in the form it is needed, remains the fundamental goal of medical recordkeeping.

Fourth, dynamic record growth must be recognized and plans made to direct it. The information explosion in medicine includes more data on the diagnosis and treatment of illness and the results of treatment, and more and more comprehensive individual medical data. In the words of Lawrence Weed, M.D., in an address to the Georgia Medical Society on the role of the problem-oriented medical record (POMR):

> The challenge today is not only to acquire new knowledge; it is to learn how to use knowledge. That is a very profound thing to do.

Fragmented Patient Records

There simply is no comprehensive health record system. The individual is treated in phases and stages of mental, physical, and social illness.

Data are developed by health care providers who must use the patient record to carry out services. Each time the provider sees the patient, another piece of information is accumulated. Each fragment is a memory element in planning the next step. Ambulatory care is an example of data development and collection.

Physicians' offices offer ambulatory care. A mother brings her children in for routine immunizations. An entry is made on each child's record. If one child is a nursing baby, there may be a fragment of information about the mother on the child's record. Down the hall may be a surgeon who performed an appendectomy on the mother ten years ago. A women's clinic in the area may have records on the mother, showing annual Pap smears and two episodes of a fungus infection of the cervix. Additional records on the woman are kept in her ophthalmologist's office and her dentist's office. Each doctor may know nothing of the woman's other medical encounters. However, providers usually are informed of other instances of care through referrals and by the patients themselves. The actual degree of fragmentation is determined by four factors:

1. The ability of the patient to share information that will help reduce fragmentation.
2. The provider's ability to record information that will facilitate its use by other providers. Using referrals, for example, bridges a communication gap between a family physician and a specialist to the benefit of the patient.

3. The ability of the doctor or therapist to draw actively on the patient and on recorded information to plan most effectively for the patient.
4. The effectiveness of the design and operation of the various patient record systems in these applications.

Figure 3-1 illustrates the variety of information categories that are keyed on the patient information system in each case.

Health care providers still do not seem to have a concept of longitudinal health records. How many programs currently training people to provide direct health services include information on patient or client medical record systems? Of those who do receive training, how many are aware of the potential uses of the information? This means that nurses, doctors, dental hygenists, respiratory therapists, physical therapists, speech pathologists, and many others may not have analyzed information systems within their own disciplines. Inadequate attention to entering information into individual patient records may affect short-range and long-range health programs for everyone.

As physicians and other providers try to sort and select data to treat each person, they are directing their own efforts to the problem. Some physicians have centralized patient information by coordinating their health records in a centralized filing system. Others routinely request information from previous records on patients new to their practice. The use of consultation and referral among care providers greatly facilitates communication and care. How well these efforts meet the need is directly related to how well the various individual health information systems support them.

Appropriate Methods for Data Retrieval

Medical information systems range from simple paper records kept in manila folders to sophisticated computer records stored on magnetic tape and retrieved through computer terminals. The particular methods used will depend on the setting and the primary care activities in that setting. In one hospital, computers are used to store all patient records on-line, that is, by direct connection to the central processing unit.[1] Pertinent patient information is called up immediately and displayed on CRT terminals at nursing stations. Nurses, doctors, and other members of the health care team can refer to the record as needed. After patients are discharged, their records are transferred from the computer to paper printouts for final disposition. The goal of the system is to promote maximum use of patient information and more efficient service. This system clearly recognizes that the record is a dynamic memory capable of offering unique assistance to its users.

Figure 3-1 Fragmented Health Services

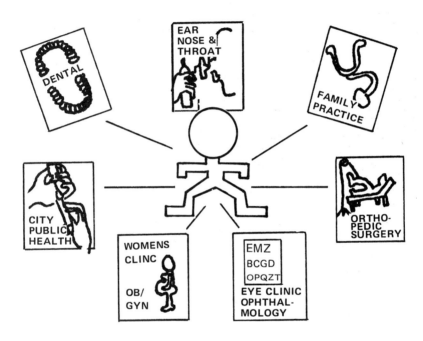

Record Linkage

The process of connecting records on the same individual that have been generated at different times and in different places is record linkage. It brings together in one file all records of an individual by means of a common identification. Two or more items of information about a person recorded at different times may be of greater significance when considered together than when either item is considered alone. The advantages in genetics, research, improved patient care, and better administrative planning are clear.

Many system designers have recognized that fragmentation is a serious obstacle to maximum use of recorded information and have established record linkage programs. Within a state system of institutions for the developmentally disabled, the record is transferred along with the patient. The two are not separated. The Veterans Administration and the military also use record linkage programs.[2] When personnel are transferred from one part of the country to another, their medical records go with them. It promotes available and current use of the information. Hospitals routinely pull forward old records when patients are readmitted so that previous information is available in the present. Active use of this resource gives all members of the health care team a more complete view of the patient and allows for more comprehensive treatment planning.

The computer offers an opportunity to achieve record linkage on a far more comprehensive scale. Centralized automated information systems promote more systematic collection and comprehensive recording of patient data. Patients whose histories are taken by automated means are systematically asked to disclose the full range of physical, social, family, and emotional data, and the resulting patient profiles become a regular feature of the file, which is updated steadily as the patient remains with that care provider. This is one of the most desirable features of computer information systems—patient records that are full, up to date, easily understood, and easily linked with information from various departments and previous episodes. Longitudinal records also may be linked over time from agency to agency.

The major objective of all record linkage research programs is to connect existing records on the same person. The E. J. Meyer Memorial Hospital in Buffalo, New York, established new records designed to satisfy both the immediate need for patient management and the long-term need for a computerized health data network.

Medical record administrators and medical record technicians can make positive changes to combat the fragmentation problem. They can incorporate concrete activities into the overall management plan of their department. The sample plan in Exhibit 3-1 illustrates how the health information manager might initiate change.

Data Responsibilities of Patients and Providers

As shown in Figure 3-1, the patient is the communication link between individual health care settings. The key to the medical record system and all its memory elements is in the patient's head. As a patient you must make connections from one aspect of your health information system to another. When you enter a health care setting, your doctor or therapist first seeks existing records for information. The written record is used, and the patient is interviewed to establish the data base from which to make diagnostic and therapeutic decisions. The medical record portrays care rendered to the individual patient. On the issue of finding memory elements, the role of the patient both as the source and as a primary connecter of fragments of the record becomes more and more apparent. As patients become more aware of their health care and as doctors encourage information sharing from one location to another, more assertive participation by patients is expected.

Exhibit 3-1 Sample Management Plan to Combat Record Fragmentation

Departmental objective:	Given daily information on all admissions, transfers, and discharges, the medical record department will retrieve appropriate patient information, incorporate it into a usable format, and make it available to accompany the patient from admission through discharge or transfer to another facility.
Supporting policy:	The medical record department will pull existing records on admissions and send them to the nursing station prior to the patient's arrival. The medical record department will provide transfer information and/or discharge summaries to accompany the patient on discharge.
Procedure in department: (excerpt)	Review planned admissions for the following day. Validate previous admission information. Prepare requisitions for files, and send request. Notify unit that the information is being sent. . . .
Follow-up: (excerpt)	Poll the medical staff and patient care coordinator's staff to verify that current activities are meeting the objective. Maintain statistics on the volume and nature of activities used in carrying out the procedures. . . .

Stop for a moment and consider your own role in your health care. Do you accept and promote individual responsibility for patient information? Do you have a record of immunizations for yourself? Have you pondered the questions, "When was my last tetanus shot?" or "Have I had or been exposed to rubella, or German measles?" Can you answer these questions right now? Shouldn't we all be able to do so? As the information explosion increases, and it will, the cost and management of individual information must surely be shared by provider and consumer. Perhaps you and I will keep a medical history of ourselves on microfilm that is updated every few years. Perhaps we will authorize health professionals to consult a health data center in our community for information on our medical history. We would then periodically review our personal medical records for accuracy and adequacy. We need to begin now to develop our individual plans for assuming this responsibility.

On the other side of the coin from patient education and attitude is professional action. This is the challenge to the health record professionals. They must develop their skills as members of the health care team in identifying, selecting, managing, and evaluating methods of collecting, storing, and retrieving patient information.

Legislative Emphasis on Complete Patient Information

Legislation has significant impact on the reduction of fragmentation of individual patient records. One of the first examples is a regulation set forth in Public Law 89-97, which amended the Social Security Act to incorporate Titles XVIII and XIX in 1965, and Title V in 1965. These amendments are more commonly known as Medicare and Medicaid.[3] This legislation made specific mention of the individual medical record. Validation of medical services rendered was required for each hospitalization. Patients transferred from hospitals to extended care facilities, which are now called skilled nursing facilities, must be accompanied by a transfer form that includes the current medication, the nursing care plan at the time of discharge, and the diagnosis by the physician. This form, as part of a formal transfer agreement, requires admitting orders from the transferring physician so that the care can be continued in the new location. Since that legislation went into effect in the mid-1960s, more and more emphasis has been placed on linkage of patient information.

Today, legislative requirements state that discharge planning begin at the time of admission to a hospital.[4] The record must document discharge planning for continuity of care. The patient's record should state exactly what the plan following discharge will be. A variety of options are open to promote individual and unique adaptations to each patient's health needs:

- Patients may be transferred to skilled nursing facilities.
- Patients may be transferred to special rehabilitative medicine centers that focus on physical and occupational therapy.
- Patients may be discharged to home with daily monitoring by the visiting nurses.
- Patients may be discharged to home and directed to follow-up care through their physicians' offices.
- Patients may be transferred to intermediate care facilities for long-term custodial care.

Whatever the determination, the plan for discharge demonstrates continuity and seeks to eliminate fragmentation. It builds a longitudinal record.

Individuality As a Major Focus of Health Care Planning

The concept of an individual plan of care that is documented in the record has extended to all aspects of health care delivery. Mental health, mental retardation, developmentally disabled, and other programs call for documentation of individual care plans, as do various laws and the Joint Commission on Accreditation of Hospital Councils in mental health.[5] The objective is to include in documentation all members of the health care team who are responsible for specifying what planning must be done to accomplish specific goals or resolve certain problems. In the documentation of an individual's program of care, the recreation therapist, the physician, a mental health counselor, and even the patient may have contributions to make. This document pulls together all available information in a coordinated, individual program.

Accountability of Health Care Team Members

Valid documentation is the major requirement of a patient medical record system. Provider accountability to the consumer patient and peer review within the health professions are also current issues in documentation. The pharmacist, for example, has become an active developer and user of patient information. Since 1972, pharmacists in New Jersey have been required to maintain patient pharmacy profile records.[6] The New Jersey state administrative code contains the following description of a patient profile record system:

A patient profile record system must be maintained in all pharmacies for persons for whom prescriptions are dispensed. The patient profile record system shall be devised so as to enable the immediate retrieval of information necessary to enable the dispensing pharmacist to identify previously dispensed medication at the time a prescription is presented for dispensing. One profile card may be maintained for all members of a family living at the same address and possessing the same family name.

The statute goes on to identify what information shall be recorded.

- The family name and the first name of the person for whom the medication is intended (the patient)
- The address of the patient
- An indication of the patient's age group—infant, child, adult
- The original date the medication is dispensed pursuant to the receipt of the physician's prescription
- The number or designation identifying the prescription
- Prescriber's name
- The name, strength, and quantity of the drug dispensed
- The initials of the dispensing pharmacist and the date of dispensing medication as a renewal if these initials and date are not recorded on the back of the original prescription

This same accountability applies to pharmacists in hospitals and skilled nursing facilities. The pharmacist reviews the medical records of the patient, and the findings of the review are reported to the medical staff or pharmacy committee. Physicians use the pharmacist's training and background in medication to help them identify drug reactions and drug incompatibilities. This is just another example of the increasing accountability of health care team members for contributing particular kinds of memory elements to the patient's medical record.

Computer Solutions to Fragmentation

Computers have helped resolve some problems of fragmentation and have made access to the record more workable. Patient information is often linked through computerization in social and health or welfare programs.

The Multi-State Information System (MSIS) is an automated records system for mental patients. It is designed to serve both treatment and research purposes for participating institutions throughout the United States. The system includes demographic, administrative, and services rendered information. It will also make information available on patient progress and treatment records, including detailed tracking of psychotropic drug therapy. Participating hospitals and mental health centers may elect to use the system at various levels of application. Users communicate via computer terminals through telephone lines. One feature of MSIS is the mental health examination record and the preliminary case history data recorded on the psychiatric anamnestic record form. These data are combined and the results analyzed, offering the clinician a suggested diagnosis. (The analysis is only a tool and does not become part of the record.) The computerized diagnosis and the doctor's diagnosis were found to be highly correlated in a recent study of the system. While most physicians still prefer to take their own notes, younger doctors at the Rockland Psychiatric Center are pro-MSIS. Use of available information seems to be increasing.[7]

The PROMIS system is also developing technology to aid patients and providers. The PROMIS program uses specific computer applications to help users recall memory elements of the patient record via CRT terminals.

> The PROMIS laboratory is engaged in the solution of three major problems in American medicine: lack of effective organization of medical data, dependence on the physician's memory for patient related data and medical information and lack of coordination in the use of medical data . . . .
>
> The PROMIS laboratory uses the POMR to provide the organization required for health care delivery. This record is kept in electronic form which facilitates access to it wherever needed within the health care system.
>
> . . . The unit health record is organized so that all problems are immediately apparent and so that not only what was done for each problem, but also why it was done and the results it achieved, are all readily discernible.[8]

Here, again, users gain access to medical records through CRT terminals installed in the nursing stations. This system also offers information via the CRTs from the University of Vermont Medical Library to help clinicians formulate problem statements and select plans for patient care.

Builders of Health Information Systems

The challenge to health record professionals is the overriding need to provide patient information to a given health care provider at the time the information is needed to carry on care or institute therapy. Registered record administrators (RRAs) and accredited record technicians (ARTs) must consider medical information, social and health information, specialized mental health information—indeed, all information relating to the individual. They must recognize where the fragments of health information are originating. They must seek to develop methods for combining memory elements for all patients and make those memory elements available as rapidly as possible when the patient needs the information for care. First, identify and establish what information must be collected. Second, devise the system for collecting the information. Third, store all information on a given patient so that it is retrievable for the use of the patient.

Effective systems are needed in all settings. The professional information handler must facilitate methods that merge the existing necessary elements and direct steps toward development of future longitudinal records. More rigorous and constructive plans for health data centers must be explored. State or regional health data centers could be established to house complete health information for use by legitimate providers on the patient's request. This could afford consistent and complete data for all providers, and decisions on personal health care programs could be based on complete and up-to-date patient data.

MEMORY ELEMENTS OF COLLECTIVE CARE

The second goal of this chapter is to uncover memory elements as they reflect collective health care. Data collection for evaluation, research, education, and active use of health statistics is directed to this goal. Besides uncovering the memory for individual patient care, medical record systems must collect information on many individuals and portray the collective care that has been provided. Uncovering the memory of collective care is critical to health resources planning: existing health care practices must be evaluated; research programs that benefit both the individual and society should continue; and patients and providers all need continuing education.

Data Collection for Evaluation

Evaluation addresses the following questions:

- What services are offered to clients or patients?
- What services are actually provided?
- Is the information documented adequately?
- What is the outcome of the care?
- Are the services that are provided to the patient cost effective?
- Do those services make the most effective use of the resources in our health system?

Answering these questions and others is the primary goal of medical care appraisal programs. Program components include utilization review of services, assessment of the process of patient treatment, and examination of the end result of patient care.

There are five steps in the evaluation of medical care.

1. Evaluation begins with examination of patient information documented in patient records.
2. Evaluation of a selected diagnosis or therapy is accomplished through review of a sample of records of patients with identical problems.
3. Reports of results are reviewed.
4. Educational programs are initiated to accomplish change or modify care plans.
5. A follow-up review of patient records completes the cycle.

The patient record remains at the heart of the evaluation process. Chapter 10 focuses on evaluation and its techniques more fully.

Figure 3-2 illustrates the continuity in communication from origin of patient information to users for individual feedback and users for collective feedback. Information is continually acquired, sifted, examined, and measured against particular goals. Evaluation merges into research and research into application of statistical methods. The results of these activities are channeled back through education into planning for resources, manpower, and facilities that create more effective health care delivery.

Research for Individuals and Society As a Whole

Research is directed to education. The purpose of research is to examine the known, to uncover the unknown, and to apply new knowledge. Use of new knowledge is the educational aspect and the heart of research. Health information systems are fertile ground for research activity. Individual diseases, such as cancer, heart disease, multiple sclerosis, and muscular dystrophy, are common targets of research. Along with individual diseases, trends in health problems and effective treatment plans are subjects of study. Research activities must be supported by dynamic medical and health record programs that provide for collection of all vital memory elements.

STATISTICS AND HEALTH INFORMATION

Statistics As a Description of Health Information

Statistics can be understood by people within and outside the health care delivery system. They collapse data into a succinct and useful form. Facts can be communicated easily in numbers, and statistics about health care can

Figure 3-2 Patient Information Extends to Statisticians, Epidemiologists, and Health Planners

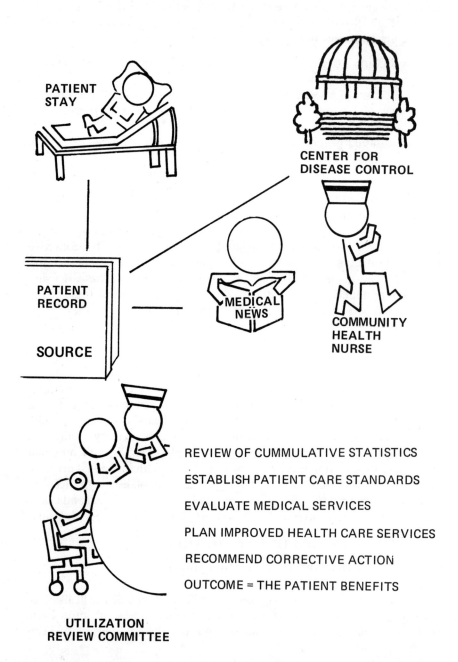

PATIENT STAY

CENTER FOR DISEASE CONTROL

PATIENT RECORD

SOURCE

MEDICAL NEWS

COMMUNITY HEALTH NURSE

REVIEW OF CUMMULATIVE STATISTICS

ESTABLISH PATIENT CARE STANDARDS

EVALUATE MEDICAL SERVICES

PLAN IMPROVED HEALTH CARE SERVICES

RECOMMEND CORRECTIVE ACTION

OUTCOME = THE PATIENT BENEFITS

UTILIZATION REVIEW COMMITTEE

facilitate communication generally and specifically with nonhealth care providers who control some aspects of health care planning. Effective management of health information systems and effective communication on behalf of the health care industry require a clear understanding of five major concepts:

1. *Descriptive statistics* are fundamental explanations of information about services, patients, and agency activity and are frequently used for planning and evaluating health services.
2. *Inferential statistics* are critical tools for retrospective and action research in medicine and provide an additional basis for planning and evaluating effective health services.
3. *Research sampling techniques* serve as a framework for statistical data.
4. *Statistical displays* facilitate understanding and appropriate application of data.
5. *Statistics in health information* are primary tools in actuating management planning, control, and evaluation of the system.

As more patient information is assembled and processed and medical services become increasingly complex, these functions of statistics move into focus. Many statistical information functions have been performed for a long time. In the past, however, such activities were merely performed, filed, or reported as the case required, and any unique use of information was the exception rather than the rule. Future delivery of health services will require relating routine statistical processes to appropriate information uses and targeting special statistical activities to justify, evaluate, and plan for patient care. Patient data comes together in the medical record and as more agencies recognize this fact, the professional who works with medical and health records in all applications must be aware of statistical techniques. Health record professionals should be able to apply statistical techniques to health data contained in their record system so that they may communicate and promote active use of the information. Perhaps the most dramatic example of the need for understanding statistics is illustrated in the growth of the accountability movement both in cost justification and in medical care appraisal programs.

Descriptive Statistics

Statistics actually describe in numerals various facets of the health care system, such as services, population activity, or use of the agency. Here are some common examples of descriptive statistics:

- Total number of patients treated in a hypertension clinic
- Total number of physicians by specialty practicing in an HMO
- Average daily census for a hospital
- Length of stay for patients with a particular diagnosis
- Total number of inpatients and outpatients using x-ray services in a hospital
- Demographic information about patients treated in a facility
- Average number of visits per patient in a diabetic clinic for a month

Quantitative analysis is another term for descriptive statistics. Quantitative analysis is a basic means of describing the population served by our health care system. There are three basic types of quantitative analysis: (1) numbers of patients and demographic information; (2) health status, which is commonly referred to as morbidity (sickness) and mortality (death) information; (3) utilization of goods and services. Population, health status, and utilization data all can be presented in numerals and in rates. Look at Exhibit 3-2.

Exhibit 3-2 The Data of Quantitative Analysis

Demographic data (describe the people)
  Geographic distribution
  Age
  Sex
  Marital status
  Ethnicity
  Income
  Education
  Employment
  Measures of social class

Numbers (quantities of conditions, individuals, events)
  1,000 births in a particular population during a year.

Rates and Ratios (*rate*, a relationship per time interval; *ratio*, a relationship per number of total relationships)
  Rate: One thousand patients in Seattle had cancer in 1975. There are one thousand cancer patients per year in Seattle in 1975.
  Ratio: One thousand out of 100,000 patients in Seattle had cancer. There are 1,000 cancer patients per 100,000 total patients in Seattle. One percent of patients in Seattle have cancer.
  Rate and ratio can be combined.
  Ratio rate: One percent of all patients in Seattle had cancer in 1975.

Hospital Use of Descriptive Statistics

Historically, medical record administrators and medical record technicians in hospitals and clinics have computed statistics that reflect patient use of the facility. They have expressed the information in numbers, rates, and percentages. Within a health facility, descriptive statistics are compiled into daily, weekly, monthly, and annual reports. This compilation may be performed manually by a statistical clerk in small facilities or automatically by in-house computers or computer service companies. A closer look at how quantitative analysis is carried out in hospitals will illustrate the compilation process.

Two major components of quantitative analysis in hospitals are the daily census and the discharge analysis carried out by the medical record service.

Statistical information and standard reports commence when the patient is admitted. At the point of admission, the patient is listed on the census report. The census is the number of inpatients present at any one time. Some patients may be admitted, treated, and discharged between the census-taking hours of the same day. The daily inpatient census must account for this to accurately reflect the activity. Daily inpatient census taking, therefore, is the number of inpatients present at the census-taking time each day, plus any patients who were *both* admitted and discharged after the census-taking time the previous day.

Census data are initiated at the point of patient care. This means that the nursing station is the place where the census is taken in hospitals. In most hospitals, however, the medical record department is responsible for compiling and using the census data. The medical record administrator makes sure that census taking is carried out consistently. This means that the census must be taken at a consistent time each day. If one consistently takes the census at the same time during any given 24-hour period or calendar day, the census data will be standard and useful. If not, errors may arise. For instance, if one counts patients at 9 A.M. one day and at 2 P.M. the next day, there is a reasonable chance that some admissions or discharges will be miscounted or missed altogether.

The location of the patient is tracked from day to day on the census. The census report provides specific daily counts of patients in the hospital as well as average daily counts and percentage of occupancy for the hospital. Census information is critical to daily management and future planning as well. Exhibits 3-3, 3-4, and 3-5 illustrate the variety of methods for computing. Notice that the information processing remains the same, though the procedures and methods differ. The census is intended to reflect current hospital activity. It can be calculated for the entire hospital population or

Exhibit 3-3 Daily Floor Census and Census Summary Sheet

DAILY FLOOR CENSUS

Admits   _____   Discharges   _____
Transfers in   _____   Transfers out   _____
                                                 Died   _____
        Total   _____   Total   _____

Summary:
                   Census from previous day   _____
                   Plus admits   _____
                   Minus discharges   _____

CENSUS SUMMARY SHEET

        Total previous day   _____
        Plus admits   _____
        Minus discharges and died   _____
        Equals daily census   _____
                Average daily census   _____
                Average daily census to date _____
                % of occupancy   _____
                % of occupancy to date   _____

PROCEDURE (manual)
1. Check in daily floor census by each floor.
2. Transfer figures to daily census summary sheet.
3. Check total admissions, discharges, and transfers against the admission, discharge, and transfer lists.
4. Balance the totals on the summary sheet.
5. Calculate and list:
   a. average daily census to date for the period.
   b. percentage of occupancy to date in the period.

Exhibit 3-4 Automated Daily Printout Showing Daily Worksheet and
Admissions, Discharges, and Transfers by Ward

PROCEDURE (manual)

1. Review the printout for accuracy.
2. Validate computations.
3. Distribute.
4. File.

```
Remaining from prev. day:        Admissions: 18 Discharges:   5
Total census:                              27Dec1977




                 Beth's DAILY WORKSHEET
                 As of 11:59pm 27Dec1977

                 Done 28Dec1977   8:29am


Previous total:              (      male,      female,      children 14 and under)
Admissions:          18  ( 12 male,   6 female,   0 children 14 and under)
Discharges:           5  (  1 male,   4 female,   0 children 14 and under)
Current total:               (      male,      female,      children 14 and under)


One day admissions:   0  (  0 male,   0 female,   0 children 14 and under)


Total discharge days:   45


Corrections for 28Dec1977:
```

Exhibit 3-4 Continued

ADMISSIONS, DISCHARGES, TRANSFERS

USPHS Hospital, Seattle WA (005)
27Dec1977

Name	ID#	Serv	Ward	Benef	Dsp	Adm date	Corr Eff
Admissions							
Axxxx,Rachel Thelma	201286	Surg	4W	AS			
Bxxxxx,Richard Tyler	413830	Surg	5E	CGEA			
Bxxx,Timothy Blair	416207	Orth	5W	SECC-CD			
Cxxxxxx,Wayne Eldon	412982	Orth	5W	AS			
Dxxx,Corey Elvin	406410	Orth	5W	CGEA			
Exxx,Rose Ann	104706	Med	4E	SEIHMNR			
Gxxxxxxxxx,Albert Thom	342452	Orth	5W	USAOR			
Hxxxx,Fred William	416075	Med	3W	AS			
Hxxxx,Hermoine	416076	Med	4E	AS			
Ixxxxxx,Clifford	254949	Orth	5W	AS			
Jxxxxxxxx,Martin R.	416230	Oto	3E	AS			
Mxxxx,Anne Agnes	400300	Orth	4E	AS			
Mxxxxxxx,Victor Lawren	077305	Oto	3W	SEIHMNR			
Nxxxxxxx,Edward Kennet	201410	Med	CCU	AS			
Oxxxx,Norma Mary	277788	Med	4E	DEPUSAR			
Sxxxxxxx,Maxine Andrea	273830	Med	4E	DEPUSNR			
Txxxxxx,Dallas Leroy	317152	Orth	5W	AS			
Vxxxxxxxxxxxxx,Anthony	400138	Orth	5W	AS			
Discharges							
Bxxxx,Marshall D	415034	Urol	5E	USAFER	A	12/19/77	
Gxxxxxx,Eva	075374	Med	4E	SEIHMNR	A	12/14/77	
Oxxxxx,Shirley Ann	416174	Med	4E	SECC-CD	A	12/23/77	
Pxxxx,Ethel Mildred	274519	Med	4E	DEPUSNR	A	12/13/77	
Sxxxxxxxx,Ponzetta	416048	Gyn	4W	SECC-CD	A	12/21/77	
Transfers							
Bxxxx,Neilie H.	037465	Surg	4W	SEIHMNR		12/13/77	

Exhibit 3-5 CRT Screen Display Showing Daily Census by Room and Bed Number

PROCEDURE (interactive)

1. Log on with user identification and password.
2. Query: for information only - census, 4 south.
3. Query: census, daily summary.
4. Review screen display:
     Census
     Admit Sheet
     Discharge Sheet
5. Key "print".
6. Key R Census to direct the program to calculate census.
7. Review screen display.
8. Validate and key "print".
9. Pick up printouts and distribute; or
0. Direct computer to print copies in appropriate locations through terminal.

INPATIENT ROSTER

As of 28Dec1977 8:33am

Name	ID#	Serv	Ward	Room	Benef.	Religion
Axxxx,Rachel Thelma	#201286	Surg	4W	402	AS	Protestant
Axxxxxx,Elizabeth Priscil	#375571	Med	4E	424	DEPUSND	Catholic
Bxxxxx,Richard Tyler	#413830	Surg	5E	523	CGEA	No Prefere
Bxxxxx,Edna Margaret	#237579	Surg	4W	401	SPECNR	Methodist
Bxxx,Timothy Blair	#416207	Orth	5W	502	SECC-CD	No Prefere
Bxxx,Joanna Mae	#415535	Med	4E	424	IND	Protestant
Bxxxxxx,Hugh Chester	#215900	Med	3E	315	AS	Catholic
Bxxx,Leo Willis	#404402	Surg	5E	524	AS	No Prefere
Bxxxxxxx,August Wilheim	#235155	Med	3E	315	AS	Protestant
Bxxxxx,Samuel Gaston	#391884	Med	3E	317	USNOR	Protestant
Bxxxxxx,Alice May	#411529	Surg	4W	402	SECC-HIP	Catholic
Bxxxxxxx,Ronald Leroy	#337612	Surg	5W	509	USAER	Protestant
Bxxxx,John Louser	#372205	Pmr	6W	602	USNOR	
Bxxxx,Neilie H.	#037465	Surg	4W	406	SEIHMNR	Catholic
Bxxxxxxx,Leroy Roald	#207455	Med	3E	315	SMSTS	Protestant
Bxxxxx,Frank Latham	#212755	Med	3E	315	USNER	
Cxxxxx,Maude	#244243	Oto	4W	406	DEPUSAR	
Cxxx,Carl Clarence	#207190	Pmr	6W	602	AS	Protestant
Cxxxxxx,Norman Matthew	#416010	Med	3W	302	IND	Presbyteri
Cxxxxxxxxxxx,Jenny Rosina	#415756	Surg	4W	402	SECC-CD	Jehovah'S
Cxxxx,Mark Steven	#415996	Orth	5W	506	AS	Baptist
Cxxxxxxxx,Clifford Hilair	#145326	Med	6W	609	SEIHMNR	Methodist
Cxxxxxx,Wayne Eldon	#412982	Orth	5W	502	AS	
Cxx,Alfred Winston	#311235	Med	3W	302	AS	No Prefere
Cxx,John Pridgeon	#243185	Med	5W	506	AS	Catholic
Cxxxx,Frank C	#415615	Med	5E	519	AS	

Exhibit 3-5 Continued

Name	ID#	Serv	Ward	Room	Benef.	Religion
D'xxx, Earl Keith	#214804	Med	3W	309	AS	Protestant
Dxxxx, George A	#333227	Med	CCU	743	IND	Presbyteri
Dxxx, Corey Elvin	#406410	Orth	5W	502	CGEA	No Prefere
Dxxxxx, Harold Arlo	#319338	Med	3E	320A	USNER	Protestant
Exxxxxx, Arthur Wendell	#415914	Med	3W	308	SPECNR	
Exxx, Rose Ann	#104706	Med	4E	424	SEIHMNR	Protestant
Exxxxxn, Sam	#405317	Med	3W	302	SECC	Protestant
Exxxxxxxx, Ada	#332604	Med	4E	418	DEPUSAD	
Fxxxx, John Van	#415969	Med	CCU	706	USAFER	Catholic
Fxxxxxx, Ovod	#366819	Surg	5E	524	USAER	
Fxxxxxxx, Peter James	#415896	Orth	5W	502	ASOCFV	No Prefere
Fxxxxxx, Albert Leonard	#226607	Med	6W	602	AS	Lutheran
Fxxxxx, William A.	#416123	Med	CCU	706	ASOCFV	No Prefere
Gxxxxxx, Mary Louise	#376587	Surg	4W	402	AS	
Gxxxxxxxx, Albert Thomas	#342452	Orth	5W	506	USAOR	Protestant
Gxxxx, Robert James Jr	#343278	Orth	5W	502	EMERNC	Baptist
Gxxxxxxx, Fredey	#416199	Surg	5E	524	AS	Catholic
Hxxxx, Fred William	#416075	Med	3W	302A	AS	Methodist
Hxxxx, Hermoine	#416076	Med	4E	424	AS	Protestant
Hxxxxx, Ernest Hugo	#325116	Med	3W	302	ASOCFV	Lutheran
Hxxxxxxx, Charles Ree	#411542	Surg	5E	518	SPECNR	No Prefere
Hxxxxxxxxxx, Herbert Fred.	#415858	Surg	4W	409	PHSOA	Protestant
Hxxxxx, Cathleen Elsinore	#053322	Med	4E	416	SEIHMNR	Protestant
Hxxx, David William	#336198	Med	3E	317	USNOR	Protestant
Ixxxxxx, Clifford	#254949	Orth	5W	502	AS	Lutheran
Jxxxxxx, Thomas Lester Jr.	#416046	Med	3W	302	IND	Protestant
Jxxxxxxxx, Martin R.	#416230	Oto	3E	320	AS	
Jxxxx, Leo D	#411262	Surg	5E	524	IND	Catholic
Jxxxxx, Ray Richard	#312939	Surg	5E	524	AS	No Prefere
Kxxxxxx, Bert George	#206423	Med	3W	302	AS	Protestant
Lxxxxx, Olav	#384218	Orth	5W	506	AS	Protestant
Lxxxxxx, Mary Anne	#415871	Surg	4W	406	SPECNR	Baptist
Mxxxxxxxe, Minerva Anna	#390192	Med	4E	418	AS	Catholic
Mxx, Kane	#390473	Surg	5E	518	USAFOR	Protestant
Mxxxx, Anne Agnes	#400300	Orth	4E	424	AS	Catholic
Mxxxxxxx, Leander Lee	#040667	Med	3W	302	SEIHMNR	Protestant
Mxxxxxxxx, Harry Pete	#416106	Surg	5E	524	IND	Protestant
Mxxxxxx, Thomas Ambrose	#402263	Med	ICU	702	AS	Catholic
Mxxxxx, Matthew John	#414494	Surg	5E	516	SPECNR	No Prefere
Mxxxxxxx, Victor Lawrence	#077305	Oto	3W	302	SEIHMNR	Catholic
Mxxxxxxx, Rolf	#409751	Med	3W	302	SECC	
Mxxxxx, Robert S	#276906	Oto	3E	320A	AS	Catholic
Mxxxxx, Juan	#232004	Surg	ICU	702	AS	Catholic
Mxxxx, John President	#228081	Surg	3W	302	AS	Methodist
Mxxxx, Sylvia Enid	#276914	Surg	4W		DEPUSAR	Catholic
Mxxxx, Ralph Angus	#231687	Med	3E	315	AS	Protestant
Mxxxx, Roger Raymond	#311820	Surg	5E	524	AS	
Nxxxxxxx, Hideaki	#349785	Med	ICU	702	USAER	Protestant
Nxxxxxxx, Edward Kenneth	#201410	Med	CCU	706	AS	Methodist
Nxxxx, Tauno William	#413442	Oto	3E	320	SPECNR	Protestant

Exhibit 3-5 Continued

Name	ID#	Serv	Ward	Room	Benef.	Religion
Oxxxx,Norma Mary	#277788	Med	4E	424	DEPUSAR	Protestant
Pxxxx,Sally Grace	#401277	Surg	4W	402	AS	Protestant
Pxxxxxxx,Francis James	#289749	Surg	5W	540	USAOR	Catholic
Pxxxxxx,Marvin Felix	#415751	Orth	5W	502	IND	Presbyteri
Pxxx,Dorothy B.	#344016	Surg	ICU	702	DEPUSAFR	Protestant
Pxxxxx,Hilda Nathalie	#260315	Med	4E	424	DEPUSND	Lutheran
Pxxx,Thomas Casio	#224526	Med	3W	305	AS	Catholic
Pxxxxr,Phyllis Ann	#415661	Oto	ICU	702	SECC	Baptist

```
3W   3W   3W   3W   3W   3W   3W   3W   3W   3W      at 08:30 on 28-Dec-77
                                                 19 beds filled out of  27
```

```
302   1    Kxxxxxx,Bert George   206423  MED  Preston, T    _____
      2    -                                                _____
      3    -                                                _____
      4    Txxxx,Joseph Levi     218326  MED  Huseby, J     _____
      5    -                                                _____
      6    Jxxxxxx,THOMAS        416046  MED  Rockey,P      _____
      7    Mxxxxxxx,Victor Lawr  077305  OTO  Clark,S       _____
      8    ExxxxxN,Sam           405317  MED  Huseby, J     _____
      9    Mxxxx,JOHN PRESIDENT  228081  SURG Thompson, A   _____
      10   Mxxxxxxx,Leander Lee  040667  MED  Griep, R      _____
      11   HxxxxN,Ernest Hugo    325116  MED  Tompkins,R    _____
      12   SxxxxxxR,Amos Sr.     416152  MED  Rockey,P      _____
      13   Cxx,Alfred Winston    311235  MED  Thompson, A   _____
      14   CxxxxxS,Norman Matth  416010  MED  Rockey,P      _____
      15   Sxxxxx,Gordon Lee     414431  MED  Paulsen,C     _____
      16   Mxxxxxxx,Rolf         409751  MED  Thompson, A   _____

302A  1    -                                                _____
      2    Rxxxxxxx,Frank Hale   408421  MED                _____
      3    -                                                _____
      4    Hxxxx,Fred William    416075  MED  Griep, R      _____
      5    -                                                _____

305   1    Pxxx,Thomas Casio     224526  MED  Huseby, J     _____

306B  1    -                                                _____

308   1    Exxxxxx,Arthur Wende  415914  MED                _____

309   1    Dxxxx k,Eareith       214804  MED  Tompkins,Rxxx _____

336   1    -                                                _____
      2    Rxxx,Clarence Frankl  416083  MED  Huseby, J     _____
```

Exhibit 3-5 Continued

```
3E   3E   3E   3E   3E   3E   3E   3E   3E   3E      at 00:30 on 28-Dec-77
                                                    16 beds filled out of  30


313  1    Pxxxx,Gary Rainer      414737 MED  Rockey,P          _____


315  1    -                                                    _____
     2    Bxxxxxxx,Leroy Roald 207455 MED  Griep, R            _____
     3    Bxxxxxx,Hugh Chester 215900 MED                      _____
     4    Bxxxxxxx,August Wilh 235155 MED  Rockey,P            _____
     5    Mxxxxx,Ralph Angus   231687 MED  Tompkins,R          _____
     6    Bxxxxx,Frank Latham  212755 MED  Huseby, J           _____


317  1    Bxxxxx,Samuel Gaston 391884 MED  Huseby,  J          _____
     2    Hxxx,David William     336198 MED  Huseby,  J        _____


320  1    -                                                    _____
     2    Jxxxxxxxx,Martin R.    416230 OTO                    _____
     3    -                                                    _____
     4    Nxxxx,Tauno William  413442 OTO  Weisberger, E       _____
     5    -                                                    _____
     6    -                                                    _____
     7    -                                                    _____
     8    -                                                    _____
     9    -                                                    _____
     10   Vxxxx,Lonn Roger       415895 OTO  Weisberger, E     _____
     11   -                                                    _____
     12   Wxxxxxx,Cecil Elwood 253539 MED                      _____
     13   -                                                    _____
     14   -                                                    _____
     15   -                                                    _____
     16   Sxxxxxx,George Helme 204030 MED  Huseby, J           _____


320A 1    -                                                    _____
     2    Mxxxxx,Robert S        276906 OTO                    _____
     3    Dxxxxx,Harold Arlo     319338 MED  Griep, R          _____
     4    Sxxxxx,Arthur Lee      217113 OTO  Weisberger, E     _____
     5    -                                                    _____
```

broken down into special populations. For example, the average daily census can be calculated for a single fiscal source such as Medicare or an individual age group of patients. Activity of each care unit or category of service, such as medical, surgical, pediatrics, and others, can also be counted. The census taking is the use of descriptive statistics in hospitals.

Let's consider how the census affects management. Within the medical record department, the census calculation usually involves receiving, checking, and balancing population information from each care unit in the hospital. Therefore, the census provides a check against other departments' activities within the hospital. For instance, total number of patients admitted to a given service for a particular time period can be determined from the census data. The admission list, usually a component of the overall census report, serves as a patient register and a number control. The census also allows for continuous listing that can be drawn on when establishing sampling for research or study.

The same census can be used beyond the medical record service. Consider some of the administrative uses of the census. First, it depicts the volume of care or the service rendered in any one period. Second, information on the census can be used by accrediting agencies and health agencies for planning. Third, census information is directly related to staffing and supply needs for the hospital. Fourth, cost accounting can be calculated according to average patient load in individual care units and for overall hospital services. Fifth, census portrays the activity of hospitals for administrative decision making. Sixth, the census affords the basis for analysis of service costs for patients.

The average daily census can also be designed to count various types of patient subgroupings. For instance, it would be quite simple with a computerized census system to routinely count Medicare patients, or male patients, and so on. A computerized census also would allow count of patients by zip code, health problem, or initial treatment plan broken down into elements, such as lab work to be performed, drugs to be taken, or diet to be started. Such sophisticated census counts might be used to track down persons involved in a natural disaster. Suspected leaking of poisonous gas in a given neighborhood or city, new information contraindicating use of a commonly ordered drug, or research interest in patients being treated currently are instances in which the lab work, drugs, or diet census counts might be helpful.

The statement, "It would be quite simple to compile census reports that reflect subgroupings of data," does imply a deviation from traditional methods of maintaining census information. However, such compilations would be simple tasks even though the practice represents a complete change from current manual census reporting methodology. Current census reports emphasize numbers of patients. Forms now used to report the number of people do not include space or designation for sex, age, address, and the like. With a computerized census system, these additional data elements could easily be transferred from an admission document. Census data could then be expanded to provide a variety of subdivisions, such as those listed previously. The limitations of the manual method (currently the most commonly used census reporting method) are that many useful and meaningful facts regarding the patient population are not available until discharge—that is, only when patients have gone home. The primary limitation with a computerized system is that of cost constraints inherent in on-line data storage and manipulation. However, such an on-line design can facilitate concurrent intervention of patient treatment. The needs and/or goals of the hospital will determine how such information will be routinely maintained.

Use of information can often be promoted and improved by the health information manager. The design and layout of the census reports, as well as other statistical reports, should be a major concern of the manager. The objectives of the health information manager should be:

1. to provide timely reports.
2. to provide accurate information.
3. to design formats to facilitate readability.
4. to lay out data that are clear and understandable.
5. to provide analysis of data upon request.

Discharge Analysis

The tabulation of data on discharged patients reflects the professional services provided in the hospital. When patients are discharged from the hospital, discharge analysis is performed by the medical record department. Patients are viewed collectively in the analysis of their use of the various services within the hospital.

The total number of patients, number of days they stay in the hospital, consultations, deaths and autopsies, and other data are all compiled according to individual care units and cross-referenced to total hospital discharges. This analysis establishes the use of the care unit within the hospital. As with the census, the discharge analysis is accomplished in a variety of ways. Manual and computerized methods are used. (See Exhibits 3-6 and 3-7.)

Hospitals view a service or care unit in three ways. First, a service or care unit can represent the various specialties of the medical staff. Surgeons, cardiologists, internists, and neurologists all admit patients. The documented reason for admission recorded for these patients usually reflects the

Exhibit 3-6 Manual Posting of Discharge Analysis

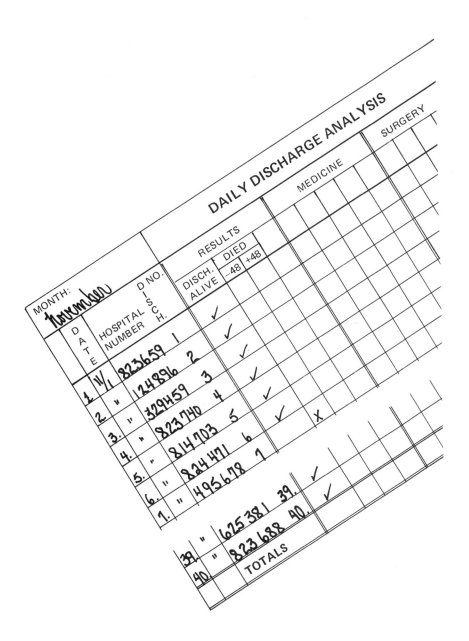

Exhibit 3-7 Sample Computer Printout of Discharge Analysis

1012 FLORIDA ULTIMATE CARE CENTER   H O S P I T A L   S E R V I C E   A N A L Y S I S   DATE PREPARED 05/26/78

FHYD040   510 - NEUROSURGERY   FOR THE MONTH OF APR. 1978   PAGE 18

	THIS MONTH	YEAR TO DATE
TOTAL PATIENTS	3	12
PERCENT OF TOTAL DISCHARGES	.32	.59
TOTAL PATIENT DAYS OF CARE	16	129
AVERAGE LENGTH OF STAY	5.33	10.75
TOTAL DAYS IN SPECIAL CARE UNITS		9
ICU		
CCU		
BOARDER		
OTHER		
ADMISSION STATUS TOTALS		
EMERGENCY	1	6
URGENT	1	2
ELECTIVE	1	4
DEATH STATISTICS		
UNDER 48 HOURS		
OVER 48 HOURS		
GROSS DEATH RATE		
NET DEATH RATE		
TOTAL AUTOPSIES		
AUTOPSY RATE		
TRANSFUSIONS		
TOTAL NUMBER		1
TOTAL REACTIONS		
TOTAL COMPLICATIONS OCCURING		2
CONSULTATIONS		
TOTAL PATIENTS RECEIVING	1	7
PERCENT RECEIVING	33.33	58.33
TOTAL CONSULTATIONS RECEIVED	2	6
AVERAGE PRE-OP DAYS		3.57
MALE PATIENTS		
TOTAL MALES	2	7
PERCENT MALES	66.67	58.33
AGE GROUP COUNTS		
0 - 13	1	1
14 - 64	2	8
65 +		3
TOTAL CHARGES	2,950	24,697
AVERAGE PATIENT CHARGE	983.33	2,058.08
AVERAGE DAILY CHARGE	184.38	191.45

1012 FLORIDA ULTIMATE CARE CENTER

FHYD045   1 - MEDICARE

PAYMENT ANALYSIS

FOR THE MONTH OF APR. 1978

DATE PREPARED 05/26/78

PAGE   1

	THIS MONTH	YEAR TO DATE
TOTAL PATIENTS	230	566
PERCENT OF TOTAL DISCHARGES	24.70	27.70
TOTAL PATIENT DAYS OF CARE	1,869	4,953
AVERAGE LENGTH OF STAY	8.13	8.75
TOTAL DAYS IN SPECIAL CARE UNITS		
ICU	20	78
CCU	75	194
BOARDER		
OTHER		
ADMISSION STATUS TOTALS		
EMERGENCY	56	158
URGENT	106	239
ELECTIVE	68	169
DISCHARGE STATUS		
ALIVE	226	545
DEAD	4	21
MALE PATIENTS		
TOTAL MALES	92	258
PERCENT MALES	40.00	45.58
AGE GROUP COUNTS		
0 - 13	18	36
14 - 64	212	530
65 +		
TOTAL CHARGES	366,338	965,156
AVERAGE PATIENT CHARGE	1,592.77	1,705.22
AVERAGE DAILY CHARGE	196.01	194.86
TOTAL PATIENTS USING SPECIAL SERVICES	222	536

specialty of the admitting physician. Hence, many medical record departments rely heavily on the specialty of the admitting physician to determine the service or unit assignment during an individual patient's hospital stay.

Second, a service unit can mean a group of patients who have related diagnoses and/or treatments. This approach also often coincides with the specialty of the admitting physician. However, the analysis and assignment of service are based on a more critical look at the patient's problems.

Third, a service unit can mean a group of inpatient beds designated as a department. Urology as a care unit may be designated as sixth floor, south wing, for example. Patients treated for urological problems are usually admitted, treated, and discharged from that location.

Hospitals may elect to use one of these definitions of service unit or a combination of them. Patients who enter the hospital for one condition and encounter complications may actually utilize the services of more than one physician. They may be treated for several problems that are not related. They may be transferred from one bed to another. With increasing emphasis on standardization of health statistics for valid comparison and analysis, the current trend is to define hospital service as a "care unit" according to predetermined assigned beds so that assigning units by location in the hospital would be an effective and consistent means of service activity assessment. The *Glossary of Hospital Terms*, published by the American Medical Record Association, supports this approach. The more consistently health information professionals elect to use standard hospital terms, the more reliable the reporting will be. The reader is directed to Huffman for detailed references to manual methods. Some hospital statistical terms, definitions, and formulas are shown in Exhibit 3-8. Review the information there and see if you can answer the questions that follow.

Exhibit 3-8 Selected Statistical Hospital Formulas and Terms

Inpatient service day is a unit of measure denoting the services received by one inpatient in one 24-hour period.

Total inpatient service days is the sum of all inpatient service days for each patient or the days in the period under consideration.

$$\text{Average daily inpatient census} = \frac{\text{Total inpatient service days for period (excluding newborn)}}{\text{Total number of days for the period}}$$

Discharge day is the sum of the days of care received by the patient for one continuous stay in the facility. It is figured by subtracting the date of admission from the date of discharge.

Exhibit 3-8 Continued

Note: Discharge days are used only for computing length of stay formulas. These may include average length of stay for all patients listed in the hospital or may be calculated for particular services or patient categories, such as average length of stay for Medicare patients.

Length of stay (for one inpatient) is the number of calendar days from admission to discharge.

Average length of stay is the average length of hospitalization of inpatients discharged during the period under consideration.

$$\text{Average length of stay} = \frac{\text{Total length of stay (discharge days)}}{\text{Total discharges}}$$

Inpatient bed count is the number of available hospital inpatient beds, both occupied and vacant, on any given day.

Inpatient bed count day is a unit of measure denoting the presence of one inpatient bed (either occupied or vacant) set up and staffed for use in one 24-hour period.

Inpatient bed count days (total) is the sum of inpatient bed count days for each of the days in the period under consideration.

$$\text{Percent of occupancy} = \frac{\text{Total inpatient service days for a period} \times 100}{\text{Total inpatient bed count days in the period}}$$

Hospital inpatient autopsy is a postmortem examination performed in a hospital facility, by a hospital pathologist or a physician of the medical staff to whom the responsibility has been delegated, on the body of a patient who died during inpatient hospitalization.

$$\text{Gross autopsy rate} = \frac{\text{Total inpatient autopsies for a given period} \times 100}{\text{Total inpatient deaths for the period}}$$

$$\text{New autopsy rate} = \frac{\text{Total inpatient autopsies for a given period} \times 100}{\text{Total inpatient deaths minus unautopsied coroner's or medical examiner's cases for the period}}$$

Exhibit 3-8 Continued

Complication is an additional diagnosis that describes a condition arising after the beginning of hospital observation and treatment and modifying the course of the patient's illness or the medical care required.

Hospital fetal death rate is the ratio of fetal deaths to total births in a given period. Usually only intermediate and late fetal deaths are included.

$$\text{Hospital fetal death rate} = \frac{\text{Total number of intermediate and/or late fetal deaths for a period} \times 100}{\text{Total number of births (including intermediate and late fetal deaths) for the period}}$$

Would computation of the percentage of occupancy in a 300-bed hospital and a 600-bed hospital provide consistent information to a hospital planning board?

How would the average length of stay differ in a 200-bed community hospital, a large teaching hospital, and a skilled nursing facility? What are some reasons for the differences?

From examining the formulas, can you tell why gross and net figures would be important to identify?

What is implied by the term *complication*? What departments within the hospital might be interested in these data? How might they be used?

Would it be helpful to compute a separate daily census for each service in the hospital?

What kind of information might be used in reporting statistics to community epidemiological agencies?

The list in Exhibit 3-9 is a composite reference for statistical terms and formulas commonly used in maintaining hospital statistics.

Exhibit 3-9 Statistical Terms and Formulas

Terms	Formulas
ADMISSION	
Hospital patient	
An individual receiving, in person, hospital-based or coordinated medical services for which the hospital is responsible.	
Inpatient admission	
The formal acceptance by a hospital of a patient who is to be provided with room, board, and continuous nursing service in an area of the hospital where patients generally stay at least overnight.	Number of patients in the hospital at midnight April 29 535
	Plus . . . . . . Number of patients admitted April 30 . +30
	565
Hospital inpatient	
A hospital patient who is provided with room, board, and continuous general nursing service in an area of the hospital where patients generally stay at least overnight.	Minus . . . . Patients discharged (including deaths) April 30 . . . . −18
	Patients in hospital at 12 p.m. (midnight) April 30 547
Inpatient census	
The number of inpatients present at any one time.	Plus . . . . . . Patients both admitted and discharged (including deaths) on April 30 . . . . . +3
Daily inpatient census	
The number of inpatients present at the census-taking time each day, plus any inpatients who were both admit-	Inpatient census (inpatient service days) April 30 550

Exhibit 3-9 Continued

Terms	Formulas
ted and discharged after the census-taking time the previous day.	**Example of Care Unit Breakdown:**

Terms

ted and discharged after the census-taking time the previous day.

Inpatient service day (also called Census day)
A unit of measure denoting the services received by one inpatient in one 24-hour period.

Formulas

Example of Care Unit Breakdown:

Intensive Care Unit
Inpatient Service Days
(Inpatient Census)

	Patients remaining midnight April 29 .	8
Plus	Patients admitted April 30	+1
Plus	Patients transferred on unit from another unit in hospital	+1
Minus ...	Patients discharged	−0
Minus ...	Patients died	−2
Minus ...	Patients transferred off unit to another unit in hospital	−1
	Midnight census April 30	7
Plus	Patients both admitted and discharged on April 30	+1

(These patients have already been counted as admission and discharges or deaths. However, since their patient days have been canceled out by adding them as admissions and subtracting them as discharges, they must be added again to determine the inpatient service days on this unit.)

Total inpatient service days (also called Census days)
The sum of all inpatient service days for each of the days in the period under consideration. Notice it is the numerator in the formula.

Average daily inpatient census
Average number of inpatients present each day for a given period of time. This is always calculated by a formula as indicated in the example.

Inpatient bed occupancy ratio
The proportion of inpatient beds occupied, defined as the ratio of inpatient service days to inpatient bed count days in the period under consideration.

Synonymous terms: percent occupancy, occupancy percent, percentage of occupancy, occupancy ratio

The formula to obtain the average daily inpatient census for a whole hospital is:

$$\frac{\text{Total inpatient service days for a period}}{\text{Total number of days in the period}}$$

The average daily inpatient census (average daily census) for newborn inpatients is generally reported separately. When it is, the following formula is used to determine the average daily inpatient census excluding newborn:

$$\frac{\text{Total inpatient service days (excluding newborn) for a period}}{\text{Total number of days in the period}}$$

$$\frac{\text{Total inpatient service days for a period} \times 100}{\text{Total inpatient bed count days} \times \text{number of days in the period}}$$

Example: A hospital has an inpatient bed count (bed complement) of 150 (excluding the newborn bassinet count of 15). During April, the hospital rendered 3,650 inpatient service days to adults and children. April has

Exhibit 3-9 Continued

Terms	Formulas

EVENTS DURING HOSPITAL STAY

Transfer (intrahospital)

A change in medical care unit, medical staff unit, or responsible physician of an inpatient during hospitalization. → Not applicable

Adjunct diagnostic or therapeutic unit (ancillary unit) → Not applicable

An organized unit of a hospital, other than an operating room, delivery room, or medical care unit, with facilities and personnel to aid physicians in the diagnosis and treatment of patients through the performance of diagnostic or therapeutic procedures.

Medical consultation

The response by one member of the medical staff to a request for consultation by another member of the medical staff, characterized by review of the patient's history, examination of the patient, and completion of a consultation report giving recommendations and/or opinions.

Formulas column:

30 days. According to the formula, this is $3,650 \times 100 \div 150 \times 30 = 365,000 \div 4,500 = 81.11\%$. Therefore, the inpatient bed occupancy percentage for April was 81.1%, or 81%.

Consultations may be viewed from two perspectives.

1. Total consultations rendered. This may be used to show specialty activity, such as the total number of psychiatric consultations rendered by the psychiatric service.

2. The percentage of consultations rendered per patients treated in the hospital. The formula for this would be:

$$\frac{\text{Total number of patients receiving consultations} \times 100}{\text{Total number of patients discharged and died for the period}}$$

Surgical operation
One or more surgical procedures performed at one time for one patient via a common approach or for a common purpose.

Complication
An additional diagnosis that describes a condition arising after the beginning of hospital observation and treatment and modifying the course of the patient's illness or the medical care required.

Hospital live birth
The complete expulsion or extraction from the mother, in a hospital facility, of a product of conception, irrespective of the duration of pregnancy, which after such separation, breathes or shows any other evidence of life such as beating of the heart, pulsation of the umbilical cord, or definite movement of voluntary muscles, whether or not the umbilical cord has been cut or the placenta is attached; each product of such a birth is considered live born.

The formula approved by the Joint Commission on Accreditation of Hospitals for computing the post-operative infection rate is:

$$\frac{\text{Number of infections in clean surgical cases for a period} \times 100}{\text{Number of surgical operations for the period}}$$

Usually calculated in a rate only in infection cases, since the formula above clearly assigns the source of the complication.

Live births may be classified according to the birth weight:

1,000 grams (2 pounds, 3 ounces) or less;
1,001 grams to 2,500 grams (5 pounds, 8 ounces);
over 2,500 grams.

Exhibit 3-9 Continued

Terms	Formulas
Hospital cesarean section rate	Formula:
Hospital cesarean section rate is the ratio of cesarean sections performed to deliveries. For statistical purposes, when a delivery results in a multiple birth, it is counted as one delivery.	$$\frac{\text{Total number of cesarean sections performed in a period} \times 100}{\text{Total number of deliveries in the period}}$$
Inpatient discharge	Admit Jan 20 or Calculation:
The termination of a period of inpatient hospitalization through the formal release of the inpatient by the hospital.	Disch Jan 24
Discharge transfer	
The disposition of an inpatient to another health care institution at the time of discharge.	
Length of stay (for one inpatient)	
The number of calendar days from admission to discharge.	

Calculation:

Disch days	24
	24
	− 20
	4

or

Admit Jan 20

Disch Feb 14

Total days in Jan	31
	− 20
days in Jan	= 11
days in Feb	+ 14
Disch days	= 25

The length of an inpatient's hospitalization is considered to be one day if he is admitted and discharged the same day and also if he is admitted one day and discharged the next day.

Total length of stay (for all inpatients) ⟶ Total duration (discharge days) of inpatient hospitalization (including deaths; excluding newborn)

The sum-of-the-days stay of any group of inpatients discharged during a specified period of time.

Average length of stay ⟶ Total discharges (including deaths; excluding newborn)

The average length of hospitalization of inpatients discharged during the period under consideration.

Gross death rate

$$= \frac{\text{Total number of deaths (including newborn)}\ \times\ 100}{\text{Total number of discharges (including deaths and newborn deaths) for the period}}$$
for a period

Net death rate (also called Institutional death rate)

$$= \frac{\text{Total number of deaths (including newborn) minus those under 48 hours for a period}\ \times\ 100}{\text{Total number of discharges (including deaths and newborn) minus deaths under 48 hours for the period}}$$

Postoperative death rate

$$= \frac{\text{Total number of deaths within 10 days postoperative for a period}\ \times\ 100}{\text{Total number of patients operated on for the period}}$$

Exhibit 3-9 Continued

Terms	Formulas
Maternal death rate	Total number of maternal deaths for a period × 100 / Total number of maternal (obstetrical) discharges (including deaths) for the period
Anesthesia death rate	Total number of deaths caused by anesthetic agents for a period × 100 / Total number of anesthetics administered for the period
Hospital fetal death Death prior to the complete expulsion or extraction from its mother, in a hospital facility, of a product of conception, irrespective of the duration of pregnancy; death is indicated by the fact that after such separation, the fetus does not breathe or show any other evidence of life such as beating of the heart, pulsation of the umbilical cord, or definite movement of voluntary muscles.	Early: Less than 20 complete weeks of gestation (500 grams or less)
	Intermediate: 20 completed weeks of gestation, but less than 28 (501 to 1,000 grams)
	Late: 28 completed weeks of gestation and over (1,001 grams and over)
	Usually only intermediate and late fetal deaths are included.
	Formula: Total number of intermediate and/or late fetal deaths for a period × 100 / Total number of births (including intermediate and late fetal deaths) for the period
Abortion Abortion is the expulsion or extraction of all (complete) or any part (incomplete) of the placenta or membranes, without an identifiable fetus or with a live-born infant or a stillborn infant weighing less than 500 gm. In the absence of known weight, an estimated length of gestation of less than 20 completed weeks (139 days) is calculated from the first day of the last normal menstrual period.	

Gross autopsy rate $= \dfrac{\text{Total inpatient autopsies for a given period} \times 100}{\text{Total inpatient deaths for the period}}$

The ratio during any given period of time of all inpatient autopsies of all inpatient deaths.

Net autopsy rate $= \dfrac{\text{Total inpatient autopsies for a given period} \times 100}{\text{Total inpatient deaths minus unautopsied coroner's or medical examiner's cases}}$

The ratio during any given period of time of all inpatient autopsies to all inpatient deaths minus unautopsied coroner's or medical examiner's cases.

Hospital autopsy rate (adjusted) $= \dfrac{\text{Total hospital autopsies} \times 100}{\text{Number of deaths of hospital patients whose bodies are available for hospital autopsy}}$

The proportion of deaths of hospital patients following which the bodies of the deceased persons are available for autopsy and hospital autopsies are performed.

SPECIAL NEEDS

Psychiatric survival rates*

The monthly statistics provided to staff gave no information as to how long a patient was able to function independently.

Admission date – Discharge date of last visit = Survival time

This formula was created when it became evident that staff was being discouraged by the high reported readmission rate, in spite of additions to staff and improved therapy programs.

Exhibit 3-9 Continued

Terms	Formulas
The use of survival time statistics demonstrated two factors to administration that were then used to revise procedures:	$$\frac{\text{Cumulative survival time for all patients for the period utilizing outpatient clinics}}{\text{Total number of admissions for the period}} =$$ Average survival rate of patients utilizing clinics
• The survival time for which patients were functioning without support was increased with each discharge.	
• There was no evidence that outpatient visits increased the survival time between hospitalizations. (Patients were returning due to attachments to staff.)	$$\frac{\text{Cumulative survival time for all patients for the period not utilizing outpatient clinics}}{\text{Total number of admissions for the period}} =$$ Average survival rate of patients *not* utilizing clinics
A program was developed to introduce outpatient clinic staff to patients and create attachments to the appropriate staff prior to discharge to reduce dependency on the patient facility.	

Source: Medical Record Management, Edna K. Huffman, Physicians Record Company Publisher, 1972; *Glossary of Hospital Terms*, American Medical Record Association, 1974.

*Designed for use in Alaska Psychiatric Institute, 1976-77 by Candace Dillman, RRA

Discharge Abstracting

The most widely used medical record computer applications today are discharge abstracting services offered through shared computer service companies. The following partial listing is representative of these programs:

- Shared Computer Systems (SCS)
- Medical Dimensions (SNAP)
- Med-Art Program
- Childrens' Hospitals' Automated Medical Program (CHAMP)
- Professional Activities Study (PAS) of the Commission on Professional Hospital Activities (CPHA)
- Hospital Utilization Program (HUP)

These companies offer medical record managers a variety of abstracting, standard reporting, and special study options. Review Figure 3-3. It illustrates the growth of the CPHA since its inception in 1953. Note the report contents available today. Expanded applications include emergency room reporting and outpatient reporting systems. Careful review of the options is a key process in determining the most effective program for any given institution.

As hospital information systems develop, the activities handled through the discharge abstracting programs are being incorporated into in-house computer systems. On-line data entry via CRT terminals and provisions for magnetic tape transmittal of discharge data to PSRO for reporting purposes are featured. Some systems include automatic coding of procedures to facilitate fiscal reporting to third-party payers such as Blue Cross and Blue Shield. The continuum from manual methods through contracted computer services to on-line, in-house hospital computer applications is well established. The challenge for medical record professionals is to select the most effective point along this continuum in which to fit their hospital's needs.

Uniform hospital discharge data set was identified in Chapter 2. It is one example of an attempt to organize and coordinate reporting requirements so that consistent health information analysis can be performed. The manager of any health information system in any of a variety of settings will need to perform the following tasks:

- Review the mandatory accrediting or certifying statistical reporting requirements for the facility. This would include local vital statistics and epidemiology reporting, state licensing, and federal certification for Medicare and Medicaid.
- Identify the need for any additional statistical reports required by

Figure 3-3 CPHA Growth Reflects Technological Change

CPHA [COMMISSION ON PROFESSIONAL AND HOSPITAL ACTIVITIES]

1950

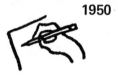

- Manual comparison of individual, non-standardized reports

- Interhospital study of routine, traditional statistical reports

1953

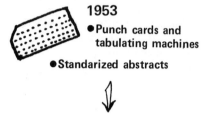

- Punch cards and tabulating machines

- Standarized abstracts

- Simple interhospital studies Monthly statistical reports

- Disease, operations and physicians indices

- 13 hospitals participating

1977

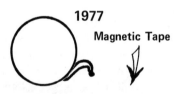

Magnetic Tape

- Quality Assurance Monitor
- Length of Stay Study
  Study of Patient Charges
- PAS Profiles
- Concurrent Review Study
- Medical Audit Program
- Medical Care Evaluation
- Special Studies

- 2200 hospitals
- 150,000,000 cases
- 17,000,000 added annually

1990's

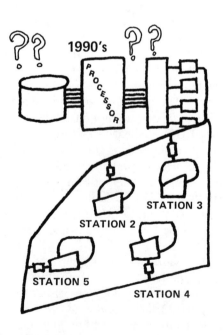

facility participation in voluntary accreditation processes. This includes the JCAH.
- Validate current statistical reporting activities against the above requirements.
- Assess any additional statistical reporting needs through systems analysis within the organization and careful investigation of its data needs.
- Coordinate required, preferred, and special statistical needs into a statistical unit in the department. This coordination should incorporate planning for data handling, maintaining required statistical items, and monitoring use of preferred or special statistical procedures for relevancy and appropriateness.

All health care facilities require basic descriptive statistical reporting. The role of the health information professional is to research, recognize, and promote active use of the statistical unit within the organization.

Descriptive statistics are used within the health facility and are also used to report information to outside agencies. Information on births and deaths would be reported to local departments of vital statistics. Information on percentage of occupancy would be reported to planning commissions. We have identified and discussed planning agencies and their effect on health services in other parts of the book. When focusing on statistical reporting, the first principle must be: Statistical reporting will be uniformly based on commonly accepted definitions of terms. This principle is the basis for the publication of *Glossary of Hospital Terms* by the AMRA. The objective of the AMRA was to help practitioners identify common definitions and report descriptive statistical information in those terms. Today, uniform reporting is a concept applied to hospitals, ambulatory care clinics, emergency rooms, and other health care settings.

The significance of uniform statistical reporting can be seen in the activities of the National Center for Health Statistics mandated under Public Law 93-353 for the design and implementation of a cooperative health statistics system for producing comparable and uniform health information figures at the federal, state, and local levels.

In a meeting of the United States National Committee on Vital and Health Statistics (USNCVHS) on January 11-12, 1978, the USNCVHS passed the following motion:[9]

> The USNCVHS endorses, in principle, the draft annual report of the USNCVHS incorporating a statement of principles for a National Statistical System.

The USNCVHS uncovers the collective memory of health records by establishing technical consulting panels (TCPs) to work in specific areas, such as the following:

- National Death Index
- Cooperative Health Statistics Advisory Group
- National Health Insurance
- National Health Interview Survey
- Manpower and Facilities
- Long-Term Care
- Ambulatory Medical Care
- Hospital Discharge Data Set
- Cooperative Health Statistics System/Mental Health

The USNCVHS committee is also concerned with monitoring and reviewing the various disease classifications and disease coding systems. It reports findings on such activities and tries to maintain some awareness of the problem in duplicative data collection in the health care delivery system. It is important for medical record administrators and technicians to understand the functions of statistics in uncovering the collective memory of patient care within individual organizations and within overall data collection systems. While we have focused our attention on hospitals, Figure 3-4 clearly demonstrates how patient information actually extends far beyond the hospital.

EXPANDED USE OF DESCRIPTIVE STATISTICS FOR RRA AND ART

Scales of Measurement

Descriptive statistics are used to illustrate findings in research. It is helpful to the student to review the concepts covered in a basic statistics course and raise the question, "How do these tools relate to health information systems?" The techniques of descriptive statistics in the form of tabular and graphic summaries are indispensable for organizing and understanding collections of sample data. Medical Audit result displays, research studies, and management reporting depend on this principle.

We will now look at a few specific applications drawn from statistical resources. Review and consider the following basic tools from the point of view of a health information manager working with statistical and research units.

Figure 3-4 The Health Data Broker Concept

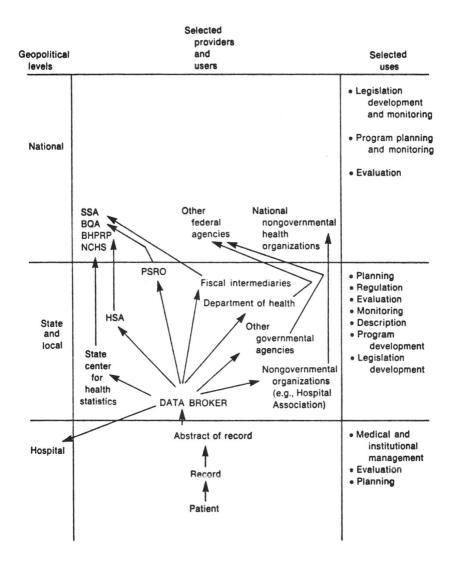

Source: Reprinted with permission from *The Information Bonus—Audit Action Letter*, June 15, 1977.

Nominal scales refer to enumeration of attribute data. Survival status is the most common example. The summary measure is the proportion of cases that exhibit the attribute. The example in Table 3-1 illustrates this.

Ordered classifications change a scale to reflect a predetermined order among the measured classifications. This is best illustrated by Table 3-2, in which the classifications indicate a particular order of complications in categorized female patients.

Table 3-1 Nominal Scale Data

Complications noted at initial evaluation and during followup in hypertensivewomen, by obesity status

Complication	Initial evaluation		New complications	
	Obese (N = 75)	*Nonobese (N = 106)*	*Obese (N = 75)*	*Nonobese (N = 106)*
Coronary heart disease	12	20	6	2
Cardiomegaly	24	23	5	3
Renal disease	3	10	5	3
Stroke	0	2	4	1
Total complications	39	55	20	9

Table 3-2   Ordered Classification Data

Dental treatment needs per 1,000 active duty personnel for total sample, by age group

Treatment	Needs per 1,000 persons, age group						Significant difference (P < .01)	Average, total
	17–19	*20–24*	*25–29*	*30–34*	*35–39*	*40 and over*		
Restorations	5,604	4,702	3,851	2,864	2,366	1,855	Yes	3,442
Crowns	274	232	253	238	246	264	NS	248
Bridge abutments	481	450	494	499	527	440	NS	481
Full dentures	10	16	31	53	66	101	Yes	47
Partial dentures	128	140	174	230	255	275	Yes	203
Endodontic, number of teeth ...	201	187	124	120	86	98	Yes	133
Extractions	1,439	1,200	734	539	417	480	Yes	767
Periodontal care	151	176	272	395	440	542	Yes	281
Oral prophylaxis	933	914	900	893	877	857	Yes	894
Calculus removal	850	810	814	832	818	797	Yes	817
Plaque control therapy	845	797	799	794	769	732	Yes	786

[1] A one-way analysis of variance was performed.
Note: NS—not significant.

Source for Tables 3-1 and 3-2: Public Health Reports, Volume 94, Number 2, March-April 1979. Published by Health Resources Administration, Public Health Service, U.S. Department of Health, Education, and Welfare, page 184.

Notice the increasing factors in Table 3-2. What additional items of information are available about the patients in this group? Can you identify a basic limitation on the information in this table?

If ranking is added, then specific statistical rules enter the picture. Instead of arbitrary descriptive terms, such as good or fair, whose precise meanings are known only to the researcher, the results are ranked first, second, third, and so on, along some dimension. The addition of ranking can generate an entirely different kind of table by clearly displaying the rank of the value or groups of values. Cancer survival rates are often ranked. Cancer sites are listed in order of largest survival rate following diagnosis confirmation. Look at Table 3-3 and decide whether the data displayed are nominal, ordered, or ranked.

The common scales of measurement also include the *numerical continuous scale*. Each observation theoretically falls along a continuum. There is no restriction to the sole use of integers, as in a discrete scale in which all classifications are mutually exclusive. Clinical measurements such as blood pressure, height, and weight are numerical continuous scales. Notice the example in Table 3-4, which represents an investigation of the initial blood pressure readings on patients with hypertension.

Frequency of Occurrences

A *frequency distribution* is a set of numbers describing the number of cases or observations that fall within each interval on a scale of measurement. Table 3-4 illustrates the percentage frequency of disease coding systems in hospitals. Frequency distributions may be displayed in a number of ways. When the distribution is illustrated in the form of a histogram, the values and their frequencies are represented by rectangles. Notice the example in Figure 3-5.

Table 3-3 *Cause of death*	*Total*	*12-15 years*	*16-17 years*
	Percent of deaths due to specified cause		
All causes	100.0	100.0	100.0
Accidents and violence	69.9	62.5	76.8
Accidents	56.5	52.5	60.4
Suicide.............................	5.4	4.0	6.7
Homicide...........................	6.5	4.5	8.3
Diseases and conditions	30.1	37.5	23.2
Neoplasms	8.9	11.2	6.8
Congenital anomalies	2.5	3.4	1.6
Heart	1.3	1.7	0.8
Nervous system	3.3	4.1	2.6
Respiratory system	2.9	3.8	2.1
Circulatory system...................	4.5	5.4	3.7
Infective and parasitic	1.4	1.9	0.9

Source: Public Health Reports, Volume 94, Number 2, March-April 1979. Published by Health Resources Administration, Public Health Service, U.S. Department of Health, Education, and Welfare, page 117.

Table 3-4   Numerical Continuous Data

Patients' blood pressures (BP) after treatment for hypertension, by initial BP class

Initial BP class	Total		BP level after treatment			
	Number	Percent	Normal	Improved	Unchanged	Worse
90–104	135	63	62	..	64	9
105–114	54	25	15	26	10	3
115–124	19	9	3	14	1	1
125 and over	7	3	0	5	2	..
Total	215	100	80	45	77	13

Source: Public Health Reports, Volume 94, Number 2, March-April 1979. Published by Health Resources Administration, Public Health Service, HEW, p. 132.

Table 3-5   Distribution of Hospitals by Type of Coding System

Type of System	Proportion of Hospitals
All systems	115%
ICDA-8	54
H-ICDA	28
Standard Nominclature	15
ICDA-7	6
CMT	4
SNOP	3
CPT	1
Other	4

Source: Common Data Set for Hospital Management, U.S. Dept. of Health, Education, and Welfare, Public Health Service Health Resources Administration, Bureau of Health Research and Evaluation, DHEW Pub. No. (HRA 74-3026), p. 19.

The vertical side of the graph, called the ordinate axis, is usually used to designate the frequency. The horizontal side, called the abscissa axis, is used for the values. In Figure 3-5, what is the direction of increase of the values on the abscissa axis (left to right)? What is the direction of increase of the frequency on the ordinate axis (upward)?

A polygon is another way of displaying frequency. Figure 3-6 is a frequency polygon showing the same information as that given in Table 3-5.

After values have been tabulated into a frequency distribution, a measure of central tendency or central position can be calculated. This affords a concise description of the performance of the group as a whole.

Figure 3-5   Histogram for the Depiction of the Frequency Distribution of
Serum Uric Acid Levels among 267 Healthy Males

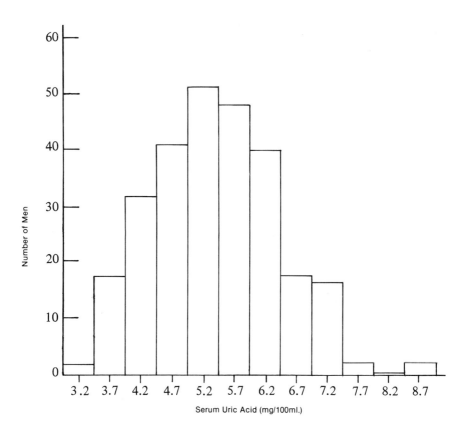

Source: Reprinted with permission from STATISTICS IN MEDICINE, Theodore Colton, Sc.D.; published by Little Brown and Company, Boston, p. 22.

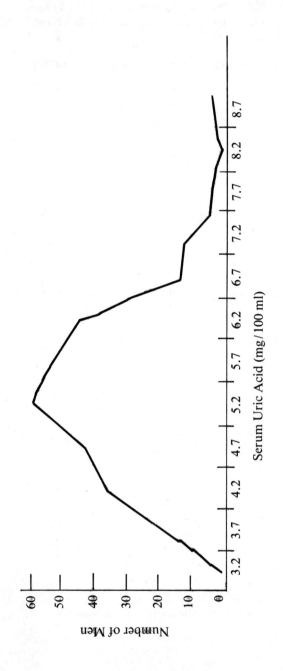

Figure 3-6 Serum Uric Acid Levels among 267 Normal Males

Source: Reprinted with permission from STATISTICS IN MEDICINE, Theodore Colton, Sc.D.; published by Little Brown and Company, Boston, p. 22.

Measures of Central Tendency

Mode, mean, and median are all measures of *central tendency*. The *mode* is the one value in the sample that occurs with the most frequency. The *mean*, generally the most familiar, is the arithmetic average of the sample values. The point in the distribution that divides the values exactly in half is the *median*.

The mean can be greatly affected by the presence of extreme values in the sampling. Therefore, as a purely descriptive measure its value can be limited. The greatest asset of the mean is its use in statistical inference tests based on the mathematical theory of probability. The median is unaffected by extreme observations of the value.

In unimodal (one peak) symmetrical distributions, the mean, median, and mode are identical. When unimodal distributions are skewed, so that the longer tail is to the left of the distribution, the mean, median, and mode occur in the order just listed, which is also alphabetical order. The three measures of central tendency occur in reverse alphabetical order when the longer tail is to the right of the distribution. For purposes of inferential statistical analysis, the mean is the most applicable tool. Let's consider the role of the mean in the normal curve.

The bell-shaped curve in Figure 3-7 approximates what statisticians call a *normal curve*. The normal curve is symmetrical. In this example, mean, median, and mode have the same value (70). There is an equal number of scores on either side of the mean (central axis). The normal curve is composed of infinitely large numbers of samples. The tails of the curve are asymptotic, that is, the tails approach but never touch the baseline.

The normal curve directs our discussion toward inferential statistics. However, let us conclude our review of descriptive statistics by targeting a

Figure 3-7 Bell-Shaped Curve

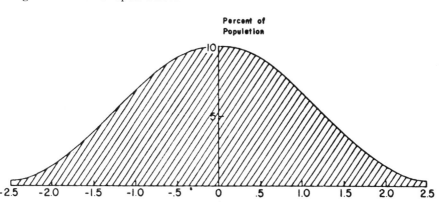

few additional terms and concepts that health information managers should incorporate in their resource files.

Working with the normal curve, there are two points at which the curve begins to change from convex to concave. These occur on either side of the curve. Using the unit of distance established by dropping a perpendicular line from that point on the curve to the abscissa, we can divide the curve into equal units. These units become *standard deviations* from the central axis. Reference can then be made to specific counts of units away from the mean as plus or minus so many standard deviations from the mean. Since the normal curve is a mathematical representation of the population, standard deviation is used in statistics. Standard deviation is a way of measuring variability of samples or values. *Variance* is a useful term and concept that can be used with measures of central tendency. The following questions, based on questions from *Statistics in Medicine*,[10] illustrate the roles of these terms in descriptive statistics. The physician or other provider must ask three statistical questions when analyzing individual patient data or research data on many patients.

1. Is the observation reproducible? Would repeated observations by the same physician, by another physician, or by the same or a different laboratory yield the same result? In other words, how much do the effect and magnitude of measurement error vary? If the error is large and the observation is not reproducible, then the observation is of little value.
2. How do the measurement values distribute among normal and abnormal individuals? What is normal, and what is abnormal? One must know the true biological variation if the observation is to be interpreted properly.
3. Are there any unusual occurrences or untoward events that might explain the observation? For example, might the observation be affected by the patient's anxiety, the degree of physical activity, the time of day? Here the focus is on temporal variation in addition to all other possible explanations for what may appear to be an aberrant result.

Clearly clinicians and other health professionals must have a working knowledge of basic statistical principles, because the use of descriptive statistics is fundamental in medical and health record department operations. Morbidity and mortality rates are the essential ingredients in vital statistics. Take another look at the formulas and terms in Exhibit 3-8. Can you think of ways to extend the calculations beyond simple expression of rates and summary totals? How would you go about comparing the statistics of a particular institution with those of other institutions? Questions of this kind will be asked of health information managers. In addition to handling the collection, processing, retention, and retrieval of data, managers must understand health information expressed in statistical terms. Descriptive statistics go far beyond elementary counts of patient days and lengths of stay.

Inferential Statistics

Medical research, patient care appraisal, utilization review, length of stay by selected diagnosis, projected effects of new therapy, and studies on effects of nutrition on underprivileged children are all examples of inferential statistics. Inferential statistics are concerned with probability. Health information managers who are working actively in research related fields will need to review probability. The mathematical theory of probability provides the foundation on which inferential statistics are based. Moreover, practitioners interested in computerization should take a close look at Bayes' theorem:[11]

> For physicians, Bayes' theorem plays a key role in recent developments in automated and computer assisted diagnosis; it pertains directly to the logic system underlying the process of performing a medical diagnosis. For theoretical statisticians, Bayes' theorem forms the cornerstone for a new structure of statistical inference. . . .

Normal distribution is the most important concept in dealing with inferential statistics. Normal distribution, or the bell-shaped curve, is a method of mathematically explaining the frequency of occurrences. This particular method includes test scores and results representative of a given population. Medicine has used these statistical concepts to establish normal values for measurements, such as red blood count, uric acid level, and amount of protein in the blood. Remember that the normal distribution is unimodal, bell-shaped, and symmetrical. Recall, also, that calculations are based on the mean value within the normal curve. Calculations on the mean are used to show that a specific sample population approximates a normal distribution and, therefore, is representative of an overall population.

The Role of the Null Hypothesis

Once a particular sample has been validated as representative of a total population, the researcher tests research findings statistically to determine if such results could have occurred by chance. This represents the fundamental step in inferential statistics. Can the results of a research project be considered statistically significant? The researcher tests the null hypothesis. Can the differences in the means derived from research data be explained by chance fluctuation about a common mean representing the population? Exhibit 3-10 shows the process and possible outcomes of null hypothesis testing. All health research is based on work with samples of populations. Health information managers need to understand sampling and hypothesis testing.[12]

From this point, researchers build their case. Results are stated in specific terms of significance. For example, an investigator states that the level of significance will be 5 percent. This means the risk of erroneously rejecting the null hypothesis is 1 chance in 20. Or, at 5 percent, there is a 95 percent chance the results are statistically significant. The reader can see the appropriateness of noting such measurement levels when reading health and medical research data. The RRA must be able to assist in analysis of data, and this includes evaluating the appropriateness of measurement levels.

Research Sampling Techniques

Research sampling techniques are used in medical and clinical research. The following list of types of samples is adapted from *Probability Sampling of Hospitals and Patients* by Hess, Riedel, and Fitzpatrick.[13]

- *Nonprobability sampling* permits the researcher at some stage in the study to select some samples and reject others arbitrarily.
- *Probability sampling* depends on the design of a study and affords the investigator a variety of choices in design. Some probability samples are simple, and some more complex.

Exhibit 3-10 Testing Statistical Significance

Statistically significant	=	Reject the null hypothesis	=	Sample value not compatible with null hypothesis value	=	Sampling variation is an unlikely explanation of discrepancy between null hypothesis and sample values
Not statistically significant	=	Do not reject the null hypothesis	=	Sample value compatible with a null hypothesis value	=	Sampling variation is a likely explanation of discrepancy between null hypothesis and sample values

- In *simple random sampling*, every unit in the population has an equal and independent chance of being selected. Researchers often arbitrarily assign numbers to patients in the population under study and then use a table of random numbers to guide their selection of a sample from that population, such as in follow-up research of hypertension clinic patients.
- *Stratified sampling* is dividing the patient population into homogenous groups according to some characteristic, such as type of service received (surgery or cardiology) or source of payment (Medicare), and then selecting a separate sample from within each group. For example, within the category of Medicare patients, one might select all those treated for hip fractures, or within the category of psychiatric patients, one might select all those treated for drug overdose.
- *Systematic sampling* is the selection of every nth individual from a list or card file of patients. For instance, one might choose every fifth entry on a register or index or all patients admitted on a certain day or at certain intervals during a month. Systematic sampling can reduce the clerical time and effort inherently involved in the previously defined methods.
- *Cluster sampling* applies to the selection of population elements in groups or clusters. Medical record administrators may cluster sample from a master patient index file to ascertain particular growth patterns of cards.
- The *control selection* technique increases the likelihood (over that of random sampling) that a preferred combination of sampling units will be chosen while probability methods are maintained.

Certainly, it is useful for health information managers to understand research sampling techniques and the application of statistics in the health care field. The difference between assertive, forthright assistance in medical research and simple clerical acquiescence depends on the comfort level of the health information manager in dealing with sampling techniques and their implications in research.

COMMUNICATION THROUGH STATISTICAL DISPLAYS

The way statistical data are displayed can determine whether they will be understood and applied by appropriate people. Consider the role of monthly and annual reports prepared by medical record departments in hospitals. Each month, the daily discharge analysis reports are compiled, and total statistical data for the month are calculated. The data must be summarized in an organized, readable, and useful format. The display should have eye appeal so that the reader will be inclined to cogitate on the data offered. Key items should be flagged for immediate attention. Comparative reports, such as information for the current month compared with information for the same month the previous year, are often useful. Effective use of statistical displays involves several steps:

1. A recapitulation of work sheets to organize the data.
2. The selection of a format to be used in the report itself. This may be a standard or a specialized format.
3. The transfer of statistical information from work sheet to the final statistical report.
4. A review of the completed report.

Report review is often the most critical step in the preparation of statistical displays. Health information managers need to be familiar with statistical information that is produced in their departments. Review of these data should reveal trends and indicators that direct the reviewer to further action. Review might suggest that the manager take one of the following steps:

• Include more detailed studies.
• Collect additional data.
• Rearrange data for emphasis.
• Notify other users to review the data.

Statistical reports should be reviewed for logic and consistency so that an infection rate is not listed as .9 percent when it should be listed as .09 percent. By reading statistical reports for logic and comparing them with reports from previous months, practitioners gain a general understanding of the data contained in the report. Verification procedures should always be followed, and routine audits of overall statistical processes should be a continuing part of the individual management plan for the department.

One recent development in statistical displays is the increased emphasis on patient care appraisal. Many health information managers deal with data display based on medical audit. Utilization review and medical care evaluation studies are often displayed in table and graph forms.

Table 3-6 and Figures 3-8 and 3-9 represent different ways to display data. Each shows the results of a study or health care topic survey. Look at them carefully and see how well they comply with the following criteria:

• Is the message in the display clear to the viewer?
• Is the chart or graph used for the display the most effective possible?

Table 3-6 Frequency of Respiratory Symptoms among the 898 Respondents

Symptoms status	Cough		Sputum or phlegm		Wheeze		Shortness of breath	
	Number	*Percent*	*Number*	*Percent*	*Number*	*Percent*	*Number*	*Percent*
Claimed symptom	308	34.3	277	30.8	122	13.6	198	22.0
Denied symptom	559	62.2	536	59.7	713	79.4	630	70.2
Other	0	0.0	1	0.1	0	0.0	0	0.0
Undeterminable	31	3.5	84	9.4	63	7.0	70	7.8

Source: Public Health Reports, Volume 92, Number 6, November-December 1977. Published by Health Resources Administration, Public Health Service, HEW, p. 547.

- Is the display attractive to the eye?
- Does the layout add to or detract from the message of the display?
- Are there unnecessary words or distracting details in the display?

Review of these displays and analysis of their content should lead the reader to consider the use of graphs, charts, and techniques of data display in effective communication of statistical information. There are four basic types of charts: (1) *Bar charts*; (2) *Line charts* which are more commonly called graphs (these depict movement); (3) *Pie charts* for relationships such as percentages; and (4) *Step charts* which are often used in place of line charts to convey patterns of motion. Histograms are illustrative of both line and step charts. Figure 3-5 is an example of a histogram.

Tables are another way to display data. Several examples are included in this chapter. Tables should be concise. They are useful because they present a change in the formatting of information on reports. Both tables and charts can be used to track project developments in a medical record department. For example, in the computerization of the master patient index, a GANTT chart could be used to monitor project activities and display information on progress toward scheduled target dates.

Statistical displays, including graphs, tables, reports, and analyses highlighting key information, are all useful to the health information practitioner.

- They help explain health services planning and research both within and outside the organization.
- They provide an effective medium for display of provider services.
- They help uncover the collective memory of patient information.

Over and above their use in health information and medical research, effective displays can reinforce the use of statistics in management activ-

Figure 3-8 Sample Distribution of Systolic Blood Pressure in Males and Females

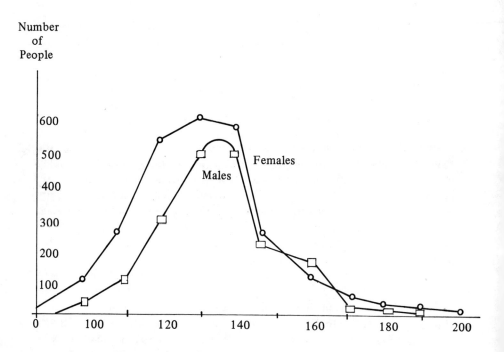

Systolic blood pressure (mm Hg)

Figure 3-9 Sources of Payment for Nursing Homes and Extended Care Facilities for Cerebrovascular Disease Cases, Orleans Parish, 1971

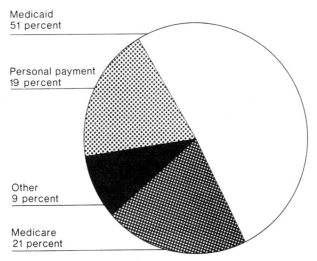

Medicaid
51 percent

Personal payment
19 percent

Other
9 percent

Medicare
21 percent

NOTE: Percentages based on data obtained from 9 participating nursing homes and 2 extended care facilities.

Source: Public Health Reports, Volume 92, Number 3, May-June 1977. Health Resources Administration, U.S. Department of Health, Education, and Welfare, p. 277.

ities. Planning, controlling, and evaluating health information systems require effective statistical applications.

Statistical information is the result of fact finding. It identifies current data and operations within a system in a given institution. Statistics describe activities within that system and provide an analysis of trends. Trend analysis can direct changes in procedures and objectives in medical record departments and their associated hospitals. In working with medical staff committees in hospitals, the record administrator should analyze exceptional items on statistical reports. Such analysis can affect changes in objectives in the services provided by the agency.

Statistical analysis is necessary for justification of the budget. Suppose that the medical record administrator wishes to computerize the master patient index in the hospital. Statistics could be used to describe the current activity involving the master patient index. Such statistics might include number of admissions and readmissions during a given time period. To calculate the costs of computerizing the index and to relate those costs to the cost of the present system necessitate calculations based on available statistical data.

The cost justification concept also applies in long-range planning, such as constructing five-year plans for health care delivery systems. It is used in long-range planning for departmental growth. Statistical data are involved in overall agency planning, staffing, recognition of the need for health manpower, service personnel for agencies, and the services provided. For instance, ambulatory care services may be expanded on the basis of statistical analysis of current service activity load. Computer technology may be given the go-ahead if statistical analysis reveals high current activity.

All validation or evaluation of activities involves statistics. Evidence of statistical use in planning that is external to the organization is also important. In 1965, regional medical programs were created to concentrate on the three major causes of death: heart disease, cancer, and stroke. Today, Health Systems Agencies, national PSROs, Social Security, HEW, National Health Insurance, and National Cooperative Health Statistics are all targeted by health information statistics. Not only are these agencies and programs targeted, but they are supported and justified by current health statistics. The medical record, both individually and within a given medical information system, is the source for all of this health information. The data that are abstracted from the patient record must be cross-balanced against statistical data kept on particular services provided in the health care delivery system.

The reader is urged to view statistics as a useful tool in planning within and beyond the individual department. It is a measure of health care services. It can be used to justify the use of improved methods in health care delivery. Promotion of responsible, effective use of health statistics is a current and vital challenge to medical record practitioners today.

NOTES

1. Melville Hodge, *Medical Information Systems* (Germantown, Md.: Aspen Systems Corp., 1977), p. 14.

2. Lorraine Gay, RRA, "Record Linkage in Community Health and Hospital Services," paper prepared for delivery at 6th International Congress on Medical Records, Sydney, Australia, May 2, 1972, (Chicago: AMRA, 1972).

3. P.L. 89-97, Medicare/Medicaid Amendments to the Social Security Act, 1965.

4. Sharon Van Sell Davidson, ed., *PSRO Utilization and Audit in Patient Care* (Saint Louis, Mo.: C. V. Mosby Co., 1976), p. 111.

5. Joint Commission on Accreditation of Hospitals, *Standards for Programs for Mental Health and Developmentally Disabled Persons* (Chicago: JCAH, 1978).

6. Alan Westin, *Computers, Health Records and Citizens' Rights* (Dept. of HEW, National Bureau of Standards, 1976), p. 187.

7. PB-263 578, *Automation of a Problem Oriented Medical Record* (Rockville, Md.: National Center for Health Services Research, 1976), p. 179.

8. Report from the U.S. National Committee on Vital and Health Statistics, National Center for Health Statistics, January 11-12, 1978.

9. Theodore Colton, *Statistics in Medicine* (Boston: Little, Brown & Co., 1974), p. 43.

10. Ibid., p. 71.

11. Ibid., p. 116.

12. Irene Hess, Donald Riedel, and Thomas B. Fitzpatrick, *Probability Sampling of Hospitals and Patients* (Ann Arbor, Mich.: Health Administration Press, 1975), p. 7.

13. Ibid.

REFERENCES

Colton, Theodore. *Statistics in Medicine*. Boston: Little, Brown & Co., 1974.

Duncan, Robert C.; Knapp, Rebecca G.; and Miller, M. Clinton III. *Introductory Biostatistics for the Health Sciences*. New York: John Wiley & Sons, 1977.

Hess, Irene; Riedel, Donald C.; and Fitzpatrick, Thomas B. *Probability Sampling of Hospitals and Patients*. Ann Arbor: Health Administration Press, 1975.

Huffman, Edna K. *Medical Record Management*. Berwyn, Ill.: Physicians' Record Co., 1972.

American Medical Record Association. *Glossary of Hospital Terms*. Chicago: AMRA, 1974.

Pierce, Patricia J., RRA. *Commonly Computed Rates & Percentages for Hospital Inpatients*. Chicago: AMRA, 1975.

Chapter 4

Designing Forms and Formats for Data Collection and Use

CHAPTER OBJECTIVES

1. Relate the principles of forms design to forms used in the collection and retention of patient records
2. Identify appropriate guidelines for design of particular patient care forms
3. Recognize the significance of forms design in directing data users and providers
4. Understand the rationale for changing record form sequences from inpatient to outpatient and inpatient to discharged patient record.
5. Relate record formats to computer technology
6. Differentiate between chronological, source-oriented, and problem-oriented record formats

Health information professionals employ analytical skills in designing forms and formats for data collection and use. When taking a systems look at forms and formats for the many areas where data will be collected for future use, we must consider the whole system. Forms and formats are used at the onset of treatment for health care encounters. They aid in collecting all types of data for patient care, research, education, and the many other needs. Forms and formats are also a useful communication link for the health professionals during the treatment of the patient. Later, data from initial reports is compiled into secondary documents (indexes, registers, and so on) and used by those who need certain elements from specific forms and formats. In this chapter, we will explore how the design of forms and formats affects their uses.

PROVIDING THE FOUNDATION

The purpose of the form designates its design. In design, our concern is with the following terms and their meanings: standardized, multipurpose, preprinted, handwritten, and computer generated. We have not included single-purpose forms in the listing above because there are none in the processing of health information. Every data element and every form used in the health record has potential multiple uses and is categorized as multipurpose. This is true whether the form is a single original filed in one place or one of many copies distributed to a variety of places. For our purposes, therefore, every form used in health records is a multipurpose form.

Some forms used in processing health information contain narrative content. Patient history and nurses' notes are examples. Other forms summarize particular events or record data compiled from other forms, such as work sheets. For example, nurses' notes that provide a cumulative, 48-hour record of fluid intake and output serve as summary entries. Diagnostic test results are also examples of data entries in summary form whereas physiological and laboratory findings are usually reported in an abbreviated or numerical form.

It might be helpful at this point to become familiar with the traditional contents of a hospital record. Exhibit 4-1 gives a brief descriptive overview of the titles and contents of common hospital forms.

Many parts of health information are recorded through coded information that can be alphabetical, numerical, or a combination of alphanumerical coded data entries. Many records are still being handwritten; others are designed for typing; and more and more computer printout forms are being seen in medical and health information systems. Special forms are used for scheduling, others are designed specifically for auditing. Indexes and registers illustrate the various forms used by different types of health care facilities.

Patient care is primarily reflected in the patient record forms. These, in turn, reflect individual patient care settings. Physicians' office records are vastly different from a mental health center's records, which are also different from dental records, and so on. Exhibit 4-2 shows the differences in a form when it is seen in three different media.

Specific things must be considered in designing forms. In English, we are familiar with reading from left to right and from the top of a page to the bottom. This should be a primary consideration in design. The readability component, along with the purpose of the form, is a major concern. While other factors are involved, we must bear in mind the following primary questions:

Exhibit 4-1 Common Hospital Forms

1. Identification Data and Consent Forms
2. Provisional Diagnosis. There should be an admitting problem identified on every patient at the time of admission. If a patient requires hospitalization, the hospital staff needs this information to proceed intelligently.
3. History: Chief Complaint, Present Illness, Past History, Present History, and Family History
4. Physical Examination.
5. Consultations. Consultations imply an examination of the patient and the patient's record. The consultation note should be recorded and either signed or authenticated by the consultant.
6. Clinical Laboratory Reports. The original signed laboratory report is entered in the patient's record. Duplicates are filed in the laboratory.
7. X-ray Reports. The original signed radiological report is entered in the patient's record. Duplicates are filed in the x-ray department.
8. Tissue (Pathological Specimen) Report. Since all tissues removed in surgery are sent to the laboratory, acknowledgment that the tissue has been received and a gross description should be entered in the record. If a microscopic examination is done, a description of the findings should be made a part of the record. The decision to do a microscopic examination is determined by the medical staff and the pathologist according to the rules and regulations of the hospital.
9. Physician's Diagnostic and Therapeutic Orders
10. Treatment: Medical and Surgical. All treatment procedures are in the medical record. Except in cases of grave emergency, the patient should receive a complete diagnostic workup before surgery. Operative notes should be dictated immediately after surgery and should contain both a description of the findings and a detailed account of the technique used and tissue removed.
11. Progress Notes. Provide a chronological picture and analysis of the clinical course of the patient. The frequency with which they are made is determined by the condition of the patient, the complexity of the treatment, and the need for information exchange among the medical team providers.
12. Nurses' Notes. Provide a description of daily objective and subjective findings.
13. Final Diagnosis. A definitive final diagnosis or a complete problem list is entered on each record.
14. Summary. A summary of the patient's condition on discharge and course in the hospital is valuable as a recapitulation of the patient's hospitalization.
15. Autopsy Findings. When an autopsy is performed, a complete protocol of the findings should be made a part of the record.

Exhibit 4-2 Examples of Patient Record Forms

CARDIOVASCULAR CLINIC	ENCOUNTER #21	BACK-N OTHER	160 :SAME *169

PATIENT NO: _N 08000_   DOCTOR: _R_

PATIENT NAME: _JOHN NONAME_

APPT. DATE: _12/27/74_   APPT. TIME: _____

APPT. TYPE: OC   O/CM (N/CM) OTHER: _____

LEGS-N	170	:SAME
EDEMA	171 LRB 1234 :
FEM-PULSE	172 LRB 1234 :
POP-PULSE	173 LRB 1234 :
DOR-PULSE	(172) LRB 1234 :
TIB-PULSE	(175) LRB 1234 :
THROMBO	176 LRB :
VARICOSE	177 LRB :
FEM-BRU	(178) LRB :
OTHER	*179

WEIGHT(LB) (001) : _180_
HEIGHT(IN) (002) : _72_
BODY BUILD (003) 1/3: ____
PULSE 004 :
BP(LYING) 005L :
 (005R) :
BP(SIT) (006L) : _190/120_
 (006R) : _180/124_
BP(STAND) 007L : _184/126_
 (007R) : _160/130_
TEMP 008 :

HEART-N 070 :SAME
ENLARGED 071 :
LIFT (072) LRB:
EJECT CL 073 EML:
OPEN SNAP 074 :
S1 075 ID :
S2 076 ID :
S3 (077) ID : _GALLOP_
S4 (078) ID :
MURMURS
SYS-APEX 091 EMLH 123456 :
SYS-AORT 092 EMLH 123456 :
SYS-PUL 093 EMLH 123456 :
SYS-TRI 094 EMLH 123456 :
DIA-APEX 095 EML 1234 :
DIA-AORT 096 EML 1234 :
DIA-PUL 097 EML 1234 :
DIA-TRI 098 EML 1234 :
OTHER *099

ARMS-N (190) :SAME
EDEMA 191 LRB 1234 :
BRA-PULSE 192 LRB 1234 :
RAD-PULSE 193 LRB 1234 :
ULN-PULSE 194 LRB 1234 :
OTHER *199

NEURO-N 200 :SAME
PARKINSON 201 :
PARALYSIS 202 LRB:
OTHER *209

X-RAY-N 500 :SAME
CARD-ENL 501 :
RV-ENL 502 :
LA-ENL 503 :
LV-ENL (504) : _MINIMAL_
AO-DIL 505 :
CORARC 506 :
PA-DIL 507 :
LUNGS
CONGEST 511 LRB:
EFFUSION 512 LRB:
FIBROSIS 513 LRB:
NODULE 514 LRB:
OTHER *519

EYES-N 010 :SAME
GRADE (011) LRB 1234 :
CATARACT 012 LRB.
OTHER *019

HENT-N 020 :SAME
EDENTU 021 ULB:
OTHER *029

THYROID-N (030) :SAME
ENLARGED 031 :
NODULE 032 LRB:
OTHER *039

NECK-N 040 :SAME
BRUIT (041) LRB: _FAINT_
VEINS 042 LRB:
OTHER *049

BREASTS-N 050 :SAME
FIBRO 051 LRB:
NODULE 052 LRB:
OTHER *059

CHEST-N (060) :SAME
RALES 061 LRB:
RHONCHI 062 LRB:
DIM-BS 063 LRB:
WHEEZE 064 LRB:
DULLNESS 065 LRB:
TENDER 066 LRB:
OTHER *069

ABDOMEN-N 110 :SAME
AOR-BRU (111) :
FLANK-BRU 112 LRB:
LIVER-ENL 113 :
TENDER 114 ABCDEF:
OBESE 115 :
MASS 116 ABCDEF:
HERNIA (117) LRB: _Small_
SCAR (118) ABCDEF:
OTHER *119

REC/GEN-N (130) :SAME
HEMOR 131 :
OTHER *139

PROSTATE-N 140 :SAME
ENL-SM (141) : _Slight_
ENL-IRR 142 :
SOFT-BOG 143 :
NODULE 144 :
TENDER 145 :
OTHER *149

PELVIC-N 150
DOCTOR 151 :
DATE 152 :
OTHER *159

TREAD-N 520
LEVEL 521 123456789:
ANGINA 522 :
ST-ABN 523 :
HR-MAX 524 :
BP-MAX 525 :
OTHER *529

PUL/FUNC-N 530
VC-OBS 531 :
VC-PRED 532 :
BC-OBS 533 :
BC-PRED 534 :
1-VC 535 :
2-VC 536 :
3-VC 537 :
OTHER *539

DIG: _BILATERAL XANTHELASMAS_

Exhibit 4-2 Continued

EKG

NORMAL   V-RATE: **94**   A-RATE: **94**   PM-RATE:_____   AXIS:_____
          PR:___**.13**   QRS:___**.09**   QT:___**.40**   NC:_____

RHYTHM   SR ST SB JR AFL AFB VT PAT PAC PVC PJC PACE-DM PACE-FX

COND.   AVB-1 AVB-2 MOB-I MOB-II AVB-3 RBBB RBBB-I LBBB LAHB LPHB . TFB

          WPW LGL LVH RVH CVH LAE RAE STT-DIG STT-NS STT-LI STT-AI STT-II

          ASMI ASMI-A ASMI-O ALMI ALMI-A ALMI-O ISMI (ISMI-A) ISMI-O LMI

          LMI-A LMI-O SEMI SEMI-A

FTA:_____
FTB:_____

PLAN

OC CM WK:____ MN:____ LAB:_____
(FTA) **BAPTIST HOSPITAL FOR ACUTE MI.**
FTB:_____

RISK FACTORS		INFARCTION			CVA	HYP	HD	DM	CAB	CAC	MAL	AGES	
		1-39	40-50	51-								EXP	ALIVE
MOTHER	01												
FATHER	02												
BROTHERS	03												
SISTERS	04												
OTHER	05												

SMOKER   11: CIG   QUIT OTHER NONE   WORK   15: SED   NORM LABOR
PERSON   12: I   II   III   IV   EXERC PG 16: NONE   MOD   VIG
MARITAL 13: S   M   W   D   HOME   17: ALONE   N-A
ECON.   14: W   L   M   H   DISABLE   18: R ABCD Z   1234

PROBLEMS: **U GI (Duodenal Ulcer 1968)   DRUG (PENICILLIN)**
          HCL   HYP
          FPD
          M I (acute)

MEDICATIONS:_____
_____
_____

PRESENT ILLNESS: *Acute onset of substernal burning*
pain 2 hours ago with radiation to
left arm and associated nausea,
vomiting, and sweating. Definite history
of anaphylaxis after penicillin
injection 3 years ago. Prior history
of hypertension.

Reprinted with permission: Jenkin, M.A., M.D.,
A Manual of Computers in Medical Practice,
The Society of Computer Medicine, 1977.

Exhibit 4-2 Continued

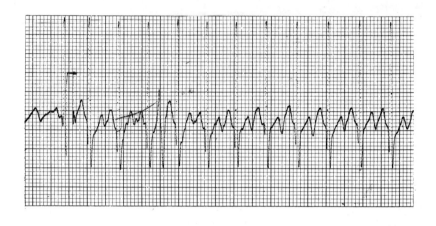

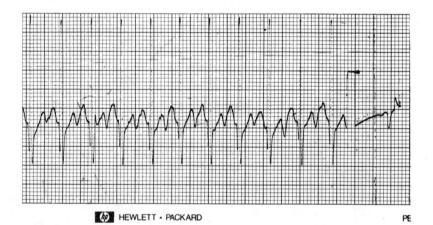

(hp) HEWLETT · PACKARD   PE

Electrocardiogram Tracing—Machine-Made Graph or Tracing

- Why is the information being recorded?
- What will it be used for?
- Who will be using it?
- How will they use it?
- How long do we want to retain the information?

Fetal monitoring strips, comprised of scans or tracings, are a current example of forms that raise questions regarding their design and use. Fetal monitoring strips have joined the electrocardiogram and the electroencephalogram tracings. Intrapartum fetal monitoring strips can run up to 30 feet in an eight-hour chart pack. Although there are no standard requirements, federal regulations are now being proposed that would require retention of the entire fetal monitoring chart until age 21. Currently, some hospitals retain a short portion of the strip and attach it to a summary report. Other facilities keep the entire strip, while some throw it away. Each facility determines how these and other forms will be incorporated into the record.

Guidelines for Designing Forms

One of the most important things in designing forms is considering a design that will facilitate ease in data collection, data completeness, and error control. Data can be collected several ways. They can be entered on a form through handwriting or dictated and transcribed on reports for inclusion in patient records. They can be collected for computer processing by keypunching cards, by being keyed directly to magnetic tape, and by being entered directly into CRT terminals.

Exhibit 4-3 lists guidelines that are helpful in knowing where to begin and what steps to take in designing a form.

The more opportunities there are for copying and reentering information, the greater the chance of error. It is important to design forms that will capture data at the most propitious time. That is, data should be recorded during or immediately after an encounter and collected on an instrument that provides permanency. This will reduce the possibility of transposing and making other errors when the data are copied.

Another important consideration is grouping similar types of data on one form. Identification data, for instance, can be grouped in one section of a form, as can patient provider entries. Other ways of identifying data are through the use of shaded coloring, boldface print, or underscoring particular items. Information managers should review various forms to illustrate these characteristics and others when developing forms design programs.

Exhibit 4-3 Guidelines for Designing Forms

1. Assess each form individually to
   a. insure its necessity.
   b. avoid duplicate recording.
   c. insure it integrates with the existing records system.
2. Determine the purpose of the form, which will determine information to be included.
3. Identify benefits that will be derived from introduction of the form into the record.
4. Design forms as simply as possible; do not clutter them with headings, captions, or instructions.
5. Consider use of unstructured, multipurpose flow sheets. They will eliminate the need for several special forms to monitor special care factors and reduce chart bulk.
6. Plan all forms in the record to be a uniform size.
7. Place form titles and patient identification consistently on every form.
8. Include space for at least
   a. full patient name.
   b. medical, health, or client record file number.
9. Consider printing headings and captions in bold print.
10. Line up headings to provide an uncluttered appearance and to promote ease in locating desired information.
11. Consider logical sequence of subject headings.
12. Use white paper with color-coded borders for quick identification of different forms; colored paper may be difficult to read or photocopy.
13. Select captions that clearly state what information is to be entered.
14. Use a box arrangement to save time in checklists.
15. Plan spacing according to the specific method of documentation.
    a. Typewritten entries: set lines according to number of lines per inch on a typewriter and to accommodate vertical spacing.
    b. Handwritten entries: set lines far enough apart to insure readability.
    c. CRT or computer printout format: set margin, spacing, and punctuation clearly.
    d. Consider the period of time each side of the form covers.
16. Identify certain portions that are restricted for use by designated staff or groups (for example, medical record service, infection control committee, utilization review committee); those areas should be surrounded with bold lines.
17. Consider printing on both sides of the sheet to maximize paper use and reduce chart bulk.

Exhibit 4-3 Continued

18. Consider printing on reverse side to facilitate reference when form is in chart holder and/or fastened at top as a closed record.
19. When possible, eliminate the need for a special form by utilizing a rubber stamp on an existing form.
20. Allow sufficient space for signatures of those making entries.
21. Because newly designed forms often need revisions, mimeograph or photocopy a small supply for trial use.
22. Use good, quality paper stock in final printing to avoid dog-earring and tearing, and to insure permanency; 20-pound paper weight stock is recommended for long-term use.
23. Card stock should be avoided since it creates bulk, is difficult to handle, and may complicate photocopy technique.
24. Stock only a six-month supply of the form to prevent waste in the event of a revision or change in documentation procedures.
25. Always introduce a proposed new form before implementation and preferably during initial design phases; this promotes input by those making entries and using the data.
26. Complete final review and approval of the draft form prior to implementation; this is accomplished by a multidisciplinary forms committee that includes the medical record administrator.
27. Simple printed instructions will insure uniformity, if a form is to be used by various departments.
28. If instructions are detailed, prepare separate directions regarding
    a. purpose.
    b. use.
    c. instructions for completion.
    d. staff responsibilities.
    e. references, if any.
29. Include the name, address, and city of the facility on forms that are likely to be sent elsewhere.
30. Identify all forms by
    a. a descriptive and simple title.
    b. a stock control number.
    c. the month and year of first, revised, or last printing.

Establishing Forms Committees

In most health information organizations, a forms committee is organized to facilitate a systems approach to design. In some instances, the
purpose of the committee is more than participation in the design process. It
serves not only as a source of input when forms are being designed, but also
as an organizational means for continual recognition that new data elements
will be introduced and old data elements reviewed and periodically discarded from forms. In Chapter 8 we will discuss in detail some of the
controls of the health information system and in Chapter 7 some of the
controls needed for a retention and retrieval system. Both of these directly
relate to controls needed in the design of forms. The following list suggests
a few policies necessary in controlling forms design.

- There should be a forms inventory that outlines the most recent revision dates.
- There should be policies established by a forms review committee that
  clearly delineate parameters for entry.
- There should be procedures specifying the steps necessary to redesign a
  form, enter a new form, or revise or remove a current form from the
  inventory.

These policies are necessary to prevent individual departments or providers from proliferating forms in the system and causing unnecessary bulk
for the total document. In some organizations, forms design is so controlled
that physicians and other health care providers are not allowed to work or
maintain staff privileges in a facility unless they agree to utilize and comply
with policies established by the organization and monitored by the records
manager or forms control committee. Another method of controlling forms
is to purchase preprinted, packaged forms from commercial printers who
specialize in health and medical records. This illustrates a method of stan-
dardizing and fostering control of forms and formats. Any form that is not
preprinted is not allowed in the record and can be discarded.

Providing Forms Directions

The design of the form can facilitate or obstruct the ease of data entry as
well as the understanding of the data entered on that form. It is difficult to
prepare a summary or an abstract or even to read a medical record if data
entries are scattered and not standardized. If a medical record contains
mixed forms of entry, it is difficult to read and understand. For instance, if
the record contains some forms that are handwritten, others that are type-

written, and still others of various sizes and colors, it is most difficult to try to abstract or summarize information from that record. Forms design, then, provides the direction for all of these important activities. Effective forms design requires awareness of the flow of information in individual settings. The following questions summarize the targets used in creating effective documents through forms design.

- Where does the form originate; that is, what department originally enters data onto the form or enters the form into the system to be used by others?
- What individual enters data on the form?
- What information should be on the form?
- What information is currently being entered on the form?
- Who ascertains the completeness of the data entries?
- Where will the form finally be filed?
- Who will use the information on the form?
- Who will receive copies of the form?
- How long should the form be retained?

Notice that many of the questions are similar to those applied in considering data entries.[1] This is a continuation of working with data entries by grouping and organizing them into useful patient documents for particular settings. Exhibit 4-4 portrays organized descriptions of patient records in individual settings by means of the forms order or arrangement. Read through each example and consider the following questions:

- How do the examples portray types of care provided the patient?
- Does the information listed on the form title clearly indicate the nature of the data entries in the form?
- Is the complexity of patient care services suggested?
- Do the examples provide an organized approach to the order of arrangement?

Computer technology has made significant contributions to individual forms as well as forms sequence. Let's examine two aspects. An extensive development project was carried out at Holy Family Hospital in Spokane, Washington, from 1968 to 1973. Roger Shannon, M.D., developed automated medical histories and reviewed the results in the *Journal of Clinical Computing* in 1977. He identified history acquisition and record review as two key elements that have direct impact on the patient history.

At Holy Family Hospital the standard on-line device was the IBM 2260 CRT. All frames were automatically generated from coding sheets. Each frame provided for instructional material and up to nine one-line questions.

Exhibit 4-4 Comparison of Forms Sequence within Patient Records

Acute Care Hospital	Long-Term Care Skilled Nursing Facility	Ambulatory Care Family Practice Clinic
Identification sheet	Identification sheet	Identification sheet
Medical section	Transfer report from hospital	Data-base section
• Autopsy report	Consent forms	• History
• Discharge summary	Admission certification/Medicare	• Physical examination
• Emergency room (ER) report	History and physical examination	• Admission lab data
• Medical history	Nursing history and assessment	Problem list
• Physical examination	Laboratory reports	• Active problems, numbers, and titles
• Progress notes	X-ray reports	• Inactive problem list, numbers, and titles
• Consultations	Doctors' order sheet	• Plans for each problem
Diagnostic section	Medication record	Orders to collect more data
• Laboratory reports	Treatment record	• X-ray
• X-ray	Medication destruction form	• Electrocardiogram
• Electrocardiograms	Patient care plan	• Kidney scan
• Electroencephalograms	Nurses' notes	• Monitoring of blood pressure and weight
• Brain scan		Treatment plans for each problem
• Liver scan		• Medication order
• Kidney scan		• Physical medicine therapy
• Block transfusion report		Education of patient plans
Treatment section		• Patient to attend hypertension class
• Anesthesia report		
• Operative report		
• Pathology report		

- Physical therapy
- Occupational therapy
- Respiratory therapy
- Radiation therapy

Orders

- Physicians' orders

Nurses' section

- Medication report
- Graphic charts
- Intake and output record
- Nurses' observations

Miscellaneous

- Consent forms
- Patient transfer record
- Death card

Progress follow up to problems

- Progress notes, number, and title for each problem

Flow sheet indicating medication, blood pressure, and weight at daily intervals

Yes and no answers to questions were usually indicated by depressing single appropriate keys on a standard typewriter keyboard, such as Y for yes and N for no. For the unusual question requiring a numerical or text answer, responses could be entered normally through the keyboard.

Several initial history questionnaires were devised to be used by two groups—patients and medical personnel. Patients were instructed to use the Y and N answer keys and allowed to proceed at their own pace through the questionnaire presented on the CRT. At the end of the questionnaire, a notice asked the patient to call for an attendant.

The initial patient questionnaire was approximately 160 questions. It was presented in the rather brusque terminology used by the physician who had volunteered to participate in the pilot study. Once the early questionnaires were revised and refined, several other physicians volunteered to test their use. Because some physicians wanted fewer details than others, the branching instructions were modified to provide only those details the physicians themselves desired. The questionnaire proved successful.

Ambulatory care settings, like hospitals, also illustrate how computers use formats and forms sequence. Computer Stored Ambulatory Record (COSTAR) is an excellent example of a computer-based medical information system. COSTAR originated at Massachusetts General Hospital's Laboratory of Computer Science in collaboration with the Harvard Community Health Plan (HCHP). HCHP is a prepaid group practice and has been in operation since 1969. COSTAR 4, currently being revised and expanded under the designation COSTAR 5, replaces the traditional document-based patient medical record with a comprehensive, centralized, and integrated information system to meet the needs of the medical care and financial/administrative needs of a fee-for-service or a prepaid group practice.

Three formats used to display COSTAR medical information are:

1. *The encounter report*: a single-visit note that includes diagnoses with associated free text, objective data, medications, test results, and consultation requests concerned with that visit.
2. *The status report*: a complete index to, and summary of, the patient's current medical status.
3. *Flowcharts*: a list of specific parameters or types of data along a horizontal axis with date of event along the vertical axis.

These reports can be produced on a schedule basis or on demand, as printed material or on the CRT display at the time of inquiry. The unique ability to create dynamic, up-to-date summaries and to extract only relevant information means that less time is spent reviewing records and that there is less chance that the provider might miss vital data.

We can expect acute, ambulatory, and long-term care facilities to be affected by developing technology and will need to direct these effects positively.

FORMATS FOR MEDICAL RECORDS

We are concerned with the structure that the final document takes when all forms have been compiled, sequenced, and somehow fastened together in a permanent document. Format, however, is more than an arrangement or an organization of forms in a permanent file folder. Format of medical and health records directs the type of entries, the way entries are made, and the future use of those entries. Formats must be considered in the total systems approach to health information management. Like forms and data entries, formats can either facilitate or prove detrimental to patient care and future use of the patient's record. An important aspect of a record's format is the sequence of forms in the total document. This sequence varies as the document progresses through developmental stages.

Care Facility Affects Record Format

When we look at records at their various locations and in their various usages, it becomes evident that there is a wide variety of formats available. For example, the record in a physician's office often needs to be in an entirely different format than one in an acute care facility. The record in the acute care facility will have at least two formats during its development and retention. During the acute stages of a patient's illness, the record is in the developmental stage. At the end of the patient's treatment when there are no further developmental entries going into the record, the format will change. During treatment, the patient's record is kept in a format that facilitates the needs of those who are giving care to the patient and those who must use the record as the communication link to know what others have done for the patient. Therefore, the sequence of the record during the acute care phase of the patient may begin with a listing of physician's orders, then nurses' notes, laboratory reports, progress notes, and so on. When the patient has been discharged and the record is being compiled for its many secondary uses, the information will often be resequenced into an entirely different format. This is true in many areas of recordkeeping. Work records and information flow reports often take a different format when they are reorganized and sent to the medical record department. The following list includes facilities that compile records in formats that are unique to each facility.

- General acute hospitals
- Psychiatric facilities
- Health maintenance organizations
- Pharmacies that develop drug profiles
- Private practice records
- Clinic records
- Statistical records

Exhibit 4-5 identifies forms and their titles. It categorizes forms according to treatment functions. This sample list is from an acute care medical center and outlines the sequence of the forms in the completed medical record.

Exhibit 4-5 Acute Care Medical Forms

1. *Face sheet*
2. *Medical section*
   Autopsy report
   Discharge summary
   Emergency room report
   Short-stay form
   History and physical
   Prenatal history
   Maternal record
   Newborn record
   Newborn nurses' notes
   Progress notes (includes dietary, OT, PT)
   PT discharge summary
   Physical therapy
   Consultations
   Social service reports
   Speech pathology
3. *Diagnostic section*
   Urinalysis
   Hematology
   Coagulation
   Chemistry
   Microbiology
   Clinical virology
   Laboratory
   LDH isoenzyme (table)
   LDH isoenzyme (graph)
   Protein electrophoresis

Exhibit 4-5 Continued

Thyroid profile
Lipid profile
Send-out labs, PKU
Secretin test
X-ray, radiation therapy reports
EKG
Copy of EKG tracings
EEG
EEG echogram
Brain scan
Liver scan
Kidney scan
Lung scan
Other nuclear medicine reports
Gastroenterology (GI) lab
Clinical physiology department
Gastric function test
Blood gas analysis
Diffusion capacity
Ventilatory function
Ventilation
Volemetron determination
Blood volume determination
4. *Treatment section*
Electroshock treatment (EST)
Labor room nurses' notes
Anesthesia report
Delivery record
Cesarean section record
Hip data
Operative report
Operative information record
Postanesthesia report
Surgical pathology
Leukemia pathology
Blood sheets
Heart sheets:
  Cardiovascular laboratory
  Coronary arteriography
  Heart sketch

Exhibit 4-5 Continued

      Oxygen content data
      Pump prime
      The heart center
      Open-heart flow sheets
   Respiratory therapy routine treatment
   Continuous respiratory care form
   Dialysis
   Peritoneal dialysis
   Electromuscular diagnosis (EMG)

5. *Orders*
   Rehabilitative medicine department prescription
   Physician's orders

6. *Nurses' section*
   Medication administration
   Initial identification
   Intravenous infusions and blood transfusions
   Anticoagulant sheet
   Diabetic chart
   Graphic chart
   Blood pressure record
   Fluid chart
   Parenteral fluid chart
   Caloric intake record
   Neurologic nursing notes
   Cardiac arrest sheet
   Nurses' notes (includes coronary care unit and intensive care unit)
   Newborn supervision score (attach Coombs and bilirubin report here)
   Master problem sheet

7. *Miscellaneous*
   Consent and authorization forms
   Death card
   Patient transfer form
   Transfer records

8. *Correspondence*
   Medic-1/fire department report
   Notes from psychiatric patients
   Other correspondence

A careful analysis of record formats can help streamline the structure so that a shift in format is facilitated. For instance, ambulatory care records can be structured according to a standard format. In skilled nursing facilities and other long-term care applications the order of forms is established in reverse chronology so that the most recent information is seen first. This format can be maintained with minimal reordering following completion of care. The critical concern is to design the structure for maximum accessibility by the users. In these cases, reformatting can be reduced markedly. Health information managers must analyze information flow of data entries as they evolve within the record to make format determinations.

Record Order Affects Record Format

Some records are divided by the content of the record, so that all nursing notes are kept in one area, all laboratory reports are kept in another area, and all diagnostic work is kept in another area of the record. These sections can be divided by either color-coded borders, tabs, or other methods devised by the facility. Some records are divided into inpatient and outpatient reports; others are kept in straight chronological order with the most recent entry on top.

The particular format that seems most useful to the provider often determines the format the record takes. In determining the format of the record, consideration should be given to all users of the data, the length of time the data will be kept, and the interrelationship between the forms, the data entries, the users, and providers of health information. Refer to Exhibit 4-4 and examine the format implied in these comparisons. Notice how some are formatted according to sections. As we begin examining the problem-oriented medical record system, we will see how the record order for the family practice clinic offers a very specific format.

PROBLEM-ORIENTED MEDICAL RECORDS

The first thing to recognize in looking at the problem-oriented medical record (POMR) is that it is more than a method of recording information. It includes a unique approach to the practice of medicine. The POMR is structured for a total approach to patient care and those who use this type of form in the delivery of medical care are assisted by the record. The POMR directs them to take a more comprehensive and structured look at patients and their treatment.

The concept of POMR was developed by Dr. Lawrence Weed in the late 1950s and has been described and extensively developed since then. One of Dr. Weed's contentions has always been that the chart and the medical record should be more than just a source of documentation. In fact, on many occasions, Weed has been known to state that the medical record is the practice of medicine, because without an organized, logical format to direct those who provide care, there can be no adequate diagnosis and treatment. POMR is structured to provide a total approach to patient care. It is designed to enumerate patient problems as single entities, list the diagnostic and therapeutic steps for each problem, indicate the progress of each, pointing to the conclusion or outcome of each, and thereby present a total picture of the patient's state of health. As such, it brings all the problems the patient has into focus for the doctor or the practitioner and indicates that all of these problems should be treated in relationship to each other.

Unique characteristics of a POMR include its ability to unify the data and prevent fragmentation of diagnostic and therapeutic information. Unlike other record formats, it brings into focus the patient as the primary source of information. It provides the strongest possible format for unifying the patient and the information that reflects the patient's feelings, thoughts, complaints, ideas, questions, and all other elements of patient involvement in the development of the medical record. Physicians and other providers who use the POMR start with the patient presentation of the problem in the patient's words. This is very different from traditional formats. It provides a focus for all diagnostic and therapeutic work that will follow. By beginning from the patient's statement of the problem, a course of action is determined that will include the social, psychological, economic, and physical factors that are involved in the stated complaint of the patient. This means that patients participate in constructing a complete picture of themselves when the problem-oriented approach is used. A traditional format is one in which patients state their complaint and the physician interprets it into medical terminology and attempts to find out the cause of that particular complaint.

The problem-oriented approach starts with patients' expression of their problems stated in their own terms. Each particular problem is titled, given a number, and dated. Every order, every plan, every diagnostic or therapeutic activity that takes place to bring that problem to a conclusion is then coded with the same number and can always be directly linked to that problem. In many ways the POMR reads like a book. The problem list functions as a table of contents that indicates what is contained in the book and identifies titles and page numbers. One can then immediately refer to titled chapters indicated by their page number and read exactly what is indicated by the chapter. At the end of the book an index is cross referenced to all of the ideas or definitions expressed in the book. The POMR, through its problem list, provides a similar format for the patient's record. No other existing medical record format does this.

There are four major parts to the POMR:

1. Data base
2. Problem list
3. Initial plan
4. Progress notes/Discharge summary

Let's look first at the data base. The data base should be predicated on age group and appropriate questions on all systems of the body, as well as such broad categories as social, psychological, and occupational elements. Data bases vary from group to group. The data base on a pediatric patient will be different from that on a young adult female patient. The data base on a 45-year-old man will be different from that on a geriatrics patient. Much of the information gathered in the data base is traditionally known as history and physical information, but the data base of the POMR is far more comprehensive than any traditional format. The data base in the POMR includes information on all problems as stated by the patient, as well as the physician's perception of the problems.

The data base in the POMR is initiated with fact-finding and information-gathering from the patient. Since it uses an ongoing approach that looks at the whole picture rather than one episode of an illness, it includes some of the traditional elements that we have mentioned. Present complaints, present illness, past history, review of systems, family history, and physical examination factors are some of these. In addition, however, it includes what can be called a patient profile, which is an account of how the patient spends his routine day. This patient profile provides the physician with a better understanding of the whole patient in his life situation.

The data base also includes laboratory and other diagnostic findings, such as EEGs, EKGs, x-rays, or lab work. Review of the systems section in the data base may raise questions about illness or treatment for the following systems, conditions, or parts of the body.

- Eye
- Ear
- Nose
- Mouth, throat, larynx
- Teeth
- Skin and/or breast
- Endocrine system
- Respiratory system
- Cardiovascular system
- Gastrointestinal system
- Genitourinary system

- Musculoskeletal system
- Obstetrical condition
- Psychiatric condition
- Gynecology
- Hematology
- Neurology

All of this information, then, is compiled in a data base and used by all members of the health care team in the diagnosis and treatment of the patient.

The problem list is the next section to consider. From the information collected in the data base and the patient's description of problems, the physician or other health care provider pulls together all of the information into a problem list. There are two sources for the problem list: what the patient states as *his or her perception* of the reason for coming to see a health care provider and the health care provider's assessments based on the completed data already described. The problem list then becomes the source that gives direction to all the parties involved in treating the patient. For example, the patient may describe something that disturbs or endangers health, which may be physical, mental, social, or a combination of these. The patient may describe something that doesn't seem to fall into any of those categories, or if it falls into only one of those categories, it does not necessarily seem that other parts of the body and mind are involved. The patient possibly perceives the problem as a simple physical complaint, when the health care provider perceives a complex, multisystem problem.

In a traditional record, if a patient came to the physician's office and reported having had a stomachache for the last two weeks, this would be interpreted by the physician, translated into medical terminology, and documented on the record in words different from those used by the patient. The admitting diagnosis might be gastrointestinal upset or gastritis, or it might rule out gastroenteritis. The diagnosis would be based solely on the patient's complaint of stomach pains for two weeks. It would then be pursued with diagnostic and therapeutic methods focused, in most cases, without exception, on the fact that the patient had stomach complaints.

In the problem-oriented system, however, the methods of both documenting and treating this patient would be quite different. The physician would take the patient's complaint and put it together with the completed data base that includes the details previously described. The physician or other provider would take the patient's initial problem, record it in the same words the patient used, and add other data problems identified in the development of a comprehensive data base. This means that lab work and other diagnostic screening functions will be incorporated in the record and used in identifying problems. In compiling the problem list, no part of the data base should be ignored. The problem list, when carefully titled and numbered, should be the first part of the medical record. It serves as an index to all of the information that is recorded thereafter. Everything else in the record will be recorded according to those titles and numbers in the problem list.

Problems recorded should not be restated in medical terms until enough investigation is carried out to make the problems more precise. The practice of translating patients' complaints or statements of problems into medical terminology or translating them into possible diseases that the physician feels may be the generic cause of the disease is no longer sufficient. A sample problem list for our patient with the stomachache might look like this:

1. Gastric distress
2. History of diarrhea
3. Anxiety about recent job loss
4. Excessive alcohol intake
5. History of cancer of the stomach in the father

In summary, then, the problem is simply an aspect of the patient that disturbs or endangers the patient's health and that requires further attention for diagnosis, treatment, or observation. It can also be something that concerns the physician when the physician has had an opportunity to review all of the information in the data base. The record can include diagnoses, physiological findings, symptoms or physical findings, and results of tests that reveal abnormalities. It should include a complete problem list on the record of the patient who has been treated in a particular facility over a period of time and every problem in the patient's history, past and present. As old problems are resolved, new ones are added, and they are identified accordingly. Each problem is dated, numbered, and titled. It is stated clearly, and there are no guesses or comments that this problem will be ruled out. It is stated at a level of understanding for both the patient and the provider of care. The doctor determines the list of problems based on the information contained in the data base.

In an alternative setting, such as in the Fircrest School for the Developmentally Disabled in Seattle, Washington, the interdisciplinary team reviews the resident's data base and mutually determines the problem list. Exhibit 4-6 is a problem list in this application.

The next part of the POMR is the plan. A complete problem list is the starting point for the doctor. A coordinated plan considers all problems individually, as well as their interactions. Each problem identified by title, date, and number will have a concomitant plan consisting of three parts: the plan for collecting further data, the plan for treatment, and the plan for

Exhibit 4-6 Sample Problem List for a Developmentally Disabled Resident

Date Noted	Problem Number	Problem Title
Adm 4/12/79	1	Head banging to objects; i.e., floor, wall, table, etc.
Adm 4/12/79	2	Hair pulling: — other peoples
Adm 4/12/79	3	Hitting sides of head with fists
Adm 4/12/79	4	Questionable seizure disorder: — abnormal EEG
Adm 4/12/79	5	Inadequate eating skills: — refuses to eat

patient education. The patient will be educated in the nature of the problem and his or her own activities in the management of that problem. The education plan will define the results of the tests and explain to the patient exactly what has taken place and any prognosis that is available. The patient will be told about life-style changes that may have to be made if the patient is to recover fully or live comfortably with a particular problem. With the POMR, the assessment of physicians, nurses, and other health care providers and the explanations of those assessments are recorded for everyone to see. Patients can obtain a copy of the POMR or receive an accurate description of what needs to be done to live a full life regardless of the problem. Look again at the forms sequences in Exhibit 4-4. Can you identify the elements of the POMR?

Exhibit 4-7 illustrates how the plan is applied to the problem. (Exhibit 4-7 is a continuation of the record shown in Exhibit 4-6.)

In conventional records, the patient care plan is primarily centered in the nursing care plan. While many facilities have not retained this form as a permanent part of the record in the past, the need to do so today is clearly recognized. In many cases the nursing care plan documents the overall coordination of care activities while the patient is in the hospital and is used as a basis for formulating discharge plans to carry on the level of care required for improving the health status of the patient.

Exhibits 4-8 and 4-9 are examples of the nursing care plan forms used during hospitalization and the subsequent discharge plan that follows. In conventional record systems, patient care plans and/or nursing care plans should be considered a permanent part of the record and retained accordingly. In POMR systems, the plan would be incorporated as a major component of the system of which nursing elements are a part.

Progress note and discharge summaries are the fourth major part of the POMR. The progress notes include notations by all persons who care for the patient. They are entered in one standard format that is used by all health care providers. It is interesting to note that the nurses now take a far more active role in recording information than they did in the past. This is particularly true in acute general hospitals and even more so in specialty hospitals such as psychiatric or long-term care facilities. Nurses traditionally recorded their information in one separate part of the record. Conventional medical records have never functioned as one-source documents where all health care providers integrated their information about the patient in one place. The SOAP format of the POMR provides the communication link for all members of the health care provider team. S stands for subjective data, and the subjective progress notes include such entries as symptomatic complaints that arise as the patient is treated. These items cannot necessarily be measured or strictly defined and are considered sub-

Exhibit 4-7 Sample Management Plan for a Developmentally Disabled Resident

Date Noted	Problem Number	Problem Title	Management Plan	Start Date	Completed or Stop Date
Adm 4/79	6	Mild spastic quadriplegia	*Asset: Relatively normal range of motion has little affect on ambulation.* — Follow physical therapy plan. — RN will monitor. — Physician to track every 2 months.	4/79	
4/79	7	Questionable conductive hearing	*Asset: Hearing within normal limits in at least one ear.* — Audiology evaluations as determined by audiologist's reports. — Communication Development Department responsible for tracking.	6/79	
4/79	8	Inadequate dressing skills	*Asset: Can remove clothes and cooperates while being dressed.* — See program under Resident Staffing Tab 7/26/79. — Implement by Resident Life staff. — Track quarterly progress.	7/79	

Exhibit 4-8 Sample Nursing Care Plan

PATIENT'S NAME				NICKNAME		AGE	
ADMIT DATE		TIME		MODE	VALUABLES/PROSTHESIS		
VITAL SIGNS: T	P		R	B P	HT	WT	OFC
LAST FLUID, FOOD OR DRUGS				PREVIOUS BLOOD TRANSFUSION			DEX
ALLERGIES				PARENTS/GUARDIANS			
				PHONE			

I. SUBJECTIVE

A. PATIENT PROFILE:

  1. CONCEPT OF CONDITION (LENGTH OF PRESENT PROBLEMS THAT LED TO ADMISSION.)

  2. PAST HOSPITALIZATIONS, SURGERIES, ILLNESSES, CHRONIC AILMENTS, REC. EXPOSURE.

  3. DRUG HISTORY: DRUG, DOSAGE, PURPOSE, HOW LONG?, DRUGS TO HOSPITAL?

B. NURSING ADMISSION EVALUATION:

  1. EENT

         BRUISE

  2. CARDIOVASCULAR (HEART TONES, PULSES, PERFUSION, NECK VEINS, EDEMA, PAIN.)

         CONTUSION

         LACERATION

  3. RESPIRATORY (B.S., RALES, DYSPNEA, RETRACTING, WHEEZING, CROUP, COUGH.) *RASH*

         BREAKDOWN

  4. NEUROLOGICAL (LOC, PUPILS, SPEECH, GAIT, SEIZURES, HEADACHE, SYNCOPE, REFLEXES.)

         MOLDING

         FORCEP MARKS

  5. GI/ABDOMEN (N/V, DIARRHEA, DISTENSION, ANOREXIA, PAIN, CONSTIPATION.)

  6. GU (MENSES, DISCHARGES, APPLIANCES.)

  7. SKIN (COLOR, TURGOR, LESIONS, ITCHING.)

  8. MUSCULOSKETETAL (DEFORMITIES, HANDICAPS, SWELLING, PAIN, STIFFNESS.)

  9. BEHAVIOR

THE CHILDREN'S ORTHOPEDIC HOSPITAL AND MEDICAL CENTER SEATTLE, WASHINGTON 90105	PATIENT
NURSING ADMISSION ASSESSMENT	

Exhibit 4-8 Continued

C. SOCIAL HISTORY (LIVING SITUTATION, HOME, MOM?, DAD?, NUMBER OF SIBLINGS.)

_____

_____

_____

_____

_____

D. DIETARY NEEDS: TYPE OF DIET: (STRAINED, CHOPPED, TABLE, FORMULA)

_____

FAVORITE SNACKS _____

SCHEDULE _____

BOTTLE_____ CUP_____ SPOON_____ FORK_____

FEEDS SELF_____ NEEDS HELP_____ SWALLOWS PILLS_____

E. ELIMINATION NEEDS: DIAPER: DAY_____ NIGHT_____ TOILET TRAINED_____

EXPRESSION OF TOILET NEEDS _____

F. SLEEP HABITS: NAPS_____ BEDTIME_____ BEDTIME RITUALS_____

FAVORITE TOY OR BLANKET_____

G. SPIRITUAL NEEDS: RELIGION_____

BAPTIZE, IN EMERGENCY? _____

H. SPECIAL NEEDS_____

_____

_____

_____

_____

_____

_____

_____

_____

II. OBJECTIVE

A. SEE VITAL SIGN AREA.

B. OTHER: E.G. X–RAYS, LAB WORK, PROCEDURES PRIOR TO ADMISSION.

_____

_____

_____

_____

III. ASSESSMENT_____

_____

_____

_____

IV. PLAN (MEASURES TO RX. NURSING PROBS., SPECIAL TEACHING NEEDS, ETC.)

_____

_____

_____

_____

_____

ORIENTATION TO UNIT_____ SIGNATURE_____ R.N.

Exhibit 4-8 Continued
Patient Flow Sheet

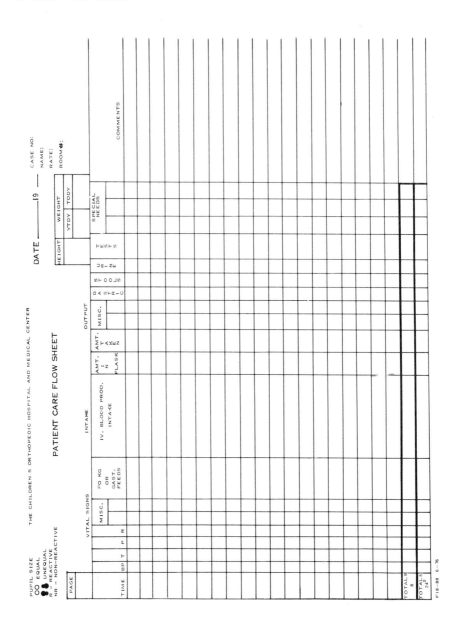

Exhibit 4-9 Sample Discharge Plan

FORM SO-222A REV. 11-76 COAST 11-76

DISCHARGE ORDER SHEET   DISCHARGE DATE

DISCHARGE DIAGNOSES AND/OR PROBLEMS

PRIMARY

1. OTHER

2.

3.

4.

5.

OPERATIONS

DIET INSTRUCTIONS, IF ANY:

DIETITIAN TO INSTRUCT: ☐ BEFORE DISCHARGE ☐ RETURN OFFICE APPOINTMENT | INSTRUCTION GIVEN: YES ☐ NO ☐

OTHER INSTRUCTIONS TO PATIENT:

PLANS FOR FOLLOW-UP CARE

1. CLINIC

2. REFERRING M.D.

3. OTHER

CHART TO DR.   OFFICE FOLLOWING DISCHARGE YES ☐ NO ☐

SUMMARY DICTATED YES NO INITIALS   DATE   PHARMACY TO FILL | PATIENT HAS OWN

MEDICATIONS   DATE
PLEASE LIST STRENGTH, NUMBER, SIG.

PATIENT   1ST LETTER   LAST NAME

APPROXIMATE DISCHARGE TIME: AM PM   OTHER

CODE	CHARGE	CHARGE
430 060 940 PP	1 4	2 5	3 6

ANOTHER BRAND OF DRUG IDENTICAL IN FORM AND CONTENT MAY BE DISPENSED UNLESS CHECKED ☐

Signature: Resident/Intern   Controlled Substance Number (BNDD)   Attending Physician   Controlled Substance Number (BNDD)

jective. Objective data (O) are those progress notes that are observable and measurable—such entries as laboratory findings, color of skin, results of tests, blood pressure, pulse rate, and any other observable activity determined by a health care provider. Assessment (A) is simply a statement of what is currently going on with that patient. It is an account of the severity of the illness, any changes or conclusions to be drawn about diagnoses, prognosis, or change in the patient's description of the problems. The plan (P) specifies action to be taken on the basis of that assessment. It can be a short-range plan, a diagnostic plan, a patient-education plan, or a long-range plan. Notice the example of the SOAP progress notes in Exhibit 4-10.

Another key element in the POMR system that is also used in conventional medical records is flow sheets. Consider a patient who has hypertension. Many variables have to be followed carefully at the same time. These items can be mapped out on a flow sheet so that the doctor and other care providers can view these variables together at any point in time. Flow sheets are useful in a wide variety of applications. Exhibits 4-11 through 4-13 are examples. Exhibit 4-11 is a prenatal physical examination record in a flow sheet format. Exhibit 4-12 is an example of a special care flow sheet, which is a general-purpose flow sheet that can be used whenever a patient requires monitoring at a special-care level. Postoperative patients would be an example. Exhibit 4-13 is an excellent illustration of the principles of flow sheets as they are applied to nursing care records in a conventional record system. The ability to view various items of information at specific time intervals, which facilitates efficient use of patient data, should be a primary goal for designers of medical record systems.

The POMR provides a logical, ordered, structured, and sequenced report of the patient's state of health and treatment. It is a logical step-by-step system that views a patient as an entity by systematically solving each problem and recording that problem in a logical sequence. There are many advantages to the POMR.

- It requires the health care provider to consider all problems of the patient.
- It requires providers to treat each problem individually and consider their interrelationships in the whole picture.
- The decision pathway and logical structure used by doctors in defining and handling each problem should be clear and easily read, followed, and evaluated.
- From the information provided in the problem-oriented format, members of the health care team can pick up a medical record of a patient they have never seen, assess what has happened, and proceed in a logical direction.

Exhibit 4-10 Sample SOAP Progress Notes

EXAMPLE 1

PROGRESS NOTES

NAME: 38-year-old executive

OFFICE VISIT: May 2, 1979

#1   EPIGASTRIC DISTRESS
   Subjective data:
      Has had only one episode of "hungry sensation" since last visit, one
      month ago. No success in decreasing smoking; if anything, it has
      increased. Has decreased coffee intake to five to six cups a week.
      Continues to drink two beers a day, eats two square meals a day but
      has succeeded in adding a midafternoon feeding of whole milk.
   PLAN:
      For more information:
         No change from outline under Initial Plan under Problem #1.
      For therapy:
         To see nurse practitioner on next visit one month from now.

#2   HISTORY OF INTERMITTENT LIQUID STOOLS
   Subjective data:
      No diarrhea whatever during past interval.

#3   OVERWEIGHT
   Subjective data:
      No effort at caloric restriction or regular exercise; in fact, extra
      meals have involved the use of whole rather than skimmed milk and
      beer intake has not significantly decreased overall calories.
   PLAN:
      For therapy:
         Use skimmed milk for between-meal feedings; attempt again to
         reduce regular beer intake.

#4   FAMILY HISTORY OF LUNG CANCER

#5   EXCESSIVE SMOKING
   PLAN:
      For more information:
         Screening chest x-ray today per patient's request. WNL CT 14/36

Exhibit 4-11 Prenatal Physical Exam Record

(PATIENT ID STAMPED HERE)	PRENATAL PHYSICAL EXAM, LAB. DATA, EDUCATION RECORD		DATE OF EXAM	
	PULSE	BLOOD PRESSURE	USUAL WEIGHT	
	HEIGHT	CURRENT WEIGHT	PREFERRED WEIGHT	

PHYSICAL EXAMINATION	Check if normal	Describe if abnormal
Nutritional status		
Skin		
Eyes, vision, fundi		
Ears, nose, throat		
Mouth, teeth, gums		
Neck, thyroid		
Breasts		
Heart		
Lungs		
Abdomen		
Extremities; veins		
edema		
reflexes		
Vulva, perineum		
Vagina,		
Cervix		
Fundus		
Adnexae		
Rectum		

PELVIC MEASUREMENTS		ASSESSMENT OF PELVIS	
Diag. conj.	Post. sag. diam.	Adequate	☐
Arch	Shape sacrum	Borderline	☐
Ischial spines	SS notch	Inadequate	☐
IT diam.	Coccyx		

LABORATORY EXAMINATIONS

REQUIRED TESTS	DATE	RESULT	SUGGESTED TESTS	DATE	RESULT
Blood type & Rh: patient			Rh & other antibodies		
baby's father					
Hemoglobin/hematocrit					
at 36 weeks			Rubella titer		
			Sickle cell screen		
Urinalysis micro:			Urine culture		
Pap smear					
Gonorrhea culture			Tuberculin test		
Serology					

PATIENT EDUCATION	Date initiated	By whom	Comments
Breast feeding & breast care			
Hygiene in pregnancy			
Nutrition in pregnancy (WIC?)			
Anesthesia & analgesia			
Labor & delivery			
Family planning			

INITIAL ASSESSMENT, PROBLEMS	DELIVERY PLAN	OTHER PLANS, ORDERS

Signature of examiner

HSA-358-5 (9-77)

Exhibit 4-12 Special Care Flow Sheet

VIRGINIA MASON HOSPITAL

SPECIAL CARE

NAME_____

WT____

DATE_____
HOUR_____
NURSE_____

VITAL SIGNS							FLUID BALANCE							REMARKS	LAB VALUES
Time	BP	P	CVP	Temp	R	Pupils R	L	Response	Blood Loss	Blood Given	Plasma Given	IV	R	Oral Intake	Urine Output	Gastric Output		

8 hr

24 hrs

RESPONSE GRADING SYSTEM
4+ Normal: Requires no arousal.
3+ Rouses to alertness c̄ minimal stimulation
2+ Needs greater stimulation and/or does not ... full alertness.
1+ Deep coma or only reflex activity.

Form #3a Rev 2 75

Exhibit 4-13 Nursing Summary Sheet

VIRGINIA MASON HOSPITAL
SEATTLE

NURSING SUMMARY SHEET

Date _____

PUPILS

Equality

(Rt) (Left)

o – o = Equal

o < ◯ = Unequal

Reaction:

(+) Reacts

(−) Does not react

Example: (+) < (−)

(Left does not react
and is larger)

RESPONSE GRADING SYSTEM

4+   Normal: Requires no arousal.

3+   Rouses to alertness c minimal stimulation

2+   Needs greater stimulation and/or does
not reach full alertness.

1+   Deep coma or only reflex activity.

MISCELLANEOUS

Expansion and qualification of
response grading.

Fluids

Hourly urines

Medications as applicable

Etc.

DATE	HOUR	CONSCIOUSNESS	PUPILS		LYING BP	STANDING BP	LYING P.	STNDG P.	R	TEMP	MISCELLANEOUS
			RIGHT	LEFT							

Purpose: 1. Neurological Nursing Summary
2. Frequent B.P. and P. Record
3. Supine and Standing B.P.
4. Vital signs post surgery.

The POMR is particularly valuable in a teaching hospital. Here, many students are involved in the day-to-day care of the patient in the absence of professors or attending physicians who only make one visit a day to the institution. It is extremely important for nurses who provide round-the-clock treatment to patients. The POMR is of ultimate importance to all health care providers because its format is the only one that provides an information link between those who will use the document to learn exactly what is going on with that patient.

Another advantage of the POMR is its use as an accessible document for peer review, patient care appraisal, audit, and even new physicians taking over in the middle of a case. The POMR, as has been pointed out, does include a table of contents known as the problem list. It is numbered, dated, titled, and is used to index the treatment and conclusions so that each problem can be followed individually and easily. The POMR enhances continuing education for all persons involved in a patient's care.

As in any system, there are some disadvantages to the POMR. Because of the logical sequence and structure of the notes, it may be more easily reviewed by such outsiders as insurance agents, insurance reviewers, and attorneys. A similar problem lies with confidentiality in that there is almost too much information present in a POMR, at least from the point of view of readability. POMRs contain more information, which is a confidentiality problem, and require the copying of more pages, which is a cost problem. This is usually solved by summarizing records rather than sending out copies. Unresolved problems may be interpreted by outside reviewers incorrectly and prevent payment by some insurance companies. Let's take a look at an assessment of the POMR by J. Willis Hurst, M.D. He points out that there are ten reasons why Lawrence Weed is right about POMR.[2]

1. He has devised a medical-record system that encourages the student, house officer, and practicing physician to use sound logic in his thoughts about patients. In this sense, his system is the essence of education itself.
2. The display system that he has created for medical data enables one to use the record as efficiently as one uses a dictionary.
3. He has devised a medical record system that allows physicians to communicate their thoughts to nurses and other personnel who are assisting in the immediate care of the patient. This makes it possible for the physician to be the director of the health care team involved in the care of the patient.
4. He has designed a medical record system that enhances the continuing education of physicians and all who assist in the care of patients.
5. The logic system and display of it prepare the student and physician

for the computer world. The system teaches those who use the computer how it can help us.

6. Group practices are increasing daily. The medical record will be the common bond between several doctors and a patient. If the medical record is of poor quality, or if the data cannot be found quickly, the group may be inefficient and could, after much effort, deliver less than the best medical care. Weed's system will improve the medical care given by a group.

7. Certain types of clinical investigation require excellent records. Weed's system of recordkeeping will improve patient care by making more accurate clinical research possible.

8. The attendant on a teaching service has, in years past, felt compelled to give an irrelevant lecture during ward rounds. Now—with Weed's display system—lectures on ward rounds will be eliminated. The Weed system makes it possible for the attendant to not only check a patient's medical problems, but also check the student's and house officer's ability to collect and interpret data, to develop a proper plan of treatment, and to observe patients properly. Ward rounds can become patient rounds and not lecture rounds.

9. The traditional method of presenting the patient's medical history, the results of the physical examination and laboratory data, has run its course. The Weed system encourages a more meaningful way of communicating information about patients.

10. Patient care is improved directly or indirectly by each of these nine reasons. This is the goal of all our efforts.

Included in Dr. Hurst's comments on the POMR is that it was designed to facilitate computer development, which is taking place rapidly. Since the late 1950s, when the POMR was first presented, individual physicians and groups of physicians, as well as hospitals, have applied computerization of the POMRs. The following are reasons why the POMR is so compatible with computers.

1. Data are standardized in such areas as the problem list, the data base, and the SOAP progress notes.

2. Information is organized in a uniform manner.

3. The POMR, particularly in the SOAP progress notes and the problem list, provides conciseness.

4. The POMR directs immediate providers; that is, members of the health care team are given directions through the communication provided by the POMR.

5. Through the problem list and the SOAP progress notes, data are far more easily computer coded for storage and retrieval than traditional elements.
6. The POMR leads to new sets of data that were never available before, and these are also computer compatible.
7. Data elements of the POMR are computer compatible particularly in the area of medical auditing.
8. The POMR limits duplications that, at the outset of establishing a computer system, provides conciseness and singularity of data entry.

There are two other kinds of records that need to be considered. One is the source-oriented record. This type of record is formatted by sectioning groups together based on the source of the data entries. For instance, all lab work is grouped together, all forms for x-rays, all nursing forms, and most physician-entered data are grouped together in one part of the record.

The other major type is the chronological format record. All data entries are kept in chronological form and therefore the different forms are integrated throughout the record. Since it is strictly a chronological listing, the most current data entries and their forms are on top of the record.

Earlier in the chapter we discussed sequence of forms within individual patient records. One difference between the problem-oriented and source-oriented record is the content and organization of the data entries, not the sequence of the data entries or forms within the record. A unique feature of the POMR is that it reflects a philosophy of patient care that, unlike traditional delivery, focuses on patient education. To become a cooperative and assertive participant in achieving optimal health, patients need to understand fully their problems and the appropriate plans established to resolve them. The POMR pulls together subjective and objective data from all sources within the record in the assessment of particular problems and construction of plans to resolve them. Assessments and plans are not found in source or chronological records. Physicians' orders and progress notes most closely approximate these elements but lack the judgmental specificity required in the assessment and plan of the POMR.

Appendix 4A features a variety of patient record forms found in health care delivery today. In Appendix 4B we have included the screen display formats from the PROMIS system to illustrate how computerization can affect forms and formats of patient records.

Forms and formats are and will continue to be the primary means of communication for and about patients. Particular health care settings will need to select those forms and formats that are the most appropriate from all of the tools available. Health information managers will need to draw on existing resources and design new resources as the various kinds of health care delivery systems continue to evolve. Organization of information will remain the primary goal.

NOTES

1. Wilmer O. Maekle, Mary F. Robek, and Gerald F. Brown, *Information & Records Management* (Beverly Hills & London: Glencoe Press, 1974), pp. 4-13.
2. J. Willis Hurst, M.D., *The Problem-Oriented System* (New York: Medcom Learning Systems, 1972).

Appendix 4A

Typical Patient Record Forms

THE MASON CLINIC
1100 Ninth Avenue - P. O. Box 900
Seattle, Washington 98111

ADVANCE PATIENT REGISTRATION

OFFICE APPOINTMENT DATE _____ TIME _____ PHYSICIAN _____

TO OUR PATIENTS: We will be able to save you time by preparing your medical record in advance of your arrival if you will complete this form and return it in the envelope provided. If you have questions about your appointment please call our New Appointment Desk, 223-6881.

Patient's Last Name	First	Middle	Social Security Number	Spouse's First Name
				Occupation

Address	Number	Street	City	State	Zip Code

Home Phone	Occupation	Business Phone	Former Mason Clinic Patient?
			Yes _____ No _____

Birth Date	Month	Day	Year	Marital Status
				Single _____ Widowed _____
Age	Birthplace			Divorced _____ Married _____ Separated _____

Local Address (If Known)	Local Phone

Name of Nearest Relative or Friend Other Than Spouse	Relationship

Address	Phone

Name of Person Responsible for Payment of Account	Relationship

Address	Number	Street	City	State	Zip Code	Phone

Occupation	Employer

Insurance Company Name and Address	Number	Street	City	State	Zip Code	Policy No.
						Group
						Individual

If your Insurance Company issues a Medical Card, please bring it with you.

Did a Physician or an Agency ask that you be seen at the Mason Clinic?	If by a Physician, His Name and Address

PLEASE RETURN IN THE ENCLOSED STAMPED ENVELOPE.

5h-141 Rev. 1-77

THE CHILDREN'S ORTHOPEDIC HOSPITAL AND MEDICAL CENTER

PATIENT CARE FLOW SHEET

DATE _____ 19 ___

CASE NO:
NAME:
RATE:
ROOM #:

HEIGHT   WEIGHT
   YTDY   TODY

PUPIL SIZE
OO EQUAL
●● UNEQUAL
R — REACTIVE
NR — NON-REACTIVE

PAGE

VITAL SIGNS
TIME   BP   T   P   R

INTAKE
MISC.   PO KG OR GAST. FEEDS   IV, BLOOD PROD. INTAKE   AMT. IN FLASK   AMT. TAKEN

OUTPUT
MISC.   GASTRIC   STOOLS   URINE   TESTS

SPECIAL NEEDS

COMMENTS

TOTALS 8
TOTALS 24°

F18-88 6-76

FORM SO-222A REV. 11-76 COAST 11-76

DISCHARGE ORDER SHEET

DISCHARGE DATE

DISCHARGE DIAGNOSES AND/OR PROBLEMS

PRIMARY

1. OTHER

2.

3.

4.

5.

OPERATIONS

DIET INSTRUCTIONS, IF ANY:

DIETITIAN TO INSTRUCT: ☐ BEFORE DISCHARGE   ☐ RETURN OFFICE APPOINTMENT   INSTRUCTION GIVEN: YES ☐ NO ☐

OTHER INSTRUCTIONS TO PATIENT:

PLANS FOR FOLLOW-UP CARE

1. CLINIC

2. REFERRING M.D.

3. OTHER

CHART TO DR.   OFFICE FOLLOWING DISCHARGE YES ☐ NO ☐

SUMMARY DICTATED	YES	NO	INITIALS	DATE	PHARMACY TO FILL	PATIENT HAS OWN

MEDICATIONS
PLEASE LIST STRENGTH, NUMBER, SIG.

DATE

PATIENT

1ST LETTER

LAST NAME

APPROXIMATE DISCHARGE TIME:

_____ AM PM

OTHER

CODE	CHARGE		CHARGE
430 060 940 PP	1	4	
	2	5	
	3	6	

ANOTHER BRAND OF DRUG IDENTICAL IN FORM AND CONTENT MAY BE DISPENSED UNLESS CHECKED ☐

Signature: Resident/Intern | Controlled Substance Number (BNDD) | Attending Physician | Controlled Substance Number (BNDD) |

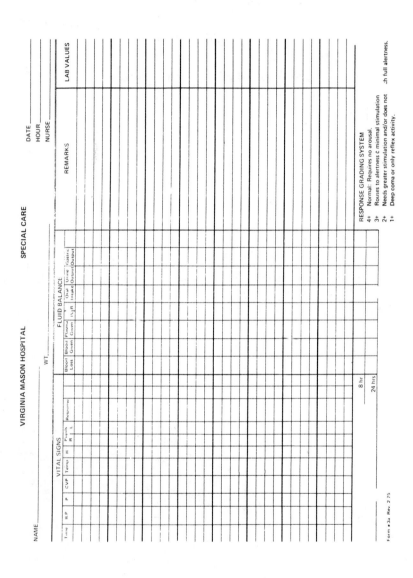

VIRGINIA MASON HOSPITAL   SPECIAL CARE

NAME_____   WT_____

DATE_____
HOUR_____
NURSE_____

RESPONSE GRADING SYSTEM
4+ Normal: Requires no arousal.
3+ Rouses to alertness c̄ minimal stimulation.
2+ Needs greater stimulation and/or does not
1+ Deep coma or only reflex activity.

...h full alertness.

Form # 34 Rev. 2/75

VIRGINIA MASON HOSPITAL
OBSTETRICAL RECOVERY RECORD

DATE _____   ROOM NO. _____

TIME	PULSE	BLOOD PRESSURE	FUNDUS	LOCHIA	COMMENTS - MEDICATIONS

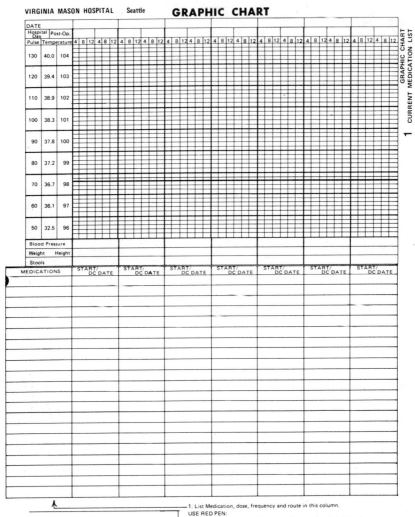

VIRGINIA MASON HOSPITAL   Seattle   **GRAPHIC CHART**

1. List Medication, dose, frequency and route in this column.
USE RED PEN:
2. Write "Start" in Start /DC Column on Start date for scheduled meds.
3. Write "Pre-op" in Start/DC Column in case of Pre-op med.
4. Write "1x" in Start/DC Column for all other 1x doses.
5. Write "DC & Time" in Start/DC Column on DC date.

FM—0001 · Rev. 6/76

PATIENT'S NAME			NICKNAME		AGE	
ADMIT DATE		TIME	MODE	VALUABLES/PROSTHESIS		
VITAL SIGNS: T	P	R	B P	HT	WT	OFC
LAST FLUID, FOOD OR DRUGS			PREVIOUS BLOOD TRANSFUSION		DEX	
ALLERGIES			PARENTS/GUARDIANS			
			PHONE			

I. SUBJECTIVE

A. PATIENT PROFILE:

   1. CONCEPT OF CONDITION (LENGTH OF PRESENT PROBLEMS THAT LED TO ADMISSION.)

   2. PAST HOSPITALIZATIONS, SURGERIES, ILLNESSES, CHRONIC AILMENTS. REC. EXPOSURE.

   3. DRUG HISTORY: DRUG, DOSAGE, PURPOSE, HOW LONG?, DRUGS TO HOSPITAL?

B. NURSING ADMISSION EVALUATION:

   1. EENT

   2. CARDIOVASCULAR (HEART TONES, PULSES, PERFUSION, NECK VEINS, EDEMA, PAIN.)

   3. RESPIRATORY (B.S., RALES, DYSPNEA, RETRACTING, WHEEZING, CROUP, COUGH.)

   4. NEUROLOGICAL (LOC, PUPILS, SPEECH, GAIT, SEIZURES, HEADACHE, SYNCOPE, REFLEXES.)

   5. GI/ABDOMEN (N/V, DIARRHEA, DISTENSION, ANOREXIA, PAIN, CONSTIPATION.)

   6. GU (MENSES, DISCHARGES, APPLIANCES.)

   7. SKIN (COLOR, TURGOR, LESIONS, ITCHING.)

   8. MUSCULOSKETETAL (DEFORMITIES, HANDICAPS, SWELLING, PAIN, STIFFNESS.)

   9. BEHAVIOR

BRUISE

CONTUSION

LACERATION

RASH

BREAKDOWN

MOLDING

FORCEP MARKS

THE CHILDREN'S ORTHOPEDIC HOSPITAL
AND MEDICAL CENTER
SEATTLE, WASHINGTON 90105

PATIENT

NURSING ADMISSION ASSESSMENT

F18–4.1 1–78

C.   SOCIAL HISTORY   (LIVING SITUTATION, HOME, MOM?, DAD?, NUMBER OF SIBLINGS.)
_____
_____
_____
_____
_____

D.   DIETARY NEEDS: TYPE OF DIET: (STRAINED, CHOPPED, TABLE, FORMULA)
_____

FAVORITE SNACKS _____
SCHEDULE _____
BOTTLE_____ CUP_____ SPOON_____ FORK_____
FEEDS SELF_____ NEEDS HELP_____ SWALLOWS PILLS_____

E.   ELIMINATION NEEDS: DIAPER: DAY_____ NIGHT_____ TOILET TRAINED_____
EXPRESSION OF TOILET NEEDS _____
F.   SLEEP HABITS: NAPS_____ BEDTIME_____ BEDTIME RITUALS_____
FAVORITE TOY OR BLANKET_____
G.   SPIRITUAL NEEDS: RELIGION_____
BAPTIZE, IN EMERGENCY?_____
H.   SPECIAL NEEDS_____
_____
_____
_____
_____
_____
_____
_____
_____

II. OBJECTIVE

A.   SEE VITAL SIGN AREA.
B.   OTHER: E.G. X–RAYS, LAB WORK, PROCEDURES PRIOR TO ADMISSION.
_____
_____
_____
_____

III. ASSESSMENT_____
_____
_____
_____

IV. PLAN (MEASURES TO RX. NURSING PROBS., SPECIAL TEACHING NEEDS, ETC.)
_____
_____
_____
_____
_____

ORIENTATION TO UNIT_____ SIGNATURE_____ R.N.

VIRGINIA MASON HOSPITAL
SEATTLE

NURSING SUMMARY SHEET

Date _____

PUPILS

Equality
(Rt) (Left)
o - o = Equal
o < ◯ = Unequal
Reaction:
(+) Reacts
(−) Does not react
Example: (+) < (−)
(Left does not react
and is larger)

RESPONSE GRADING SYSTEM
4+ Normal: Requires no arousal.
3+ Rouses to alertness c̄ minimal stimulation
2+ Needs greater stimulation and/or does
    not reach full alertness.
1+ Deep coma or only reflex activity.

MISCELLANEOUS
Expansion and qualification of
response grading.
Fluids
Hourly urines
Medications as applicable
Etc.

DATE	HOUR	CONSCIOUSNESS	PUPILS		LYING BP	STANDING BP	LYING P	STNDG P	R	TEMP	MISCELLANEOUS
			RIGHT	LEFT							

Purpose:　1. Neurological Nursing Summary
　　　　　　2. Frequent B.P. and P. Record
　　　　　　3. Supine and Standing B.P.
　　　　　　4. Vital signs post surgery.

PARENTERAL/ENTERAL NUTRITION PROFILE

DATE

BOTTLE NUMBER

SOLUTIONS / ADDITIVES	REVENUE CODE	SERV. CODE	TOTAL UNITS	UNIT PRICE	TOTAL PRICE
D-25 Amino Acids 4.25%	377-070	0001	BTL	21.00	
D-20 Amino Acids 4.25%	377-070	0001	BTL	21.00	
D-10 Amino Acids 4.25%	377-070	0001	BTL	21.00	
	377-070	0002	BTL		
	377-070	0002	BTL		
Vivonex	377-070	0003	BTL	10.50	
Vivonex HN	377-070	0003	BTL	13.70	
INTRALIPID 10%	377-070	0004	BTL	34.50	
NaCl (meq)	430-010	0300		3.00	
KCl (meq)	430-010	0300		3.00	
K Phosphate (meq)	430-010	0300		3.00	
K Acetate (meq)	430-010	0300		3.00	
Na Acetate (meq)	430-010	0300		3.00	
Ca Gluconate (meq)	430-010	0300		3.00	
Mg SO4 (meq)	430-010	0300		3.00	
Regular Insulin (units)	430-010	0300		3.00	
VIT B & C (ml)	430-010	0300		3.00	
MVI CONC (ml)	430-010	0300		3.75	
	430-010				
	430-010				
	430-010				

SOLUTIONS / ADDITIVES

TIME TO RUN

START TIME

END TIME

RECORDED BY

COMMENTS:

FIRST LETTER
LAST NAME

BOTTLE UNIT CODE:
1000 cc = 1
500 cc = .5
250 cc = .25
Other Vol. Specify

VIRGINIA MASON HOSPITAL PHARMACY

FM. 0527 Rev. 11-78

NO.	PROBLEM	DATES								
1.	HEALTH MAINTENANCE									

SPECIAL NOTES (DRUG ALLERGY ETC.)

THE CHILDREN'S ORTHOPEDIC HOSPITAL
AND MEDICAL CENTER
SEATTLE, WASH.   98105

CASE NO.

NAME

MASTER PROBLEM LIST
F-18-100 REV. 1-77

BIRTHDATE

CHECK (✔)

YES (Y), NO (N), NOT ASKED (NA)

COMMENTS

PREVIOUS MEDICAL PROBLEMS

	Y	N	NA
HOSPITALIZATIONS			
SURGERY			
MAJOR ILLS OR TRAUMA			
LONG TERM MEDICATION			
ALLERGIES			
MEDICATION REACTIONS			
BLEEDING			
OTHER MD/ CLINICS			

REVIEW OF SYSTEMS

	Y	N	NA
UNEXPLAIN FEVERS			
WEIGHT LOSS			
RASHES			
HEADACHE			
EAR / EYE PROBLEMS			
DENTAL PROBLEMS			
CHRONIC URI			
COUGH, WHEEZING			
FEED, DIET PROBLEMS			
ABD, PAIN			
VOMIT, DIARRHEA, CONSTIP.			
UTI, DYSURIA, ENURESIS			
JT. PAIN, SWELLING			
SEIZURES			
MENSES, SEXUAL ACTIVE			
BEHAVIOR, SCHOOL PROBLEMS			
OTHER			

BIRTH DEVELOPMENT

BIRTH WT. _____ LENGTH _____
NEONATAL PROBLEMS?

FEED   BREAST____BOTTLE ____
MATERNAL AGE AT BIRTH _____
PATERNAL AGE AT BIRTH _____
GRAVIDA _____ PARA _____ AB _____

LENGTH GESTATION _____
COMPLICATIONS OF PREG DELIV.?

MOTOR   SAT_____ WALK _____

LANGUAGE   WORDS____SENTENCES_____

SCHOOL _____

GRADE _____ SPECIAL CLASS? _____
PEER RELATIONS?
DPT _____   _____   _____   _____
OPV _____   _____   _____   _____
MMR _____TINE PPD_____
OTHER_____

THE CHILDREN'S ORTHOPEDIC HOSPITAL
AND MEDICAL CENTER

SEATTLE, WASHINGTON 98105

MASTER DATA BASE

F 18-123 1-1 2-79

CASE NO.

NAME

B. DATE

CHECK (✓)

YES (Y), NO (N), NOT ASKED (NA)

FAMILY PEDIGREE AND COMMENTS

FAMILY HISTORY	Y	N	NA
ALLERGIES / ASTHMA			
SEIZURES (EPILEPSY)			
HEART DISEASE / BP			
EARLY MI-CVA			
CANCER			
DIABETES MELLITUS			
RHEUMATOID ARTHRITIS			
MENTAL RETARDATION			
ALCOHOLISM			
PSYCHIATRIC PROBS			
OTHER			
RACE			

SOCIAL HISTORY

MOTHER: IN HOME____(BIRTHPLACE_____) EDUCATION _____ JOB _____

FATHER: IN HOME____(BIRTHPLACE_____) EDUCATION _____ JOB _____

(NOTE PARENTS' MARITAL STATUS, FAMILY PROBLEMS OR STRENGTHS, OTHERS INVOLVED IN CHILD'S CARE OR AVAILABLE IN CRISIS.)

DATE_____COMPLETED BY_____

MD:

THE CHILDREN'S ORTHOPEDIC HOSPITAL
AND MEDICAL CENTER
SEATTLE. WASHINGTON 98105

THE MASON CLINIC

REPORT OF FOOD ALLERGY TEST

DATE						DOCTOR		
PATIENT NAME			AGE		SEX	CLINIC NUMBER		
FOOD	S	I	FOOD	S	I	SCREENING FOODS	S	I
1. BANANA			16. PEANUT			1. CHOCOLATE		
2. BEEF			17. PECAN			2. EGG		
3. CHEESE, AMERICAN			18. PORK			3. MILK		
4. CHEESE, SWISS			19. RICE			4. ORANGE		
5. CHICKEN			20. SALMON			5. PEANUT		
6. CHOCOLATE			21. SHRIMP			6. SOY BEAN		
7. CLAMS			22. SOY BEAN			7. WHEAT		
8. COFFEE			23. STRAWBERRY					
9. CORN			24. TEA					
10. CRAB			25. TOMATO			CONTROL		
11. EGG			26. WALNUT, BLACK			HISTAMINE		
12. LAMB			27. WATERMELON			MISCELLANEOUS		
13. MILK			28. WHEAT					
14. MUSKMELON MIX			29. YEAST, BAKER'S					
15. ORANGE			30. YEAST, BREWER'S					

5e804 Rev. 2 77

CHECK (✓) NORMAL (NL), ABNORMAL (AB), NOT EXAMINED (NE)

DATE_____ HT.____ (__%/__) WT.____ (__%/__) OFC___ (__%/__) T__P__R__BP___

PHYSICAL EXAM		NL	AB	NE	COMMENTS — DESCRIBE ABNORMALITIES
SKIN	TURGER				
	CYANOSIS				
	RASH / LESIONS				
HEAD	FONTANELLES				
	SYMMETRY				
	TRANSILLUMINATION				
EYE	ACUITY				
	CONJUNCTIVA				
	EOM				
	PUPILS				
	RED REFLEX				
	PLACEMENT / SIZE				
EARS	HEARING				
	TM				
NOSE					
MOUTH	MUCOSA				
	TEETH				
	PALATE				
PHARYNX					
NODES					
THYROID					
CHEST	SYMMETRY				
	LUNGS				
	BREASTS				
HEART	RHYTHM				
	HEART SOUNDS				
	MURMUR				
	VENOUS HUM				
	PULSES				
ABDOM	BOWEL SOUNDS				
	LIVER				
	SPLEEN				
	MASSES				
	KIDNEYS				
	RECTUM				
	TENDERNESS				
GENIT.	INTROI/TEST / PENIS				
	SEXUAL DEVELOP				
	HERNIA / HYDRO				
BACK					
EXTREM					
NEURO	MENTAL STATUS				
	CRAINAL NERVES				
	CEREBELLAR				
	SENSATION				
	COORDINATION				
	STRENGTH / TONE				
	INVOLUNTRY MOVT				
	PRIMITIVE RFLXS				
	DTR				
	BABINSKI				

THE CHILDREN'S ORTHOPEDIC HOSPITAL
AND MEDICAL CENTER
SEATTLE, WASHINGTON 98105

PHYSICAL EXAMINATION

CASE NO.

NAME

B. DATE

Please Use Imprinter:

PROBLEM/ASSET/PLAN LIST

Individual Program Plan (IPP) Objectives of _____
(Date of most recent IPP)

I. _____ V. _____

II. _____ VI. _____

III. _____ VII. _____

IV. _____ VIII. _____

Date Noted	Prob. No.	Problem Title	Assets/Management Plan	Start Date	Stop Date

FS 26-52 (Rev. 1/78)

Please Use Imprinter:

PROBLEM/ASSET/PLAN LIST

Individual Program Plan (IPP) Objectives of _____
(Date of most recent IPP)

I. _____ V. _____

II. _____ VI. _____

III. _____ VII. _____

IV. _____ VIII. _____

Date Noted	Prob. No.	Problem Title	*Assets*/Management Plan	Start Date	Stop Date

FS 26-52 (Rev. 1/78)

PATIENT ID STAMPED HERE	PEDIATRIC INITIAL HISTORY		DATE	
	DATE OF BIRTH	CITY	HOSPITAL	
	AGE AT TIME OF THIS HISTORY		GRADE IN SCHOOL IF SCHOOL AGE	

MATERNAL AND BIRTH HISTORY

# PREGNANCIES	LIVE BIRTHS	SPONT. ABS.	INDUCED ABS.	WAS THIS PREGNANCY NORMAL? ☐ YES ☐ NO	LENGTH OF THIS PREGNANCY	MO. PRENATAL CARE BEGAN

ILLNESSES DURING THIS PREGNANCY (DESCRIBE EACH ONE CHECKED)
- ☐ ANEMIA
- ☐ BLEEDING
- ☐ DIABETES
- ☐ HYPERTENSION
- ☐ KIDNEY DISEASE
- ☐ RUBELLA
- ☐ DRUG ABUSE (TYPE) _____
- ☐ OTHER

LENGTH OF LABOR (HOURS)

BIRTH WEIGHT   LBS.   OZ.

DELIVERY ☐ VAG. ☐ C-SECT

FORCEPS USED? ☐ YES ☐ NO

PRESENTATION ☐ VTX ☐ BREECH

HEALTHY NEWBORN ☐ YES ☐ NO

PROBLEMS AT BIRTH (DESCRIBE)
- ☐ COLOR
- ☐ BREATHING
- ☐ MECONIUM STAINING
- ☐ DEFORMITY
- ☐ OTHER

PROBLEMS IN FIRST WEEK (DESCRIBE)
- ☐ FEEDING
- ☐ BREATHING
- ☐ ANEMIA
- ☐ JAUNDICE (MAX. BILI. ___)
- ☐ INFECTION
- ☐ OTHER

FAMILY HISTORY

FAMILY ROSTER (NAMES)	AGE	SEX	HEALTHY YES	HEALTHY NO
MOTHER		F		
FATHER		M		
CHILDREN (INCLUDING PATIENT)				
1.				
2.				
3.				
4.				
5.				
6.				
OTHERS IN HOUSEHOLD (RELATION)				

CHECK ALL MEDICAL PROBLEMS IN FAMILY AND STATE RELATIONSHIP OF FAMILY MEMBER AFFECTED:

☐ ANEMIA	☐ HEART DISEASE
☐ ARTHRITIS	☐ HYPERTENSION
☐ BLEEDING	☐ CANCER
☐ DEAFNESS	☐ TUBERCULOSIS
☐ DIABETES	☐ RETARDATION
☐ KIDNEY DISEASE	☐ EMOTIONAL
☐ THYROID DISEASE	☐ SUICIDE
☐ ASTHMA	☐ OTHER

MEDICAL HISTORY

	YES	NO
ILLNESS: (GIVE DATES)		
HOSPITALIZATIONS: (GIVE REASON, PLACE, AND DATE FOR EACH)		
SURGERY: (GIVE DATES)		
CURRENT MEDICATIONS:		
DRUG ALLERGIES:		

SOCIAL & DEVELOPMENTAL HISTORY

PROBLEMS WITH	YES	NO	GIVE DETAILS:
SLEEPING			
EATING			
TOILET TRAINING			
GROWTH			
SPEECH			
BEHAVIOR			
SCHOOL			
OTHER (SPECIFY)			

NUTRITIONAL HISTORY

BREAST FEEDING ☐ YES ☐ NO
UNTIL AGE: _____
FORMULA TYPE: _____
UNTIL AGE:

SOLIDS: TYPE AND DATE STARTED; CURRENT DIET

FOOD ALLERGIES:

CURRENTLY TAKING:
- ☐ IRON
- ☐ VITAMINS
- ☐ FLUORIDE

HSA-358-9 (9-77)   SIGNATURE OF HISTORY TAKER:

MEDICATION SUMMARY

START DATE	MEDICATION	DOSAGE SCHEDULE	PHYSICIAN	COMMENTS	STOP DATE

THE CHILDREN S ORTHOPEDIC HOSPITAL
AND MEDICAL CENTER
SEATTLE, WASHINGTON 98105

**LONG TERM MEDICATION
FLOW SHEET**

F18-71 3-77

CASE NO.

NAME

BIRTHDATE

Appendix 4B

Screen Display Formats for Patient Records from the PROMIS System

A typical progression through the computer displays as work is done and the patient's record is generated.*

Display 1

Initial Frame
Select patient group (Ward—Brown III)
Select patient group (Ward X)
Select patient group (Ward Y)

Display 1—When the user chooses one of the three patient groups listed above, display 2 appears.

---

*This series of displays . . . were presented and published as part of the November 1977 proceedings of the seventh annual conference of The Society For Computer Medicine under the title, *Effective Performance In The Dynamic Health Care Environment*, edited by Nancy S. Hill, Minneapolis, Minnesota.

Source: Lawrence Weed, M.D., *Your Health Care & How to Manage It* (Burlington, Vermont: Promis Laboratory, Essex Publishing Co., 1975).

Display 2

Brown III

Choose A Patient

Alphabetically
By Room

Problem Lists for Review
  Total Lists
  Changes Yesterday and Today

Other Groups
(Practice Ward)

Discharge: #1   #2   #3

Ward Functions
Ancillary Reports:
  Today   Yesterday   2 Days Ago
#Countersign Order   Reject Order   Review
New Order: Sign-Off   Transcribe   Review

IV List   Diet
Report RX Given
Report Tests
Retrieve Worklist

Information: Drug   Lab   Rad

Display 2—One can either get an alphabetic list of all the patients on the ward or a reverse chronological file of all the reports from the ward from the ancillary areas. Many of the other choices are self-explanatory such as touching "countersign order" would give a resident or attending physician those orders that need to be countersigned, and so forth. A nurse can touch the "IV list" and find out what IVs should be done and for what problem. A physician or nurse can retrieve a worklist on his or her patients that contains all the outstanding things that should be done at that particular time. One can use the terminal at this point to look things up about a drug or a type of tumor on a chest film independent of actions on any patient on that particular ward.

Let us assume that you touch "Alphabetically" on display 2 and you will get display 3.

Display 3

Patients, Alphabetically

FAAAAA, OAA . . . . F 92 548-371-4 3/17/77 BP3-304 (Attending's name)
GAAAA, DAAAAAAA . . . . M 79 538-311-2 4/05/77 BP3-313 (Attending's name)
GAAAA, EAA . . . . M 70 618-841-1 3/30/77 BP3-303 (Attending's name)
HAAAAAAA, MAAAAA . . . . F 56 700-087-0 3/10/77 BP3-320 (Attending's name)
KAAAAAA, OAAAA . . . . F 68 632-924-7 4/02/77 BP3-315 (Attending's name)
KAAAAAAA, GAAAAAAA . . . . F 45 687-813-6 4/06/77 BP3-309 (Attending's name)
LAAAA, JAAAAA . . . . M 55 559-924-6 4/05/77 BP3-306 (Attending's name)
NAAAAAAAA, FAAAAA . . . . F 53 824-452-7 03/30/77 BP3-319 (Attending's name)

Display 3 is a list of patients. On this display we see the patients' names, sex, age, unit number, date of admission, bed location, and attendings. We then touch one of those names and get display 4.

Display 4

4 Phases of Medical Action

Retrieve	Add to
Data Base	Data Base
Problem List	Problem List
Initial Plans	Initial Plans
Progress Notes	Progress Notes
Other Retrievals	Other Actions
Flowsheet Retrievals	Emergency Management
Graph Retrievals	Consult Reply
To Printer	Audit

Choose other ward/other functions   Choose other patient on this ward

Display 4 is a basic structural frame of the computerized problem-oriented medical record. You can either retrieve from the record or add to it. In this way, care is coordinated among many providers. Anyone who has a terminal has immediate, up-to-date access to all the information on that patient. If, for example, we touch "data base," on the Retrieve side, up will come display 5.

Display 5

Data Base Retrievals

Retrieve from Data Base	Admission Screening
Patient Profile	Patient's "Sickness"
History Data Base by System:	Complete History Data Base.
Present Illness:	All Present Illnesses.
Laboratory Data Base.	
Physical Exam Data Base by System	Complete Physical Exam Data Base

Physical Exam: Vital signs, height & weight, general appearance.

All sections, grouped by section.	All sections, chronologically.

  Administrative Data, all sections
    Audit Log
    Audit comments on major record sections

Display 5 not only immediately shows the user what the elements of a good data base are, it also allows him to retrieve any part he wishes. For example, if he touches "physical exam data base by system," display 6 pops up.

Display 6

Physical Exam Data Base, Body Systems, Retrieval

Retrieve Physical Exam Data Base System

Vital signs (& Adm Scr)	Eyes,	Breast,
Height & weight,	Ears,	Abdomen,
General appearance,	Nose/sinuses,	Costo-vertebral angle,
General skin features,	Mouth/oropharynx,	Musculoskeletal,
Skin lesions,	Neck,	Rectal,
Hair,	Lymph nodes,	Female genitalia,
Nails,	Chest and lungs,	Male genitalia,
Head,	Cardiovascular,	Neurologic.

Display 6 gives the user the opportunity to pick the system he wishes to obtain information from. In this instance, he will make the choice "cardio-vascular" and he will immediately have display 7.

Display 7

Cardiovascular (including sections below)
Heart
Peripheral artery
Peripheral vein
Cervical venous pressure and pulse

On Display 7, he will choose "heart" exam and display 8 will appear.

Display 8

Retrieve Physical Exam Data Base System Heart

Physical Exam Data Base

Heart: No entries
Cardiovascular:
  Heart exam
    Normal precordial inspection
    Normal precordial palpation
    Systolic murmur, left side, sternal border, radiates to carotid artery. Bilat,
      R L1 Grade III, middle-range of pitch, blowing
    Normal S1 heart sound
    Normal intensity and split of the S2 heart sound
    Regular heart rhythm
Normal data base peripheral artery exam
Normal data base peripheral vein exam

Display 8—If the user then touches the function pad at the lower part of display 8 marked "Return" he will go back, step by step, to his basic frame showing the 4 phases of medical action (display 9).

Display 9

4 Phases of Medical Action

Retrieve	Add to
Data Base	Data Base
Problem List	Problem List
Initial Plans	Initial Plans
Progress Notes	Progress Notes
Other Retrievals	Other Actions
Flowsheet Retrievals	Emergency Management
Graph Retrievals	Consult Reply
To Printer	Audit

Choose other ward/other functions   Choose other patient on this ward

On Display 9 he may decide to read the progress note from one of the problems and will touch "progress notes."

Display 10

Progress Note Retrievals

Retrieve progress notes
  For one active problem: For one problem:
  For an active problem with condition of concern:
  For a problem with condition worse than expected:

  For all problems, grouped by problem, with audit log & comments

SX only for one problem: SX & Obj for one problem
Obj only for one problem

Display 10 will ask him: Does he want progress notes for one problem, all problems, and so forth. If he touches "for one problem," up will come display 11.

Display 11

Choose Active/Combined Problem

Hospitalization	3/17/77
1. Abdominal cramps, onset on 03/16/17.	3/17/77
Guarded & staying same.	
2. Mass of abdomen, lower midline of abdomen, onset in 02/77	3/17/77
Guarded & getting worse.	
4. [Flexion contractures of hand bilat.] onset in 1974.	3/17/77
Satisfactory & staying same.	
5. Anemia: indeterminate onset, hypochromic, microcytic.	11/03/77
Satisfactory & staying same.	
11. H/O drug reaction: due to aspirin manifested by: with NA	3/17/77
12. Needs placement in extended care facility.	3/30/77
13. [Potential skin breakdown-coccyxgeal area.]	3/31/77
Guarded & getting worse.	
14. Location unknown by patient onset on 8/11/77, etiology unknown.	8/19/77
Guarded & staying same.	
15. Bronchogenic carcinoma, small cell anaplastic.	8/25/77
Guarded & staying same.	

Display 11 is the problem list. He will then touch the problem for which he wants the progress notes and up will come display 12.

Display 12

Retrieval Time Interval

Since	Including
16:00 (4 pm) today.	Today.
08:00 (8 am) today.	Today and yesterday.
00:00 (midnight) today.	Today and last 2 days.
	On specific date __/__/77
	From date __/__/77 to present
16:00 (4 pm) yesterday.	From date __/__/77 through
08:00 (8 am) yesterday.	Last week (today and last 7 days).
00:00 (midnight) yesterday.	Entire record.

Since 2 hours before I last stored an audit note in this record

Display 12 will ask the user over what period of time does he want the progress notes. Having made his choice, he will go to display 13.

Display 13 is just one of the many displays chosen from the progress notes on that problem and is put here to demonstrate information identified as either symptomatic, objective, assessment, or plans with the various components under that. All providers use the same progress notes whether they are physicians, practical nurses, secretaries, and so forth. On the actual computer display the date and time of each entry and the name of the provider who is adding the data is automatically shown on the right hand margin along side of the date. Having looked at the progress note, one can then touch the function pad "return" and go back, step by step, to the basic frame which is display 14.

Display 13

Sx

    [Pt. still thinking about alternatives presented yesterday by Dr. _____, with no decisions reached as yet]

Obj

    up in chair ad lib. Done at 19:00

Sx

    Nausea symptom/finding not present.
    Vomiting symptom/finding not present.
    Anorexia symptom/finding not present.
    (Pt. now eating well)

Obj

    (Abdominal exam unchanged)

Asmt

    Condition of problem: satisfactory, and staying the same. Condition is as expected considering available data.

Other Asmt:

    (Pt. is having problems deciding what to do about further RX. for

1st Page	Prev. Page	Return	Next Page

Display 14

4 Phases of Medical Action

Retrieve	Add to
Data Base	Data Base
Problem List	Problem List
Initial Plans	Initial Plans
Progress Notes	Progress Notes
Other Retrievals	Other Actions
Flowsheet Retrievals	Emergency Management
Graph Retrievals	Consult Reply
To Printer	Audit

Choose other ward/other functions   Choose other patient on this ward

Display 14—For this display we will now choose "other retrievals."

Display 15

Other Retrievals

Retrieve
Orders and reports
Procedure
Current aims for active prob
Current condition for active prob

All sections, grouped by section
All sections, chronologically
Total problem list

Pharmacy billing
Pharmacy billing, orders only

Discharge summary
Objectives during hosp., all active probs
Person coord. mgmt., all active probs
Current goal, all active probs

Abstract for active problem:
Lab data base & Obj for all probs
Drugs given for all problems
   Vital signs
Drugs given with charge code
Audit notes

Countersigned orders

Emergency room problem abstract
Emergency room recycled record

Display 15—It is apparent from the above display that there is a wide variety of choices which provide immediate coordination with other areas and other personnel in the medical care system. If we touch "orders and reports," we immediately see display 16.

Display 16

Order Related Retrievals

Review current orders:
   Short form— Treatment Test Drugs
   Long form— For one active prob For all problems
Select orders from following lists to retrieve all data on the same procedure
   Pharmacy (only occurrences of same dosage form will be included)

   Rad/Lab/Spec DX Consult notes by same service

Select orders from following lists to retrieve data for the specific order only:
   All studies/drugs ever ordered All studies/drugs outstanding
   Pharmacy Rad/Nuc Med studies Chemistry Hematology Consults
Urinalysis Microbiology Serology Administrative functions

Retrieve countersigned orders

Display 16—One can touch any of the above choices on this display and be in immediate contact with that category on a particular patient or group of patients. Returning to the basic display, we have display 17.

Display 17—On this display, we will now touch the choice "flowsheet retrievals" and display 18 will appear.

Display 17

4 Phases of Medical Action

Retrieve	Add to
Data Base	Data Base
Problem List	Problem List
Initial Plans	Initial Plans
Progress Notes	Progress Notes
Other Retrievals	Other Actions
Flowsheet Retrievals	Emergency Management
Graph Retrievals	Consult Reply
To Printer	Audit

Choose other ward/other functions   Choose other patient on this ward

Display 18

From Patient Orders	Standard Flowsheets
Lab procedures, all	Routine vital signs (BP/T/P/R)
Chemistry Hematology Serology	Neuro vital signs
Urine/stool Microbiology	Venous pressure
Radiology procedures, all	Fluid & electrolyte
X-rays Ultrasound Radioisotope	Bone marrow exam
Pharmacy procedures, all	

Oral/parenteral   Topical/EENT

Pharmacy procedures, current
Oral/parenteral   Topical/EENT

Physical Exam Procedures, All

Flowsheets on this page cover the last 10 days of admission with one column per day, for other time spans, touch here.
Flowsheet Information

Single Lab Procedure

Display 18—One can retrieve many parameters in flow sheet form, as the above display suggests.

If, for example, one touches "routine vital signs", one gets a display in the form of display 19, with the appropriate values inserted in the blanks for a given patient. Problem-oriented flow sheets and systems-oriented flow sheets are also possible in the PROMIS system. The former are useful when one wants to follow the course of a given problem, see the logic of the actions taken, and eventually correct that logic with "outcome" data. The latter are useful when a new problem arises in a given body system and one would like to have immediately available in flow sheet form all the data pertaining to that system regardless of the original context and problem that led to its acquisition. (See step 4 of the plan.) Efficient use of information energy requires multiple retrievals that act on large bodies of data which were acquired over long periods of time. Paper systems do not allow this, and the patient therefore risks either actions taken in ignorance of useful data already in existence or unnecessary duplication of tests and questions.

Display 19

Routine Vital Signs

Period: 11/14/77 00:00 to 11/24/77 00:00
Resolution: 1 Day

	11/18/77 00:00	11/19/77 00:00	11/20/77 00:00	11/21/77 00:00	11/22/77 00:00	11/23/77 00:00
BP	. . . .	. . . .	. . . .	. . . .	. . . .	. . . .
Temperature	. . . .	. . . .	. . . .	. . . .	. . . .	. . . .
Pulse	. . . .	. . . .	. . . .	. . . .	. . . .	. . . .
Respirations	. . . .	. . . .	. . . .	. . . .	. . . .	. . . .

Left 4   Return

Display 19—If there is more than one value for a given day, then one can touch that particular date and immediately one will have a flow sheet of all the values on that particular day. If one wants to know values on the days before those designated, he can touch "left 4" at the bottom of the display and get the flow sheet from an earlier period. We will touch "return" now and go back to the basic display.

Display 20

4 Phases of Medical Action

Retrieve	Add to
Data Base	Data Base
Problem List	Problem List
Initial Plans	Initial Plans
Progress Notes	Progress Notes
Other Retrievals	Other Actions
Flowsheet Retrievals	Emergency Management
Graph Retrievals	Consult Reply
To Printer	Audit

Choose other ward/other functions   Choose other patient on this ward

Display 20—If we touch "graph retrievals," we then get display 21.

Display 21

GRAPH FLOW SHEETS

Electrolytes:	Vital signs:
NA K CL CO2	T P R BP
Arterial "gases"	
PO2 PCO2 PH	WGT

Blood counts:
HCT HGB WBC RETIC
Coagulation:
PTT Pro Time

Plasma glucose:
Spot 2 Hr PC FASTING   Graph Information
Bun Creatinine

Display 21 provides us with a series of choices for parameters to appear in graphic form.

Display 22

4 Phases of Medical Action

Retrieve	Add to
Data Base	Data Base
Problem List	Problem List
Initial Plans	Initial Plans
Progress Notes	Progress Notes
Other Retrievals	Other Actions
Flowsheet Retrievals	Emergency Management
Graph Retrievals	Consult Reply
To Printer	Audit

Choose other ward/other functions	Choose other patient on this ward

Display 22—Having discussed briefly some of the various types of retrievals, we can now go to the "Add to" side of the above display. For example, we may want to enter a present illness on diabetes. We do that by touching "data base" and going on display 23.

Display 23

Add to Data Base

Admission Screening
Patient's "sickness" (major complaints)
Patient profile
History data base, questionnaire   History data base, additions
Physical exam data base
Laboratory data base
Begin new present illness   Add to existing present illness

Display 23—This immediately educates us as to what are the basic components of a data base. We will choose "begin a new present illness" and up will come display 24.

Display 24

Begin a New Present Illness

A primary finding
  Symptom
  Habit/life style finding
  Social problem
  Environmental problem
  Physical exam finding
  Lab/X-ray/other test finding
  Family H/O
  H/O problem

Drug/surgery/other procedure
S/P drug/surgery/other procedure

A synthesis of findings
  Psychiatric/Behavioral problem
  Physiological abnormality
  Medical/surgical diagnosis

Display 24—The user is immediately forced to think logically as to how he should classify his present illness. Diabetes is a defined diagnosis. He would touch "medical/surgical diagnosis" which would lead him directly to display 25.

Display 25

Diagnostic Entities by Body System

General/Systemic	Respiratory	Endocrine/Metabolic
Skin and appendages	Cardiovascular	Male reproductive
Eye	Gastrointestinal	Female reproductive
Ear	Urinary	Breast
Nose, nasopharynx,	Musculoskeletal	Obstetrical
sinuses	Hematological	Neurological
Mouth and oropharynx		Psychiatric/Behavioral
Hypopharynx and larynx		

Display 25—Since diabetes is an endocrine/metabolic disorder, he would enter that group of known diagnoses, leading to display 26.

Display 26

Endocrine/Metabolic

Common problems
- Diabetes mellitus
- Gout
- Pseudogout
- Hyperlipoproteinemia
- Metabolic acidosis
- Obesity
- Water/Electrolyte/Acid-base

Problems by anatomic site
- Systemic (entire body)
- Adenohypophysis
- Adrenal cortex
- Adrenal medulla
- Neurohypophysis
- Ovaries
- Pancreas
- Parathyroid
- Testes
- Thyroid
- Multiple endocrine organs

Display 26—Since diabetes is a common disease, it would be immediately available on the side of the screen saying "common problems." More unusual diagnoses would require going through a more detailed classification scheme. It is with these techniques that very large volumes of information can be accessed with great speed if one can be very specific and logical about what he is trying to do. It is this demand for specificity and logic at each step that is so beneficial to the patient and so beneficial to medical science in that feedback loops can be very rigorous with such well-defined input. We would then progress to display 27.

Display 27

Diabetes Mellitus
Adult diabetes mellitus,
Juvenile diabetes mellitus,
Nonketotic hyperosmolar coma,
Diabetic ketoacidosis.

Display 27—One would, at this point, choose the appropriate choice which, in our case, will be "adult diabetes mellitus", progressing to display 28.

Display 28

Adult Diabetes Mellitus
(Not specified)
Prediabetes, -Def-
Overt diabetes mellitus, -Def-

"Subclinical diabetes" -Def-
"Latent diabetes" -Def-

Display 28—It will be noted that opposite each of the terms is -Def-. If one touches -Def-, one gets a definition of each term. For example, if we touch -Def- opposite "overt diabetes mellitus" on display 28, we will get display 29.

Display 29

Overt Diabetes Mellitus
Overt diabetes mellitus is the persistent elevation of the fasting blood sugar (FBS 140 MG/DL serum or plasma or 120 MG/DL blood) in the absence of pancreatitis. Cushing's disease, pheochromocytoma and hyperlipidemia, a 2 hour plasma glucose, as during a glucose tolerance test. 200 MG/DL is evidence of probable diabetes mellitus.

Display 29 is a definition of overt diabetes mellitus. We can then return from that frame to display 28 and actually touch "overt diabetes mellitus" and proceed to get the present illness as seen on display 30.

Display 30

Overt Diabetes
Well-controlled
Poorly controlled
Uncontrolled
Insulin-dependent
Insulin-independent

Display 30—One would make the appropriate choice on display 30 and go to display 31.

Display 31

Problem Descriptors and Associations

Amount at worst	Relieved by/not relieved by
Severity	Made worse by
Quality	Onset associated with
Location	Associated with
Radiation	
Time relationships	Objective information

Serial Reporting

Display 31 is an outline of how one should really think about any problem. It is a logical grouping of choices as you obtain a present illness from a patient. For example, if we touch "associated with," we will come up with display 32.

Display 32

Associated with:
  Symptoms/findings
  Problems
  Concurrent medications
  Social-environmental problems
  Genetic factors
  Constitutional symptoms

Could not determine.
Did not determine.
Nothing.

Display 32—One should think in terms of associated findings in another set of groups as defined above. Let us choose "symptoms/findings" and we will get display 33.

Display 33

SX, Signs, Findings

Associated symptoms/findings:
  Obesity,
  Weight gain,
  Weight loss,
  Polyuria/nocturia
  Vaginal pruritis
  Neurological SX/signs:
  Eye SX signs:
  Infections:

  Ketoacidosis,
  Hypoglycemic episodes:
  Cardiovascular SX/signs
  Peripheal vascular SX/signs
  Renal S/signs
  Lipid abnormalities:
  Skin disorders:
  Obstetrical complications:

Did not determine.
None.

REVIEW   PRINT

Display 33—One could make choices directly from this display such as "obesity" or "weight gain", and they would be incorporated into the record. Other choices such as "skin disorders" would lead you to another display with specific choices on it such as "necrobiosis" and other skin disorders appropriate to diabetes. It can be seen from these displays that we are depending upon the memory of the provider. We are telling him very explicitly what information he should get on a diabetic. It will be on the basis of this information that we can then build explicit guidance for plans and progress notes.

At any time, one can touch "review" at the bottom of the screen and see what he has put in thus far. For example, what you might see on display 34 as you are starting a diabetic present illness.

Display 34

FAAAAA, OAA . . . . F 92 548-371-4 . . . .
   Begin new present illness
     Diabetes mellitus, adult mellitus, overt diabetes mellitus,
      The problem is currently active. The problem has been continuous since its discovery
      It began 5 years ago. Symptoms/findings
      Associated skin signs, necrobiosis, xanthoma,
      Associated symptoms/findings: weight gain, 16 lbs. over a period of:
                  RETURN

Display 34—The above display is what comes up at a particular point in the progression as one touches review. Touching "return" on this display, we will go to display 35, our basic frame.

Display 35

4 Phases of Medical Action

Retrieve	Add to
Data Base	Data Base
Problem List	Problem List
Initial Plans	Initial Plans
Progress Notes	Progress Notes
Other Retrievals	Other Actions
Flowsheet Retrievals	Emergency Management
Graph Retrievals	Consult Reply
To Printer	Audit

Choose other ward/other functions   Choose other patient on this ward

Display 35—At this point, we may choose to add to the problem list, for example, a lipoproteinemia in a patient. We would then touch "problem list" and display 36 would appear.

Display 36

Problem List

Add a major problem
    Active problem:
    Inactive problem:

Add a temporary problem:

Activate a problem:
Review active problem list

Restate/update a major problem:
Restate/update a temporary problem:
Combine problems:

Inactivate a problem:
Discard a problem:
Review total problem list

Display 36—We are asked at this point to logically decide whether it is an active problem, inactive problem, or temporary problem, and so forth. Let us choose "active problem" and go to display 37.

Display 37

Level of Major Problem

A primary finding
    Symptom
    Habit/life style finding
    Social problem
    Environmental problem
    Physical exam finding
    Lab/x-ray/other test finding

Family history of
H/O problem

A primary finding (cont.)
    Drug/surgery/other procedure
    S/P surgery/other procedure
    Health maintenance
    Incomplete data base

A synthesis of findings
    Psychiatric/behavioral problem
    Physiological abnormality
    Medical/surgical diagnosis

Display 37—Since it is a physiological lipid abnormality we want to enter, we would touch "physiological abnormality" and go to display 38.

Display 38

Diagnostic Entities by Body System

General/Systemic	Respiratory	Endocrine/Metabolic
Skin and appendages	Cardiovascular	Male reproductive
Eye	Gastrointestinal	Female reproductive
Ear	Urinary	Breast
Nose, nasopharynx,	Musculoskeletal	Obstetrical
sinuses	Hematological	Neurological
Mouth and oropharynx		Psychiatric/Behavioral
Hypopharynx and larynx		

Display 38—At this point, we would choose "endocrine/metabolic" and proceed to display 39.

Display 39

Endocrine/Metabolic

Adenohypophysis:	Ovaries:
Neurohypophysis:	Testes:
Thyroid:	Sexual differentiation:
Parathyroid:	Inborn errors of metabolism:
Adrenal Cortex:	Lipopathies:
Adrenal Medulla:	Disorders of growth/development:
Pancreas:	Water/electrolyte/acid base

Display 39—Since one of the hyperlipoproteinemias is a lipopathy, we will make that choice and proceed to display 40.

Display 40

Lipopathies

Obesity
Hyperlipoproteinemia
Uncommon lipid disorders
Atherosclerosis
Cholelithiasis
Xanthomatosis

Display 40—At this point, we would touch "hyperlipoproteinemia" and it would be the first word of the message that now directly goes into the patient's record. The reader must be reminded that choosing is, in effect, writing the record, and at the time you are doing it, you are getting all the guidance you need to write it correctly. This is what is meant by building a non-memory dependent system. Also, since one chooses to use electronic tools such as this, one simultaneously solves both the coordination and logic problems that are plaguing medicine. Others have this available at any other terminal immediately, and we know precisely where we are because we have stated we are entering a problem and that it is an endocrine/metabolic one of this type.

We will now progress to display 41.

Display 41

Hyperlipoproteinemia

(Not specified)

Type I.	-DEF-
Type IIA.	-DEF-
Type IIB.	-DEF-
Type III.	-DEF-
Type IV.	-DEF-
Type V.	-DEF-

Display 41—Let us assume that the patient has a "Type IIA" and we want to know precisely what the definition of that is. We would touch -DEF- and go to display 42.

Display 42

Lipid Profile and Clinical Presentation of Type IIA Hyperlipoproteinemia

Type IIA—Characterized by H/O premature vascular disease and tendon tuberous xanthomas, may be noted at birth, but often not detected until vascular disease develops.

Lab data: Cholesterol—increased
Triglycerides—normal
Cholesterol/triglyceride ratio—1.5/1.0
Lipoprotein electrophoresis—increased beta
Cold serum—no creamy top, clear serum
Low density lipoprotein (LDL = cholesterol − (triglyceride + 45))
Elevated by calculation or ultracentrifugation
NL = 170 MG/DL (0-29 yr)
NL = 190 MG/DL (30-49 yr)
NL = 210 MG/DL (+ 50 yr)

Display 42—Having reviewed the definition and deciding this is appropriate for our patient, we would immediately go back to display 41 and choose "Type IIA" and it would progress to display 43.

Display 43

Type IIA Hyperlipoproteinemia
(Not specified)
Primary
Familial
Secondary

Display 43—We would then pick the choice that is appropriate above and progress, each choice making a more precise record. Having completed a problem statement, we may now want to write a plan. We would go on to display 44, our basic display.

Display 44

4 Phases of Medical Action

Retrieve	Add to
Data Base	Data Base
Problem List	Problem List
Initial Plans	Initial Plans
Progress Notes	Progress Notes
Other Retrievals	Other Actions
Flowsheet Retrievals	Emergency Management
Graph Retrievals	Consult Reply
To Printer	Audit

Choose other ward/other functions   Choose other patient on this ward

Display 44—In our effort to write a plan, we would touch "initial plans" and progress to display 45.

Display 45

Active Problems for Initial Plans:

*	**Hospitalization**	**3/17/77**
1.	Abdominal cramps, onset on 03/16/17.	3/17/77
	Guarded & staying same.	
2.	Mass of abdomen, lower midline of abdomen, onset in 02/77	3/17/77
	Guarded & getting worse.	
4.	[Flexion contractures of hand bilat.] onset in 1974.	3/17/77
	Satisfactory & staying same.	
5.	Anemia: indeterminate onset, hypochromic, microcytic.	11/03/77
	Satisfactory & staying same.	
11.	H/O drug reaction: due to aspirin manifested by: with NA	3/17/77
12.	Needs placement in extended care facility.	3/30/77
13.	[Potential skin breakdown-coccyxgeal area.]	3/31/77
	Guarded & getting worse.	
14.	Location unknown by patient onset on 8/11/77, etiology unknown.	8/19/77
	Guarded & staying same.	
15.	Bronchogenic carcinoma, small cell anaplastic.	8/25/77
	Guarded & staying same.	
16.	Hyperlipoproteinemia Type IIA	8/25/77

Display 45—It will be noted that we are immediately confronted with a problem list. In this manner, our logic is captured. We cannot write plans of any sort without first stating what our problem is. Let us pick choice number 5 "Anemia: Indeterminate onset, hypochromic, microcytic." This will immediately lead us to display 46.

Display 46

Initial Plan

1. State aims for problem management
2. Check how problem may be contributing to patient's "sickness"
3. Check for effects/disabilities produced by problem
4. Check function/status of systems that may be involved with problem
5. Assess and follow course
6. Investigate problem and its etiology
7. Watch for/prevent complications of problem
8. If indicated, institute and monitor treatment

Emergency management   Choose another problem

Display 46—It is clear from the above display that the fundamental steps in planning for a problem are immediately revealed to a user. It is not a computer-assisted instruction in the sense that we expect the user to "learn" or memorize this approach. It will always be available. The very tool that he uses to do his work provides such guidance. Let us assume he has gone through all the steps up to step number six where he wants to investigate the problem and its etiology. Having made this choice, you will go to display 47.

Display 47

Investigate Problem and Its Etiology
1. Check for previous patterns of similar problems
2. Characterize problem further (if appropriate)
3. Check problem list for possible etiologic relationships
4. Check current treatment for possible etiologic relationships
5. Investigate causes of initial concern (if appropriate)
6. Investigate other causes (if appropriate)
7. Screen for predisposing problems (if appropriate)

Display 47—Again, the user is taught how to think carefully about the pursuit of a problem. Assuming he has done the first four steps, he can touch step number five and investigate the cause of initial concern. He will be immediately confronted with display 48.

Display 48

Hypochromic, Microcytic Anemia: Causes of Initial Concern
Lead poisoning
Iron deficiency
Pyridoxine-responsive anemia
Chronic disease
Crude liver factor responsive anemia
Beta thalassemia minor

Begin/continue/resume other investigation

Display 48—Here are the choices that he must now consider as causes for his anemia. If he touches "lead poisoning," he will go on to display 49.

Display 49

Investigate for Cause
1. Screen for this cause
2. R/O this cause
   or
   suspend investigation for this cause due to "negative screen"
   Discontinue investigation due to "unacceptable risk or cost"
   Report this cause as "ruled out" (not present)
   Report this cause as present

Display 49—To screen for lead poisoning, he will touch that choice (number 1) and up will come display 50.

The distinction between "screen for" and "rule out" as used in the above display is important to the efficient and safe practice of medicine. Before plunging into expensive and even dangerous procedures to rule out a diagnostic possibility, one should examine critically facts already known about a patient, or facts harmlessly and cheaply obtained, to see if the possibility under consideration is appropriate to the context of a particular unique individual. By touching the "screen for" choice we are immediately given the guidance that allows us to do just that.

Display 50

Hypochromic, Microcytic Anemia: Cluster to Screen for Cause

Cause: Lead poisoning

Findings that suggest this cause	Sensitiv.	Conf. Rate
Pica with residence in older housing	—	—
Prolonged exposure to lead compounds	—	—
Basophilic stippling of RBCs	—	—

Order screen procedures

Contingency plan   Recommendations

Display 50—The above display is self-explanatory. If it appropriately describes his patient, he would go on to rule it out. He would do this by returning to display 51.

Display 51

Investigate for Cause

1. Screen for this cause
2. R/O this cause
   or
   Suspend investigation for this cause due to "negative screen"
   Discontinue investigation due to "unacceptable risk or cost"
   Report this cause as "ruled out" (not present)
   Report this cause as present

Display 51—Since he is now prepared to rule out lead poisoning as a cause, he would touch "rule out" and get display 52.

Display 52

R/O Lead Poisoning

1. Do   24 Hr urine lead
        or
        Blood lead
2. If urine lead concentration is approximately 300 micrograms/liter, then lead poisoning is present.
   If urine lead concentration is greater than 80 micrograms/liter in children or greater than 100 micrograms/liter in adults, then lead poisoning may be present; repeat determination indicated.
3. If blood lead concentration is greater than 80 micrograms/milliter in an adult, then lead poisoning is present.
   If blood lead concentration is greater than 60 micrograms/100 milliters in a child, poisoning may be present; repeat determination indicated.
   If blood lead concentration, is greater than 60 micrograms/100 milliters in a child, then lead poisoning is present.
   If blood lead concentration is greater than 40 micrograms/100 milliters in a child, then lead poisoning may be present; repeat determination indicated.
4. If urine lead and blood lead concentrations are equivocal or negative but suggestive clinical findings are present, then do calcium EDTA test.
5. If greater than 1000 micrograms of lead are excreted per liter of urine after 8 hours of EDTA administration, then lead poisoning is present.
   If greater than 500 micrograms of lead are excreted per liter of urine after 8 hours of EDTA administration, then an excessive lead burden is indicated and lead poisoning may be present.
   If less than 400 micrograms of lead are excreted per liter of urine after 8 hours of EDTA administration, then lead poisoning is not present.
Contingency plan   Recommendations

REFERENCES

Flink, Edmund: Heavy Metal Poisoning, pp. 57-62 in Textbook of Medicine (14th Ed.), Edited by Paul B. Beeson and Walsh McDermott, 1975.

Levine, W.G.: Heavy Metals, pp. 947-957 in The Pharmaceutical Basis of Therapeutics (4th Ed.), Edited by Goodman & Gilman, 1970.

MCHV Normal Chemistry Values, MCHV Chemistry Laboratory.

Poskanzer, David C. and Bennett, Ivan L.: Heavy metals, pp. 667-671 in Harrison's Principles of Internal Medicine (7th Ed.), Edited by Maxwell M. Wintrobe, et al., 1974.

Weissman, Norman: Laboratory Aids in Toxicological Problems, p. 19-20, (copyright: Bio-Science Laboratories, 1973.).

Display 52—The above is detailed guidance of how to rule out lead poisoning along with the references. Let us assume he went through all the causes of initial concern and they were all ruled out. He then returns to display 53.

Display 53

Investigate Problem and Its Etiology
1. Check for previous patterns of similar problems
2. Characterize problem further (if appropriate)
3. Check problem list for possible etiologic relationships
4. Check current treatment for possible etiologic relationships
5. Investigate causes of initial concern (if appropriate)
6. Investigate other causes (if appropriate)
7. Screen for predisposing problems (if appropriate)

Display 53—Now he chooses "investigate other causes" which leads him to display 54.

Display 54

Hypochromic, Microcytic Anemia: Other Causes
Copper deficiency (mostly infants)   Hemoglobin E
Sideroblastic anemia
Familial hypochromic, microcytic anemia
Congenital atransferrinemia
Hemoglobin koln
Hemoglobin lepore
Hemoglobln
Begin/continue/resume other investigation

Display 54—It is clear from the above how one can step by step be led to the most sophisticated analysis of a problem without being dependent upon memory.

Display 55

Radiology

Report of previous studies & record retrievals	Pts with outstanding radiology orders
Brown III	Brown III
Emergency Room	Emergency Room
Discharge Ward: #1 #2 #3	Discharge Ward: #1 #2 #3
E.R. Discharge	E.R. Discharge

Radiology Lockup   Drug Information   Lab Information

Display 55 shows how coordinated efforts with the radiologist are carried out. At his terminal, he would touch "Brown III" on the above display to get the x-rays ordered from that ward and display 56 would come up.

Display 56

Select Study to be Reported

Data Base
   Chest x-ray: PA/Lat (already done)   (1). 4/03

Display 56—The radiologist would then touch "chest x-ray" and display 57 would appear showing also the patient's name and the problem for each procedure that had been ordered.

Display 57

Indicate Status of Order:
Study done as ordered.
Additional study done.
Study not done.
Study done but only limited assessment possible.
Study to be redone.
Study already reported as part of other study.
Routine introductive data for nuclear medicine study.

Display 57—The radiologist would touch "study done as ordered" and display 58 would appear.

Display 58
Chest

Are there findings in the
   Soft tissues
   Thorax (bony)
   Pleura
   Diaphragm
   Lung parenchyma
   Lung vasculature
   Lung hila
   Measurement of heart and diaphragm level

   Cardiac outline
   Mediastinum
   Larynx
   Abdomen
   "Extras"

Display 58—The radiologist would touch "mediastinum" if his particular patient had a mediastinal mass. Up would come display 59.

Display 59

Mediastinum Finding
Anterior junction line, effaced.
Aortic knob, prominent.
Ascending aorta, prominent.
Azygous vein, dilated.
Calcification, aortic arch.
Calcification, superior mediastinum.
Descending aorta, prominent.
Endotracheal tube position, normal.

"Figure 3" sign, upper mediastinum.
Mass. anterior mediastinum.
Mass. middle mediastinum.
Mass. posterior mediastinum.
Mass. right cardiophrenic angle.
Mass. superior mediastinum.
Mediastinal shift.
Paratracheal stripe, right, widened.

Pneumomediastinum.
Thoracic aorta prominent.
Thickening of posterior tracheal stripe.
Trachea deviated.
Trachea narrowed.
Widened mediastinum.120

Display 59—The radiologist chooses "mass, posterior mediastinum" and immediately gets display 60.

Display 60

Posterior Mediastinal Mass
Description
Differential diagnosis of this finding

Display 60—He would first be expected to describe this finding as he saw it on the film. He would touch "description" and up would come the appropriate descriptors and would lead him through the appropriate branching logic for his description.

Display 61

Description

Number
Size
Shape
Margins
Location of lymph node chains involved
Mediastinal pleural reflections altered
Associated with tracheal narrowing
Associated with bronchial narrowing
Comparison of this finding with previous exam

Density
Distribution
Air/fluid level present

Display 61—Having completed this description for the posterior mediastinal mass, he would proceed to display 62.

Display 62

Posterior Mediastinal Mass
Description
Differential diagnosis of this finding

Display 62—From this display, the user would pick "differential diagnosis" and get display 63.

Display 63

Posterior Mediastinal Mass
This finding could fit
  Aneurysm, descending aorta
  Neural tumor gamut
  Paraspinal abscess
  Spine disease gamut

Uncommon

Display 63—At this point, the radiologist selects "neural tumor gamut" and goes to display 64.

Display 64

Neural Tumor Gamut

This finding could fit

Neural tumor type; not specified	-DEF-
Neuroblastoma	-DEF-
Neurofibroma	-DEF-
Neurilemmoma	-DEF-
Ganglioneuroma	-DEF-
Neurosarcoma	-DEF-
Pheochromocytoma	-DEF-
Chemodectoma	-DEF-
Chordoma	-DEF-

Display 64—The radiologist then, at this point, may choose to refresh his knowledge and touch -DEF- on ganglioneuroma which will lead him to display 65.

Display 65

Ganglioneuroma (Chain Ganglia)

1. Medium-large size.
2. Smooth fusiform, rarely dumbbell shaped.
3. Extrapleural sign—no sulcus.
4. Unilateral greater than Bilateral.
5. 25-35% have stippled calcification.
0. Seen in younger age than neurilemmoma.
7. Ganglioneuroma or neuroblastoma can appear as "dumbbell" shaped neurofibroma, in pediatric age group. May require emergency decompressive laminectomy.

Roentgen findings
Paraspinal mass, scoliosis, possible calcification, rib changes, pedicular erosion, posterior vertebral bodies scalloped.

General
Ganglioneuromas originate in the sympathetic ganglia, lateral to the neural canal on either side.

Display 65—Above is a detailed description of the ganglioneuroma. If this fits with the situation at hand, the radiologist would make this choice and, in the process, complete his report which would be immediately available to all of the terminal users. There would not be any typing or transmission of paper records. He could now return to display 66 for further actions.

Display 66

4 Phases of Medical Action

Retrieve	Add to
Data Base	Data Base
Problem List	Problem List
Initial Plans	Initial Plans
Progress Notes	Progress Notes
Other Retrievals	Other Actions
Flowsheet Retrievals	Emergency Management
Graph Retrievals	Consult Reply
To Printer	Audit

Choose other ward/other functions   Choose other patient on this ward

Display 66—Let us assume we wanted to give a drug for a problem. We would touch "initial plans"; and go on to display 67.

Display 67

Active Problems for Initial Plans:

*	Hospitalization	4/06/77
1.	Supraventricular tachycardia paroxysmal, onset in 1975. (Propan. . . Good & staying same.	4/05/77
2.	Hypertension, diastolic, mild, onset approximately in 1960. Good and staying same.	4/05/77
4.	Depression (& anxiety)	4/05/77
9.	(Neurogenic bladder, autonomous) onset on 3/20/75. Satisfactory & staying same.	4/05/77
11.	Renal failure chronic onset on 3/22/75, etiology unknown. Satisfactory/stability not known.	4/05/77
16.	(Polymyalgia rheumatica) onset in 12/76. (Prednisone Rx) Guarded/stability not known.	4/05/77
17.	Extremity weakness, both legs symmetrically, onset in 3/77, etio. . . Guarded and getting worse.	4/05/77
18.	Anemia: chronic, hypochromic, microcytic. Satisfactory & staying same.	9/15/77

Display 67—Then we would be asked to pick a problem. We will pick problem #2, "hypertension". We would then be confronted with display 68.

Display 68

Initial Plan

1. State aims for problem management
2. Check how problem may be contributing to patient's "sickness"
3. Check for effects/disabilities produced by problem
4. Check function/status of systems that may be involved with problem
5. Assess and follow course
6. Investigate problem and its etiology
7. Watch for/prevent complications of problem
8. If indicated, institute and monitor treatment

Emergency management   Choose another problem

Display 68—We choose to go straight to item 8 for treatment. Having touched number 8, we would get display 69.

Display 69

Institute and Monitor Treatment

1. Assess response to treatment (if any currently being done)
2. Order procedures for treatment baseline data
3. Order treatment: Supportive/nursing care
                Symptomatic treatment
                "Corrective" therapy
4. Order procedures to follow response to treatment

Enter planned treatment protocol

Display 69—We would choose to go directly to "corrective therapy" and we would get display 70.

Display 70

General Treatments for Cardiovascular Problems

Anticoagulants	Tranquilizers, minor
Antilipemic agents	Routine medications
Cardiac drugs	Ward procedures
Digitalis group	Activity Oxygen
Diuretics	Diets
Hypotensive drugs	I.V. therapy
Nitroglycerin	Drug index
Potassium chloride (oral)	Recommendations

Display 70—We would pick "hypotensive drugs" shown on the above display in our efforts to treat the hypertension. Immediately we would get display 71.

In addition to this general guidance many more detailed options (more specific guidance) are now becoming available. The present guidance is a very useful intermediate step.

Display 71

Antihypertensive Agents—By Mechanism of Action

Alpha-adrenergic blockers
  Phentolamine (regitine)

Beta-adrenergic blockers
  Propranolol (inderal)

Centrally acting
  Clonidine
  Nethyldopa

Direct arteriole dilators
  Diazoxide (hyperstat)
  Hydalazine (apresoline)
  Nitroprusside (nipride)

Ganglionic blockers
  Mecamylamine (inversive)
  Trimethaphan (arfonad)

Vasodilator (via effect on cyclic amp)
  Prazosin (minipress)

Post-ganglionic agents
  Guanethidine (ismelin)
  Reserpine (sandnl)

Diuretics, loop acting
  Ethacrynic acid (Edecrin)
  Furosemide (Lasix)

Diuretics, potassium sparing
  Spuonolactone (aldactone)
  Triameterene (dyrenium)

Diuretics, thiazides
  Hydrochlorothiazide, others

Diuretics, thiazide-like
  Chlorthalidone (hygroton)
  Quinethazone (hydromox)

Combination products
  Dyazide

Alphabetically

Display 71—We would go further in our efforts to treat by touching "diazoxide" and getting display 72.

The above set of options should be known to those making treatment decisions. Guidance as to the appropriate choice for a given individual is becoming available as each display in the present system is backed up by the next deeper level of logic. Each individual patient's unique combinations of attributes coupled with the guidance of the logic underlying each option allow the evolution of a protocol appropriate to that patient's needs. It is like coupling the details of a road map to the unique needs of a traveler to construct an efficient route to a clear goal.

"Function" pads are available at the base of each display from which one can immediately retrieve the patient's problem list or current treatments to allow the tailoring of choices to the particular individual. The coding of each choice and of all the known facts on the patients allow future studies of outcomes in a meaningful way because the same coding will make automatic guidance more and more of a reality without ignoring the unique requirements of individuals. In the above sense, the computer allows the delivery of personalized care on a scale never before possible by human specialists and generalists acting on their own with limited human memories, inadequate information tools, and unrealistic premises for medical education.

Display 72

Arteriole Dilators
Diazoxide (hyperstat)
Hydralazine (apresoline)
Nitroprusside (nipride)

Display 72—We will touch "diazoxide" and go to display 73.

Display 73

Diazoxide
Diazoxide I.V. injection 15 MG/ML = 20 ML $15.16

Display 73—It will be noted that the price of the drug is known and we can make our choice, and that single choice could be involved with updating the inventory, going on the patient's bill in addition to ordering the drug for the patient. Having made that choice, we can go on to display 74.

Display 74

General Ordering Methodology for Drugs
Explanation of this frame
1. Check "aims for problem management" for consistency
2. Check for duplicate order
3. Check for findings which may affect use of drug in patient
4. Discuss use of drug with patient
5. Check dosage and frequency
6. Continue to order

Select another procedure

Display 74—At this point, if we choose choice #3, we can find out the relationship of the drug to the patient's other problems and drugs as seen on display 75.

A more detailed discussion of the pharmacy component of PROMIS may be found in the article, "Integration of pharmacy into the computerized problem oriented medical information system (PROMIS)—a demonstration project", Gen. Gilroy, Brian J. Ellinoy, George E. Nelson, and Stephen V. Cantrill, Am. J. Hosp Pharm 34:155-162 (Feb) 1977.

Display 75

Types of Circumstances Which May Effect the Use of a Treatment
1. Drug—problem interactions
2. Drug—drug interactions
3. Drug—test interactions

Serial check

Display 75—As we pick the choices on this display, we will progress through displays 76, 77, and 78.

Display 76

Diazoxide

Drug—problem interactions

Finding	Potential adverse effect	Quantitative data/ cautions
Congestive heart failure	Fluid retention	Administer thiazide Diuretic or furosemide concomittantly
Impaired renal function	Fluid retention	Dose unchanged (unless repeated often) Administer furosemide concurrently
Diabetes	Hyperglycemic Hyperosmolar Nonketoacidotic coma	Follow plasma glucose Adjust dose of Hypoglycemic drug

Drug—problem interactions (diazoxide)

Finding	Potential adverse effect	Quantitative data/ cautions
Pregnancy (W/long term pregnancy)	Terotogenic effects	
Ischemic Cardiovascular disease, severe	Infarct (Due to poor perfusion of tissue during rapid reduction of blood pressure)	Consider alternate hypotensive, e.g. sodium nitroprusside

Display 77

Diazoxide potentiated by

Drug	Possible clinical effect	Quantitative data/cautions
Thiazide diuretics (Thiazides relax Peripheral Arterioloar Smooth muscle Initially reduce ECF, plasma volume, sodium cardiac output)	Decreased fluid retention Enhanced hypotensive effect	Therapeutic intention

Diazoxide potentiated by

Drug	Possible clinical effect	Quantitative data/cautions
Furosemide Ethacrynic acid (These drugs maintain negative sodium balance)	Enhanced hypotensive effect.	Therapeutic intention

Display 78

Diazoxide:
Drug—test interactions:
Physiologic drug effects:
    Plasma glucose elevated
    Serum uric acid elevated

It is clear from all these displays how a guidance system has been produced. Further guidance is available for monitoring drug therapy with
displays for direct ordering of blood levels etc. when appropriate.

Indeed, there are many aspects of the guidance system, the audit structure, and the population studies that are now shown by this selected
sequence of basic functions.

Chapter 5

Focusing on the Legal Properties and Uses of Medical Records

CHAPTER OBJECTIVES

1. Differentiate between confidentiality and privacy
2. Relate ownership of information to ownership of recorded information
3. Recognize the role of the health record professional in providing policies and procedures that address confidentiality of patient data
4. Relate selected legal terms and their definitions to functions of health information management
5. Understand the meaning and function of a subpoena duces tecum
6. Recognize the significant impact of computer technology on legal issues and concerns in health information

Managers of patient information systems are responsible for establishing and maintaining effective methods in providing patient information for individual care. They are also charged with the responsibility for planning, processing, and promoting collective use of patient information as discussed in Chapter 3. A third charge is to understand, inform, and establish procedures for monitoring legal issues and processes of medical and health records. Health information managers are responsible for safeguarding the information. The following statements reflect the range of concerns involved in this area:

- The medical record is the legal document of the facility. Not only does it document the health services rendered to the patient during a given period of time, but also it is viewed by law as the official recorded proof that specific patient services were provided.

- Specific components must be present in patient records that demonstrate that appropriate services were provided. This includes identification of published standards that specify what constitutes a patient record within a particular health care setting.
- In cases where evidence of health care status is required, the medical or health record can serve as a legal tool for patients. This record is also useful in personal injury cases between patients and third parties.
- In the event of malpractice suits, the medical record is used against the providers and the health facilities by individual patients.
- Standards for care are designated in hospital bylaws, established by individual departments such as surgery, obstetrics, and psychiatry, and verified through examination of patient records.
- Information abstracted from patient records for use in administrative and clinical assessment programs and incorporated into committee minutes can be a target for legal scrutiny.
- The health information manager is responsible for policy and procedure development in identifying, supporting, and maintaining appropriate legal activities involved with patient information for individual patients and the health facility.

You can see in Exhibit 5-1 that the challenge for health information managers is far-reaching.

This chapter is directed to three major concerns:

1. The current issues of legal properties of medical records are confidentiality, individual control of personal medical information, data security in patient information, computerization, and ownership of the medical record.
2. Managers of patient record systems must target legal and professional resources to meet these needs. This includes familiarizing yourself with useful legal terms and concepts, the American Medical Record Association (AMRA) Confidentiality Position, Ethical Tenets of the Joint Task Group on Patient Confidentiality in Health Data Centers, Policy Analysis and Recommendations identified in *Computers, Health Records and Citizen Rights*, and *Personal Privacy in an Information Society* from the Report of the Privacy Protection Study Commission.
3. Effective monitoring of patient information related to current legal issues requires the ability to understand and apply appropriate methods and procedures within specific medical record departments. Health information managers' responsibilities include monitoring

Exhibit 5-1 Challenges and Responsibilities of Health Information Managers

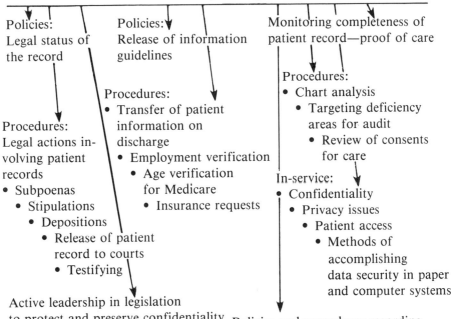

Health Facility Governing Board—Board of Trustees
. . . have the full legal responsibility for
the activities of the facility

Chief Administrative Officer
. . . responsible for carrying out policies (nonmedical)

Health Information System Manager
. . . responsible to administrator for carrying out
policies and procedures related to health information activities
as established by the organization

Policies:
Legal status of
the record

Policies:
Release of information
guidelines

Monitoring completeness of
patient record—proof of care

Procedures:
Legal actions in-
volving patient
records
• Subpoenas
  • Stipulations
    • Depositions
      • Release of patient
        record to courts
        • Testifying

Procedures:
• Transfer of patient
  information on
  discharge
  • Employment verification
    • Age verification
      for Medicare
      • Insurance requests

Procedures:
• Chart analysis
  • Targeting deficiency
    areas for audit
    • Review of consents
      for care

In-service:
• Confidentiality
  • Privacy issues
    • Patient access
      • Methods of
        accomplishing
        data security in paper
        and computer systems

Active leadership in legislation
to protect and preserve confidentiality
• Keeping informed of current laws
  • Participating on review boards
    and in public hearings on legal
    issues
    • Preparing formal responses/
      amendments
      to proposed legislation via
      professional groups

Policies and procedures regarding
care providers' access to patient records
• Physical security
  • Employee education
    • Maintaining log of users' access
      to patient records
      • Developing computer techniques
        to protect access
        • Reviewing audit records on
          access practices

authorizations for treatment, special procedures, and release of information as well as access to patient records, transfer of information, and carrying out legal activities within the department.

Medical record practitioners must build on knowledge of current legal issues and be prepared to communicate these issues to allied health professionals and service personnel within the health care delivery system. They must adapt and construct effective policies and procedures using existing resources that address ways and means of handling patient information within legal guidelines, such as the AMRA Confidentiality Position, Ethical Tenets for Health Data Centers, and recommended and proposed policies and statutes. Legal properties constitute another eclectic building block in the foundation of effective health information systems management. Let's examine the current issues involved in the legal properties of medical and health records.

CONFIDENTIALITY AS A LEGAL PROPERTY OF THE MEDICAL RECORD

Individual mental and physical health is a distinct aspect of personality. Each of us experiences health problems and relates information about these problems to someone else—usually a doctor or nurse. This information is about ourselves. Relating the information creates the record that can be a permanent representation and a unique description of an individual. We consider it private. Although there is no doctrine of confidential communications under common law, it is accepted that information contained in the medical record is private and personal, therefore confidential. This concept is widely supported by state statutes and formulated in the professional ethics of physicians and other health care professionals. In *Privacy Definition*, developed by Dr. Willis H. Ware, Rand Corporation, September 23, 1975, confidentiality is defined as:

> Status accorded to data or information indicating that it is sensitive for some reason, therefore needs to be protected against theft or improper use, and must be disseminated only to individuals or organizations authorized to have it.[1]

Privacy is a right. Declaring information confidential is formally recognizing the inherent right of patients to privacy. Confidentiality indicates that individuals have the right to say what information about them will be available to whom. This is an extension of our democratic practice of freedom. To acknowledge confidentiality of data implies that individuals have a right to control, insofar as possible, their own destiny. Awareness of this led Congress to pass Public Law 93-579, also known as the Privacy Act of 1974.[2] This law requires federal agencies that maintain records of any type on individuals to permit the person to determine what records are maintained and for what purpose. There are five major elements:

1. It allows the individual to know identifiable, personal information is available in a record or record system and what that information is used for.
2. It allows the individual access to the records, the right to have a copy made, and the right to amend or correct the records.
3. It prevents use beyond that for which the data are collected (as specified by law or regulation).
4. It requires that written consent of the individual be obtained for all other uses.
5. It requires that data be collected and used only for a necessary and lawful purpose.

Another example of an individual's right to privacy is the statute on confidentiality of alcohol and drug abuse records that became effective August 1, 1975.[3] This act severely limits the dissemination of information on persons enrolled in alcohol and drug abuse treatment programs. The purpose of this act is to prevent intentional or inadvertent disclosures of personal information, including an individual's identity as a patient. This is an extension of the patient-physician relationship. Confidential communications statutes are intended to protect the patient and encourage confidence in information sharing to better effect health care services. Many states are developing bills of rights for patients in health care settings. The statements include the standards indicated in the Privacy Act of 1974, but they also extend beyond it when they define the role of the patient in designating as confidential communication between the patient and health care providers. Appendix 5A is a patient's bill of rights developed by the American Hospital Association.

MONITORING CONFIDENTIALITY

In hospitals, medical record departments are responsible for establishing appropriate policies and procedures for safeguarding the confidential information of the patient. The medical record professional carries out in-service training for hospital employees regarding information handling and elements of confidentiality. In some large medical centers, the record department may be part of a department of information services, which includes admitting, outpatient, and social services.

Ambulatory care settings such as hospital outpatient clinics and neighborhood health centers also develop policies and procedures to insure confidential handling of patient information. Specialized areas like psychiatric outpatient clinics and drug abuse clinics also must meet state statutes and federal requirements. In any environment, the patient or client has a right to determine what particular items of information will be stored and in what manner the information will be accessible and retrievable.

INSUFFICIENT CONFIDENTIALITY LAWS

Two major concerns exist in the handling of confidential information. The first is the understanding and use of consents for release of confidential information. Information is released for a variety of reasons ranging from credit information verification to insurance or employment eligibility. In some cases, prospective employers are interested in the medical information of an employee because the company pays the insurance premiums. Consents for release of confidential information are integral elements in health insurance programs and health maintenance organizations (HMOs). The individual may sign a consent for medical information to be freely available to the insurance or HMO provider for payment of benefits. Sometimes people unknowingly sign consents for release of medical information when they apply for insurance for themselves or family. It is a requirement for persons participating in the Medicare and Medicaid program that their medical information be available to the fiscal intermediary who pays the bills for the care provided. Blue Cross and Mutual of Omaha are examples of fiscal intermediaries. They regularly receive information from hospitals on Medicare patients treated. Decisions about eligibility and the extent of benefits covered are processed through the intermediary. The intermediary pays the hospital and is reimbursed by the federal government.

Many people are unaware how much information may be made available by signing a general release form. Figure 5-1 illustrates the range of authorizations. In *Computers, Health Records and Citizen Rights*, author Alan Westin studied the use of medical records when a patient seeks help from providers, including physicians, clinics, hospitals, and medical units of an institution. Westin examined the role of informed consent as it applies to release of information by the patient.

The study found that the requirement of informed consent by patients to release of their primary care data is rarely well observed today. In part, this is because consent is often coerced

Figure 5-1 The Range of Authorizations

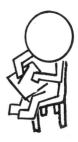

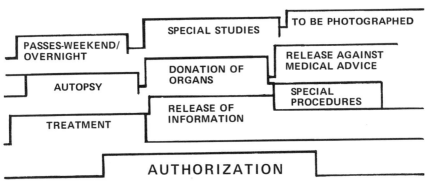

by the threat of losing services or is assumed to be implied. Informed consent is also weakened because patients do not have a general right to see what is in their records, either before the data is released to third parties or as a matter of patient interest during regular care. . . . Overall, the main finding of this section (primary care) is that identified patient information for medical records now flows regularly out of the primary care setting in ways that allow patients few controls over these disclosures.[4]

In 1979 three bills were introduced to Congress. These bills specifically address confidentiality of patient medical records, patient right to access their own medical record, and the right to make corrections in the record. These bills have significant implications for health information managers in all areas. With the exception of restrictions set forth in the confidentiality of alcohol and drug abuse records legislation, which takes precedent, regulations derived from this legislation will result in major policy changes in health information systems. See Appendixes 5C, 5D, and 5E of this chapter.

Managing health information so that it will benefit patient, provider, and society while protecting the individual's right to privacy, requires:

- Educating the consumer toward understanding the current processing of an individual's personal health information
- Recognition by the health care industry of the need to establish procedures that support current and projected legislation governing privacy and confidentiality
- Active monitoring of current and projected use of individual patient data
- Promoting concurrent developments for safeguarding patient data
- Active political support for laws dealing with violations of health information

Without consumer education, appropriate organizational policies and procedures, and informed up-to-date legislation, a comprehensive and workable plan for protecting the confidentiality of patient records will remain an unmet objective.

TECHNOLOGY AND CONFIDENTIALITY LAWS

The Potentials of Computer Technology

As in all areas of American life, computer technology is exploding into the health care environment. Computers have the power to enhance and extend the skill of providers. Patient information is collected faster and more accurately with computers. Scheduling services and reporting results of diagnostic tests are expedited. Billing and health insurance processing are simplified. Patient information, stored on magnetic tape at less cost than paper record systems, can be designed to provide doctors and other providers with faster access.

Hospitals and clinics can participate in shared computer systems that collect, process, and report statistics on patient services and needs based on diagnostic indexes, and so on. Studies comparing individual health facility performance with similar facilities are available. The Commission on Professional Hospital Activities (CPHA), Ann Arbor, Michigan, is an organization that has collected patients' data from hospitals and published epidemiological information and length-of-stay statistics since 1953. Today, similar shared computer systems like Medi-Tech Corporation offer computer system packages in which hospitals, nursing homes, and ambulatory care facilities send in statistical information that is put to a variety of uses. These include disease tracking, medical care evaluation, and audit programs. Chapter 3 introduced discharge abstract and statistical programs. Figure 5-2 illustrates many uses to which patient data are put and some of the forms they may take.

Figure 5-2 Various Uses of Patient Data

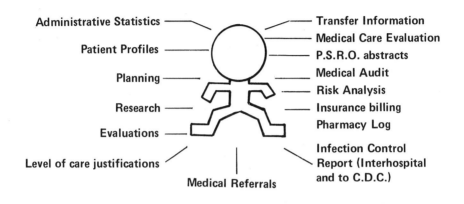

The introduction of technology in the form of computer service bureaus required an extension of the health facility responsibility to preserve confidentiality of patient information. Protectives were established for patient identification by individual profiles identified by number. The key to the patient's identity remained with the hospital. Agreements between health facilities and service bureaus included policies stated by the service bureau for treating confidentiality. When computer technology is housed within a health care facility, there is an increase in data about individual patients, and they are usually available in more locations within the organization. El Camino Hospital, for example, has computer terminals at the nursing stations where various users have access. Protection of data was also built into the technology. Monitoring confidentiality goes hand in hand with the technology. While paper printers make the printed record more readable and keep the information inquiry in one location, the use of cathode-ray tube (CRT) terminals opens up a Pandora's box for confidentiality. Machine and programming protectives need to be examined.

Potential invasion of privacy in vast information storage systems has not gone unnoticed. Concerned groups have monitored and studied the issue as the technology itself developed. *Databanks in a Free Society* is a report of the Project on Computer Data Banks which is a three-year research study done under the auspices of the Computer Science and Engineering Board of the National Academy of Sciences.[5] This report concluded a nationwide factual study on what the use of computers is actually doing to recordkeeping processes in the United States and what the growth of both manual and computerized large-scale data banks implies for the citizens' constitutional rights to privacy and due process. The report summed up the databanks and civil liberties problem as follows:

> If our empirical findings show anything, they indicate that man is still in charge of the machines. What is collected, for what purposes, with whom, information and what opportunities individuals have to see and contest records are all matters of policy choice, not technological determinism. Man cannot escape his social and moral responsibilities by murmuring feebly that "the machine made me do it."[6]

Health Professionals' Concerns

Medicine has responded to the conclusions regarding patients' rights, and individual special interest groups are assuming assertive roles in the confidentiality issue. Four significant published standards for handling confidential information in computer applications illustrate the continued commitment to this role.

The Joint Task Group was appointed in 1973 by the president of the Medical Society of the County of Erie and by the chairman of the Committee on Data Processing, Medical Society of the State of New York to form a multidisciplinary team to explore the potential use of electronic data processing and related scientific disciplines, and to examine the potential risks attached to computerization of sensitive clinical information. Exhibit 5-2 portrays the uses and risks of computerization of clinical information.

In 1975, the policies of confidentiality for professional standards review organizations (PSROs) were established by the U.S. Department of Health, Education, and Welfare (HEW) to assist PSROs in reviewing utilization of health services for patients participating in Medicare, Medicaid, and maternal or child health programs. HEW policies reflect a strong concern for maintaining personal privacy of the consumer.

In 1976, Alan Westin in his policy analysis and recommendations from *Computers, Health Records and Citizen Rights* promoted a strong role— both legislative and professional—to continue to direct and control the handling of information in large data banks and the harnessing of computer technology in medicine itself.

A fourth major publication item is from the report from the President's Commission to Study Privacy in Health Records, published July 1977. Results of this commission's study clearly revealed increasing evidence of a greater volume of medical data available to a wider spectrum of users under fewer controls than ever before. The commission focused on needs for more informed patient awareness prior to signing consents for release of personal

Exhibit 5-2 Ethical Tenets—Joint Task Group for Medical Computing, Medical Society of the County of Erie, New York

1. Adequate documentation is an essential part of clinical care. The comprehensive and accurate primary medical record shall serve as communication among those who contribute to the care of the patient. The physician and his team shall maintain an adequate primary record.
2. Primary medical records shall be handled in the same confidential manner in which the physician is obliged to keep medical information in confidence.
3. The patient shall be the owner of the information provided by him during medical care.
4. The physician should be the owner of the information generated by him during medical care.
5. Primary medical records shall be stored and handled only by the physician or his designee. The responsibility for confidentiality of the primary records shall rest with those providing for the care of the patient.
6. Computer-based data centers accepting, storing, and releasing identified medical records shall be formally considered a part of direct patient care, and they shall be designated as ethical clinical data centers.
7. Ethical clinical data centers shall provide assured confidentiality and they shall conserve the integrity of the primary medical records.
8. The patient shall be informed of the health data center maintaining his clinical records and of the center's data access policies.
9. Ethical clinical data centers shall provide adequately processed data, upon demand, to upgrade clinical medicine and to augment patient management.
10. Ethical clinical data centers shall maintain appropriate operational standards and adequate data security policies.
11. All professional members of the ethical clinical data centers shall act at all times with integrity and with professional responsibility.
12. Identified health-related information generated by the physician and his team for administrative, fiscal, epidemiologic, or other similar purposes falls into the category of secondary medical records.
13. Identified secondary medical records shall receive confidential treatment.
14. Identified secondary health-related information shall be used only for the purpose for which it is generated, and shall be destroyed, or at least disidentified, as quickly as possible.

15. Data centers handling secondary medical records shall be regulated. Such centers shall maintain explicit operational standards, approved by the reviewing agency of the State of New York, and they shall cooperate with the spirit of the regulations formulated by the reviewing agency of the State of New York.

---

information. There was also an acknowledgment of concern that patients themselves had limited access to their personal information and only rare opportunities to correct erroneous information. The results of this investigation were incorporated into the AMRA Confidentiality Position Paper reprinted in Appendix 5B.

Policy statements on confidentiality and privacy have been published by the American Orthopsychiatric Association and the American Society of Internal Medicine. A model state bill on confidentiality of health care was developed by the American Medical Association in 1976. The American Hospital Association has also published position statements on confidentiality of information related to computer technology. Health professionals in all phases of the delivery system are active consumers and assertive leaders in assessing and directing the effects of computer technology and confidentiality.

How Confidentiality Concerns Are Reflected

The data processing industry itself is working to meet the needs of citizens whose right to privacy must be protected in all segments of society. Legal records, financial information, and social information are other areas of concern. The need to develop data security is a primary force in systems design, as evidenced by the following statement by IBM.

1. Individuals should have access to information about themselves and recordkeeping systems. And there should be some procedure for individuals to find out how this information is being used.
2. There should be some way for individuals to correct or amend an inaccurate record.
3. An individual should be able to prevent information from being improperly disclosed, or used for unauthorized purposes without his or her consent unless required by law.
4. The custodian of data files containing sensitive information should take reasonable precautions to be sure that the data are reliable and not misused.[7]

These principles reflect the recognition by the data processing industry that privacy is a social and legal issue concerned with the right of the individual to exercise some control over personal information. The industry, therefore, assumes the responsibility for data security within its own organizations and in developing computer systems for its clients. Data security encompasses the policies and procedures established by an organization to protect its information from unauthorized or accidental modification, destruction, and disclosure.

Health facility administrators are responsible for their organization's information system. They are consumers and clients of computer technology. The health care industry defines data security requirements. The data processing industry designs and constructs the technology to meet those requirements. Let's look more closely at their ideas. Data processing professionals recommend policies that will assist in maintaining appropriate data security within the health care facility. The following are some suggestions:

1. Designate one person in the organization to be the security officer.
2. Make disciplinary measures for violations specific and available to all employees.
3. Establish procedures to protect data from unauthorized use.
4. Maintain records of all access to and use of data files and review them with an internal data security committee.
5. Develop and use audit programs that verify accuracy of data.

The reader recognizes issues that medicine has addressed in position papers and ethical tenets reviewed in the text. It is apparent that many are common goals. Another area the data processing industry addresses is the hardware architecture. Machine design and construction play a significant role. Some of the companies currently involved in developing these capabilities include General Electric, Honeywell, Computer and Business Equipment Manufacturing, Advanced Computer Techniques Corporation, Burroughs, IBM, and others.

The physical equipment (hardware) combines with stored programs (software) to produce methods for effectively handling data security. Users can be identified, verified, and role authorization validated through machine programs. Passwords, fingerprints, speaker verification, and ID badges are all methods that can be used. Sometimes a combination of these is used. In addition, the computer can be programmed to limit accessibility to certain files. In some cases, persons may be permitted to read files but not permitted to change any information contained in them. When badges and passwords are used, they are changed frequently. Terminals that are used for access to computer files can be locked in secure areas or equipped with key-operated power-on switches that cannot be used without the proper keys. Computers can be programmed to produce a log that records who has used the system, when, and how. This is a key element in audit control. Additional features of audit control are discussed in Chapter 9.

How Health Record Professionals Can Help

Join the team! As a professional concerned with information handling, seek and chair committees in your health facility that develop policies in confidentiality. Participate in legislative hearings in the community. Work with your professional associations to develop and submit position papers where developmental work is being done. Join the team of system planners within your facility, and participate in community data collection and health statistics programs. If you acquire knowledge about computer capabilities and exercise consumer muscle in working with data processing departments within your organization and as clients of shared computer systems, your role will be clearly defined. Computers, an extension of technology, have become common. Data handling will always be a critical support service in medical care, and the record professional must use technology to meet medical information goals. The Joint Task Force for Medical Privacy and Computer Technology has proposed a role for the medical record administrator in a health data center.[8]

1. Definition: Data Security Administrator is a specially trained medical record administrator who is proficient in information science, medical information handling and data security systems maintenance and supervision. He must be trained and/or certified by a recognized authority verifying his level of expertise.
2. The Data Security Administrator will develop the plans for the data security system. He must be proficient in all the ramifications of data security. He must be aware of the latest technology available and be able to implement and supervise the system.
3. The Data Security Administrator must be able to maintain the system once installed. We see this as a system of checks and balances whereby the security is maintained by more than one administrator with no one being aware of the entire security system and with one administrator authorizing and balancing the other.
4. The Data Security Administrator will be the only person to override the system and release information deemed necessary but not covered by specific authorization, i.e., patient in

emergency situation and unable to give authorization or an authorized user requesting information from a different terminal for an authorized function, i.e., consultations or possible emergency acts with authorization being granted after direct communication with the user.

5. The Data Security Administrator must plan an important role in educating the public as to the security of their data establishing the confidence of the consumer in the system to encourage restricted deposit of data.

6. The Data Security Administrator must maintain the ethical tenets established governing the ethical health data center and encourage the formulation and continuous updating of these tenets.

7. The Data Security Administrator must maintain a documented security system whereby he can produce reports of ongoing monitoring of security risks. One means of doing this could be the keeping of a log whereby all transactions are recorded. He would also have to keep a surveillance over all physical parameters which could be security risks, i.e., maintenance of backup files, supervision of employment policy, etc.

8. Continuous revision by the Data Security Administrator of the data security system to correct for errors detected and to enhance cost effectiveness of the security system.

OWNERSHIP OF INFORMATION

Health Facility and Patient Ownership Rights

Ownership of health information is like two sides of a coin. The health facility rights of ownership are on one side, the patient rights are on the other. The health facility owns the record of services provided. It is a legal document. This is a business record that documents the care rendered and provides the collective information necessary to justify planning for continued services. The process of recording the events and services provided and basing future planning on information accumulated from this documentation is fundamental to all health facilities.

The record gives evidence that appropriate services were provided in an appropriate manner. If an organization's practice is questioned, the record may serve as legal protection. By demonstrating that correct procedures were ordered and carried out in rendering services, it also may serve as legal protection for health care providers. The record is a means of measuring medical care within the facility. By engaging in medical care evaluation, hospitals and other health facilities develop and maintain ongoing analysis of care and develop action plans for improving care. The record documents a dynamic delivery system, and if dynamic growth occurs, it will be found in the patient records from one period to the next.

The medical record is the document of communication between providers. It is the written record of all the multidisciplinary patient care planning and treatment done in a facility. It also provides an opportunity for that multi-disciplinary planning to fit together in a total care plan for each patient. The hospital record is a written account of all services provided from the time the patient is admitted until the patient is discharged. It includes the patients' physical location, names of the physicians, nurses, and other health professionals who provided care, and documents the result of the care.

The right of the patients to information about themselves is a vital topic in the health care industry. Many hospitals and clinics are making records available to patients on request. Some will duplicate the entire record for cost. Citizens rights movements set access to health records as a legitimate goal. This issue must be considered from alternative perspectives.

In a vocational rehabilitation center, the record will document the client's date of admission to the program, medical and social history, and occupational and physical therapy assessment. It will also document the course of treatment, including medical treatment, employment counseling, and final disposition of the case.

In a community mental health center, the record would document the ongoing relationship of the client to the center; it would include both a progress report on the client's condition and a record of medication and treatment rendered during the course of therapy. The role of both patient and provider will be pointed out. This is a vital document to health organizations. Administrators need it not only to monitor and evaluate people and programs, but also to provide accountability to the patient consumer.

To justify their programs and plan for future ones, all health facilities use cumulative information from the record of services rendered. Justification may include analyzing the effectiveness of services provided and assessing the potential role of the health facility.

To assist in budget planning for the facility, hospitals use information about the number of patients seen on the surgical service, including the kind of conditions treated, the specific services required, and how long the patients stayed in the hospital. One type of data used by health systems agencies (HSAs) is information collected from a number of skilled nursing facilities (nursing homes) in a given community. This data helps to determine if a certificate of need should be issued so that additional skilled nursing facilities may be built.

The Patient's Right to Control Access to Personal Information

The patient owns information about himself. It is recognized as personal. In Dr. Ware's definition of privacy, he states it to be:

> The right of an individual to be left alone to withdraw from the influence of his environment; to be secluded, not annoyed, and not intruded upon by extension of the right to be protected against physical or psychological invasion or against the misuse or abuse of something legally owned by an individual or normally considered by society to be his property. . . .[9]

The right to personal privacy has become increasingly important to us in our advancing technological society. Information cannot be separated from the individual and is considered in lieu of the person in many instances. Prospective employers, insurance companies, the Internal Revenue Service, and many others can and do treat the information in this fashion. A capable middle manager may be passed over for promotion because he has had a heart attack in the last year. A cancer patient may not be considered for employment due to anticipated problems in attendance and health insurance benefits. Prospective adoptive parents may not be considered as candidates for adoption because the mother was treated for mental illness five years ago. Even the option of joining a prepaid HMO may be restricted because the individual exceeded the average number of physician visits over the last three years. What is more frightening, individual citizens may not even know of these situations. They may receive the result and never know the basis for a particular decision. Ownership of the information contained in medical and health records must be recognized in two ways.

First, patients are seeking increased rights to their medical and health records. Health information managers will be seeing more and more of this and will need to plan policies and procedures to accommodate the changing needs. Second, the right of patients to correct erroneous data in the record is also emerging. Again, health information managers will need to keep abreast of legislation that focuses on this area. In his twelve basic principles in *Computers, Health Records and Citizen Rights*, Alan Westin suggests establishing a specific policy for patient access and incorporating the policy into an effective confidentiality model. He includes methods for handling sensitive data that providers believe will be harmful for patients to know. The reader should view Westin's comments as indicators of societal expectations in personal information handling.

TARGETING RESOURCES FOR POLICY DEVELOPMENT

Legal Terms and Concepts

Managers of patient information systems must target legal and professional resources to help them meet the needs in policy and procedure development. This includes a careful look at legal terms and concepts and a review of the various laws and position statements prepared by professional groups. Let's look at some useful legal terms and concepts. The excerpts listed below are representative of introductory legal definitions. Many of these are related to patient records and the handling of patient information.

Battery: Unauthorized or nonconsensual touching of a person.

Common law: The great body of unwritten law founded on custom, natural justice, and reason, sanctioned by usage and judicial decisions; used to refer to rules originating in court decisions.

Confidential information: A statement made to a lawyer, physician, or clergyman, in confidence and implicitly understood that it should remain a secret.

Consent: Concurrence of wills, voluntary yielding will to proposition of another. Acquiescence or compliance.

Contestant: One contesting a decision.

Deposition: The written testimony of a sworn witness in response to interrogation. Testimony taken on oath, in writing outside of the courtroom to be used as evidence.

Defendant: A person required to make answer in an action or suit; a person to whom an action is brought. In malpractice this could be the physician and the hospital.

Emancipation: Determined by age, intelligence, maturity, training, economic independence, general adult conduct and freedom from control of parents in considering whether parental consent is required for treatment.

Evidence: Primary, that evidence that suffices for the proof of a particular fact until contradicted or overcome by other evidence.

Expert witness: Those testifying to facts within their own knowledge who may give their opinions upon assumed facts.

Hearsay rule: Statements made by one, not a party in interest, not a party to the action, and not made under oath.

In loco parentis: In the place of a parent.

Independent contractor: One who exercises an independent calling and is subject to the control of no one in his work.

Liability: State or quality of being responsible, or having a legal obligation. That which is under obligation to pay. Hospitals, nursing homes, and health care providers can all be considered responsible for services they render.

Liability insurance: Insurance to cover answerable claims such as malpractice insurance. Physicians and other direct care providers carry malpractice insurance.

Litigation: A lawsuit.

Misrepresentation of fact: A basis for suit where a physician deliberately misleads a patient in order to obtain the patient's consent.

Judicial contest: Any controversy that must be decided upon evidence.

Malpractice: Professional misconduct or unreasonable lack of skill; failure to employ that reasonable degree of learning, skill and experience which ordinarily is possessed by others of his profession.

Negligence: Inadvertent act or omission resulting in injury; willful departure from approved medical practice.

Non compos mentis: Of unsound mind; includes all forms of mental unsoundness.

Notary public: Public officer whose function is to administer oaths; attest and certify by hand or official seal certain classes of documents to give them authenticity in foreign jurisdictions.

Notary subpoena: Used as a pretrial discovery procedure. It is issued by a notary public. The medical record is taken to an attorney's office instead of to court. The purpose of this type of subpoena is to expedite the trial of cases.

Plaintiff: One who commences personal action or suit to obtain a remedy for injury to his rights. The complaining party in any litigation. A patient suing a physician for malpractice would be the plaintiff.

Prima facie: Evidence sufficient to establish the fact and if not rebutted becomes conclusive of the fact.

Privileged communication: A statutory right of patients to object to their physician's testifying in a legal proceeding about matters related to their medical treatment.

Rebuttal: Defeat or take away from the effect of something. Testimony intended to deny or contradict.

Refutation: The act of proving the falsity or error in a statement, a proposition, or an argument.

Release: A written instrument by which some claim or interest is surrendered to another person. Release of information is a term that medical record administrators and medical record technicians will use routinely.

Res ipsa loquitur: Stands for "The occurrence speaks for itself." (The proof that an accident took place.)

Respondeat superior principle: "Let the master answer." The principle applies if an employee-employer relationship exists, that is, if the person is employed by the facility, and if the action in question was carried out by the employee in the course of his or her employment. This is the doctrine that says the employer is responsible for the act of an agent or servant. When a patient sues a nurse who is employed by the hospital, they also sue the hospital.

Rules of exclusion: Evidence offered will be excluded from the record of proceedings or from being received in evidence if it is not properly qualified or not properly identified. Medical record administrators direct staff to take medical records to court and testify to their identity as medical records from the institution in which they originated.

Shop book rule: A rule of evidence allowing the admission in evidence of a party's original business records. Medical records are considered the legal account of medical services provided to patients and are covered by this rule. There must be proof that such records were made in the routine course of hospital activity, that it was a business procedure of the hospital to make such records, and that the records were made at or near the time of the event or transaction recorded.

State statutory law: Written law that is enacted by the state legislature and carried out by state administrators. It is also referred to as administrative code.

Statute of limitations: A law limiting the period of time during which an action must be brought.

Stipulation: To specify, signify in a binding agreement; as in to designate that a document is the legal medical record for the institution.

Subpoena: A notice compelling the attendance of a person in court.

Subpoena duces tecum: A notice compelling the attendance of a person in court and ordering him to bring the books, documents, or other evidence described in the writ. It is signed by a clerk of the court or a deputy. This is what directs a record administrator or employee of a medical record department to bring a particular record to court.

Suit: An action or process in a court for the recovery of a right or claim.

Summons: A process (document) served on a defendant in civil court action to secure his appearance in the action.

Tort: An injury or wrong committed with or without force to the person or property of another. Tort claims deal with civil or federal wrongs.

Trial court: The formal examination of the matter in issue in a case before competent tribunal for the purpose of determining such issues. The court before which issues of fact and law are first determined.

Verdict: The findings or decision of a jury on the matter submitted in trial decision or judgment, opinion pronounced.

Waiver: The voluntary relinquishing of a known right.

Witness: One who testifies to facts within his or her own knowledge.

Written authorization: A written statement to clothe with legal power; to empower.

Here are some examples of state laws that affect patient-provider relations and hospital record management in legal cases.

Privileged communications. The Revised Code of Washington (RCW) 5.60.060 states:

> A regular physician or surgeon shall not without the consent of his patient be examined in a civil action as to any information acquired in attending such patient which was necessary to enable him to prescribe or act for the patient.

Business records as evidence. RCW 5.45.020 refers to the admission of the medical record as evidence and the testimony by the medical record administrator or a designee of the record administrator that this is in fact a record kept in the regular course of business.

> Business records as evidence; a record of an act, condition or event shall insofar as relevant be competent evidence if the custodian or other qualified witness testifies to its identity and the mode of his preparation and if it was made in the regular course of business; at no time near the time of the act, condition, or event, and if in the opinion of the court the source of information, method, and time of preparation were such as to justify its admission.

Recorded instruments. RCW 5.44.050 states that certified copies of recorded instruments, such as a deed, conveyance, bond, mortgage, or other writings, can be accepted as evidence in a court of law.

Incident reports in health care facilities document unforeseen, unusual, or accidental events. These administrative reports record what took place, including the approximate or correct time of the incident, the date, and a description of the incident and its known results. Useful for quality control and planning for risk management, incident reports are filled and retained by administration and, on a temporary basis, by nursing. They are not a part of the patient's record.

The previous terms represent the kind of information medical record administrators and medical record technicians need to know. Record personnel may need to know more extensive terminology, depending on the particular application or department in which they work.

On the following list are topics and concepts that health information managers in each state should be aware of so that they can develop the procedures for recording and transferring information about the activities of their institutions that satisfy state statutes in these areas:

- abortion (i.e., authorizations; reporting requirements)
- addiction (addiction would relate directly to confidentiality standards on alcohol and drug abuse that prohibit release of information except in very specific and detailed informed consent formats)
- adoption
- anatomical donations
- artificial insemination
- authorization for treatment
- autopsies and postmortems
- birth and death certificates
- child abuse reporting
- commitment of the mentally ill
- consent (directed to health care)
- confidentiality
- controlled substances (directed to medication; may refer to confidentiality on alcohol and drug abuse)
- definition of death
- discharge against medical advice
- emergency aid
- informal consent
- injuries (when occurring within health facilities; area reporting requirements)
- incident reports (validation in health records: use in safety committee activities)
- liability for unauthorized treatment
- licensure: Practitioners should know of licensure for physicians and allied health professionals and be aware of the accrediting criteria used within the health care delivery system generally.
- living will
- mandatory reporting requirements for city, state, and federal bodies (i.e., uniform discharge data sets)
- physician's assistants and nurse practitioners (many states have passed nurse practitioner statutes)

- patient records: transfer or sale; retention limits of patient records; client or resident records may be used synonymously
- reportable diseases as in national, city, and medical record; this is becoming a civil issue around the country, and practitioners should be aware of the laws within their area
- right to refuse treatment (documentation in the patient record)
- state institutions
- statute of limitations (variations)
- transfer agreements as established under Medicare and Medicaid laws that provide for automatic transfer of the patient information

This list of terms is important to the health information manager. If you scan the list, you can select items that would reflect forms in the patient record; they might reflect the establishment of a registry, such as a donor registry; they may establish communication procedures between the family and nursing, medical records, and social service personnel. Certain items may involve verification that appropriate release forms have been satisfactorily completed in the record. If the concept includes recording activities, then the health information manager has to know what is required at what intervals. As discussed in Chapter 3, the role of statistics and its relationship to the collecting, processing, and retrieval of information is critical to effective management of the data system. The concepts listed above are treated individually in each state. There also may be city or county ordinances that affect them. Concerned, informed practitioners should make them part of their file.

Setting up policies and procedures, looking at the various legal terms, and targeting particular laws or statutes that need to be explained for the state that you are working in is only the beginning. Appendix 5B is the AMRA position paper on confidentiality that was drawn up in April 1978. The paper takes a comprehensive look at the health information issue and discusses primary and secondary users of health information. It gives a breakdown on social uses of the information and also indicates how that information might be misused. The reader should consider the paper a resource that outlines parameters that can be used in establishing an individual program within an organization to handle the legal issues and the matters of confidentiality.

Policy Analysis and Recommendations: Twelve Basic Principles for Health Data Systems

The following summary of policies and recommendations for health data systems is based on *Computers, Health Records and Citizen Rights* prepared by Alan Westin.[10] You will see that Westin focuses on national legislation to protect personal information. He recommends that professionals and patients alike work for confidentiality of patient information.

1. *Public Notice and Impact Statements.* Whenever an automated data system with identified personal records is to be created for health care, service payment, quality assurance, medical research, or supervisory administration over health care, a notice should be filed with an appropriate outside authority and communicated to any continuing population of individuals whose records will be affected. A procedure should be provided for interested persons and groups to appear and make their views known on the proposed data system and on adequacy of its measures to protect citizen rights. To help focus public discussion, the organization's notice should include a privacy impact statement. This statement should describe ways in which the proposed automated data system would affect existing policies and procedures relating to citizen rights in that organization's use of personal data.

2. *Limits on Collecting and Recording Personal Health Data.* An organization creating a health data system should examine whether the collection and/or recording of each element of personal health information is essential for carrying out the organization's proper functions. Socially acceptable standards of *relevance* and *propriety* should be worked out for the data systems in each of the three zones of health data use, through public discussion and appropriate policy-setting mechanisms.

Zone 1 Primary Health Care—Medical records created when a patient seeks care from a health professional-personal physician, hospital, health center or clinic, etc.

Zone 2 Supporting Activities—The use of medical records by those who pay for medical care, both private insurance companies and government programs like Medicare and Medicaid; and by private groups and government agencies that review medical records to determine whether hospitals and other health care providers are in fact delivering the health care for which they are being reimbursed.

Zone 3 Social Users of Health Data—The use of medical records in the nonmedical world in determining whether individuals are eligible for licensing, employment, education, life insurance, credit, welfare and other government benefits, and when they are subject to investigation by law enforcement agencies.

3. *Notifying Individuals of Data Policies When Their Information Is Sought.* When an individual is asked to supply personal information to be included in a health data system, he or she should be given a clear written account of how that information will be used by the collecting

organization. This account should also include procedures for obtaining consent, which will be followed before any additional uses will be made within the collecting organization or identified information is supplied to other parties.

4. *Information Release Forms for Specific and Limited Purposes.* Because the trend in automated health data systems is to record and retain personal information more fully and systematically, general release forms do not meet proper standards of citizen rights. The forms used to release personal information from a health data system should not only be for a specific purpose, but should also describe the information to be released and limit the time period for which the release applies. Adequate procedures must be followed to obtain the individual's voluntary and informed consent to any release. Provision of entire medical records under release procedures should be permitted only upon use of a special release form, reviewed by a special officer of the recordkeeping organization. Organizations seeking release of information must file a form with the record custodian indicating how they would use the data, specifying that it will not be released without the individual's consent, and indicating what the retention or destruction policies are for the information so obtained.

5. *Increasing Patient Access Rights.* Individuals should have a general right to information about their health condition, treatment, and prognosis. It is the professional's duty to protect the patient's right to choose his or her own health destiny. In health data systems, an individual should have an absolute right to inspect any recorded data that is used to make judgments about eligibility for health programs and coverages, claims payment, or other aspects of service administration. The same absolute rights, benefits, or opportunities are applicable outside primary care settings, as in insurance, employment, licensing, education, or welfare. Procedures should be provided for explaining medical terminology when necessary and for allowing the individual to challenge the accuracy or completeness of the recorded data.

Where there are sensitive judgments about the patient's emotional condition that might be upsetting to the patient and these materials are used solely within the primary care facility, a procedure should be afforded that gives the physician an opportunity to explain to the patient why access would not be desirable or to suggest disclosure to another physician of the patient's choice; but if the patient is not persuaded by these counsels, a right of access should be provided to patients in either chronic or acute care. Disclosure of the patient's record, over the advice of the psychiatrist, requires an order from a civil court.

6. *Insuring Appropriate Accuracy.* The managers and staff of a health data system must take steps to see that personal data stored are accurate, timely, and complete. The uses of data require not only assuring the individual's proper health care, but also protecting the social opportunities and benefits of individuals that may be determined through use of such data. Patient participation in reviewing their records before release to third parties and a general right of access to their own records represent helpful ways to improve accuracy in such data systems.

7. *Applying Appropriate Data Security Measures.* Because of the sensitivity of the personal information stored in a health data system, security measures must be taken to limit access to records to those persons within the organization who have a need to see particular information items. Security measures should monitor data uses against unauthorized conduct and should protect files against outside penetration.

8. *Inculcating Respect for Citizen Rights.* There is a great gap between publishing organizational rules or enacting legal rights and achieving compliance with those rules and rights in daily life. Every health data system should develop orientation programs, interpretive guidelines, continuing seminars, problem-solving sessions, special training materials, and annual reviews to foster understanding and acceptance of the system's policies on citizen rights by the organization's own personnel. Such programs should recognize and deal with the special attitudes of major occupational groups in the organization (doctors, nurses, other health workers, administrators, data processing staffs, and so on). Wherever possible, patients and public representatives should be included in the development, management, and evaluation of these educational programs.

9. *The Need for a Patient's Rights Handbook and a Patient's Rights Representative.* Every health data system in primary care should publish a clearly written guidebook on patient's rights and responsibilities. This book should be given to the individual at the earliest point of contact with the facility. Each system should also have a person who serves as a patient's rights representative. The presence of and means for contacting this representative should be described in the handbook given to every patient.

10. *Independent Auditing and Periodic Review.* The use of electronic data processing (EDP) by organizations is not a onetime decision as to what will be automated and how, but a continuous process of expanding initial computer applications to additional files, new combinations of data, and more extensive data utilization (often reflecting new technological resources). Health data systems must be subject to regular review by an independent body, which should focus not only on the continuing

adequacy of the organization's policies and data security in light of changing data processing practices, but also examine any major expansion of the data system that would have significant impact on its treatment of citizen rights.

11. *Privacy and Public-Access Interests.* There is inevitable tension between the individual's right to privacy and the public's right to examine and supervise operations of its social institutions (especially when these are heavily supported by public funds). The rules of confidentiality set by health data systems should be examined carefully to avoid adding to existing difficulties in monitoring compliance with health program requirements and assessing the quality of health care that providers give. Using medical records without unique identifiers or with potentially identifiable data removed represents the major technique for softening the conflict between privacy and public-access interests.

12. *Reviewing and Evaluating Health Data.* Securing informed, voluntary consent should cover most situations in which medical research and program evaluations need to be conducted. However, through the use of identified data from health systems, there will be situations in which this is not feasible. In those cases, a health data system should have the purpose, procedures, and safeguards of the research reviewed by a special panel. This panel, made up of representatives from the organization owning the data system, outside scholars of high reputation, and leaders of public-interest groups relevant to the research project (minority racial groups, women's groups, civil liberties groups, and so on), is capable of reviewing such research. Furthermore, securing a legal privilege against any compulsory disclosure of research records should generally be a prerequisite for a health data system's agreement to participate in a research study, disease register, or program evaluation involving highly sensitive personal information.

EFFECTIVE MONITORING OF PATIENT INFORMATION

Health information managers must monitor the handling of patient information. Previously, we focused on a variety of concerns for health information managers. We looked at legal terms and position statements that reflect the current thinking on information handling. The health information manager must determine the specific procedures that should be used in any health information department that deals with health or medical records of any kind. Notice the variety of functions that were listed in Exhibit 5-1. The policy areas on legal status, release of information, and monitoring for completeness should be well defined within the organization. Procedures carry out the policies. Exhbits 5-3 through 5-6 show condensed procedures for handling subpoenas, stipulations, depositions, and release of patient records to the court. Managers will need to prepare such procedures to carry out policies identified in this chapter that are judged pertinent to their particular organization.

Exhibit 5-3 Release of Information Log Book

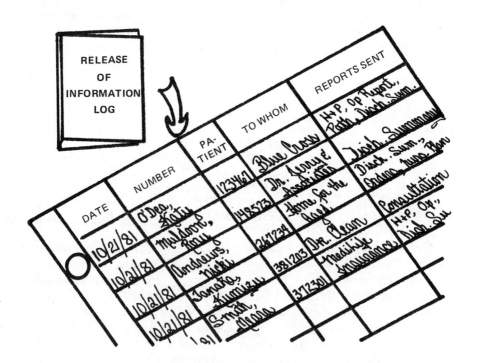

Exhibit 5-4 Procedures for Handling a Subpoena Duces Tecum

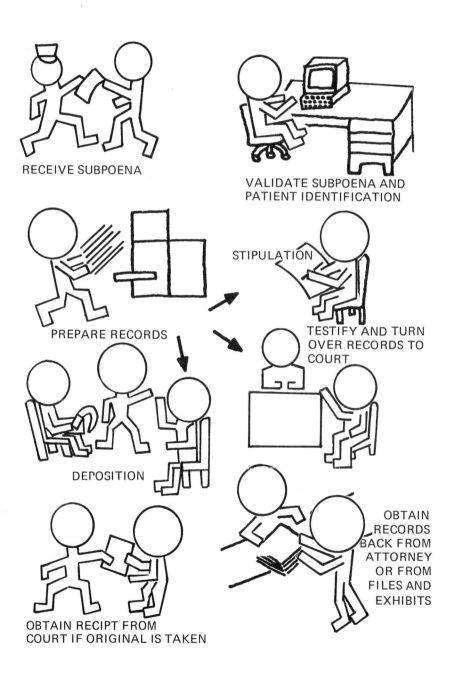

RECEIVE SUBPOENA

VALIDATE SUBPOENA AND
PATIENT IDENTIFICATION

PREPARE RECORDS

STIPULATION

TESTIFY AND TURN
OVER RECORDS TO
COURT

DEPOSITION

OBTAIN RECIPT FROM
COURT IF ORIGINAL IS TAKEN

OBTAIN
RECORDS
BACK FROM
ATTORNEY
OR FROM
FILES AND
EXHIBITS

Exhibit 5-5 Responding to a Subpoena of Records on Microfilm

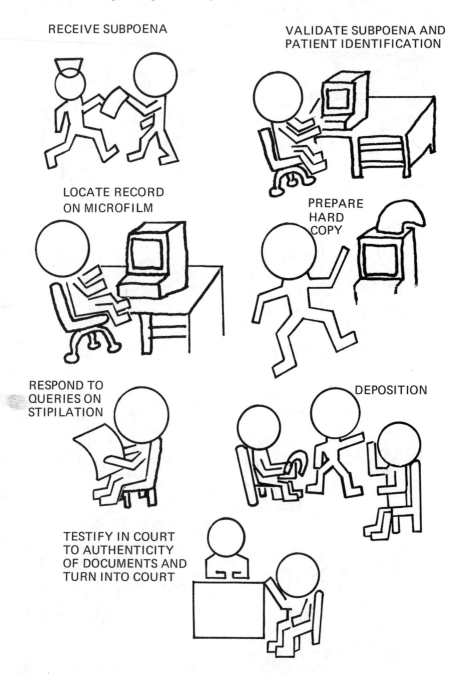

Exhibit 5-6 Responding to a Subpoena of Computerized Records

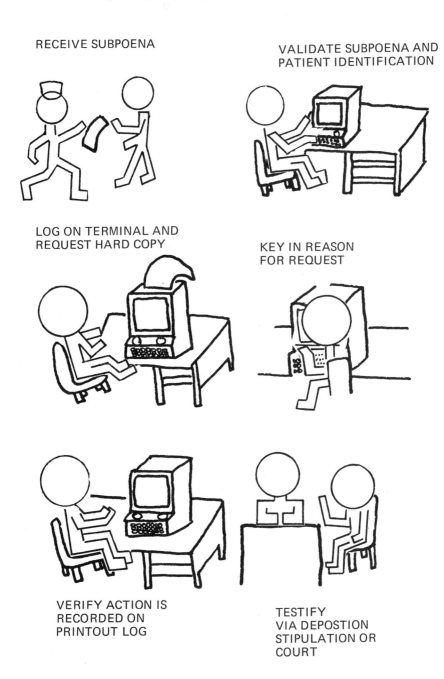

RECEIVE SUBPOENA

VALIDATE SUBPOENA AND PATIENT IDENTIFICATION

LOG ON TERMINAL AND REQUEST HARD COPY

KEY IN REASON FOR REQUEST

VERIFY ACTION IS RECORDED ON PRINTOUT LOG

TESTIFY VIA DEPOSTION STIPULATION OR COURT

NOTES

1. Alan F. Westin, *Computers, Health Records and Citizen Rights* (Washington, D.C.: Institute for Computer Sciences and Technology, National Bureau of Standards, U.S. Department of Commerce, December 1976), p. 348.
2. The Privacy Act of 1974, *P.L. 93-579* (Health, Education and Welfare, *Federal Register*, Wednesday, October 8, 1975).
3. Confidentiality of Alcohol and Drug Abuse Patient Records, *P.L. 93-282* (Health, Education and Welfare, *Federal Register*, Tuesday, July 1, 1975).
4. Alan F. Westin, op. cit., p. 12.
5. Alan F. Westin, "Databanks In a Free Society: A Summary of the Project on Computer Databanks," *Journal of Law and Computer Technology* (July/August 1973), p. 93.
6. Ibid., p. 102.
7. "IBM Reports," *U.S. News and World Report*, July 8, 1974, p. 59.
8. Gabrieli, Elmer E. "'Proposed Role of the Medical Record Administrator in an Ethical Health Data Center' Medical Privacy and Computer Technology," *Journal of Clinical Computing*, Vol. 1, 1974, p. 8.
9. Alan F. Westin, *Computers, Health Records and Citizen Rights*, p. 33.
10. Florence Isbell, Ed. and Alan F. Westin, *A Policy Analysis of Citizen Rights Issues in Health Data Systems* (Washington, D.C.: Institute for Computer Sciences and Technology, National Bureau of Standards, January, 1977), p. 28.

REFERENCES

Personal Privacy in an Information Society, Report of Privacy Protection Study Commission, July 1977.

Appendix 5A

A Patient's Bill of Rights

*The American Hospital Association Board of Trustees'
Committee on Health Care for the Disadvantaged, which has
been a consistent advocate on behalf of consumers of health care
services, developed the* Statement on a Patient's Bill of Rights,
*which was approved by the AHA House of Delegates February
6, 1973. The statement was published in several forms, one of
which was the S74 leaflet in the Association's S series. The S74
leaflet is now superseded by this reprinting of the statement.*

The American Hospital Association presents a Patient's Bill of Rights
with the expectation that observance of these rights will contribute to more
effective patient care and greater satisfaction for the patient, his physician,
and the hospital organization. Further, the Association presents these rights
in the expectation that they will be supported by the hospital on behalf of its
patients, as an integral part of the healing process. It is recognized that a
personal relationship between the physician and the patient is essential for
the provision of proper medical care. The traditional physician-patient relationship takes on a new dimension when care is rendered within an
organizational structure. Legal precedent has established that the institution
itself also has a responsibility to the patient. It is in recognition of these
factors that these rights are affirmed.

1. The patient has the right to considerate and respectful care.
2. The patient has the right to obtain from his physician complete current
information concerning his diagnosis, treatment, and prognosis in terms the
patient can be reasonably expected to understand. When it is not medically
advisable to give such information to the patient, the information should be
made available to an appropriate person in his behalf. He has the right to
know, by name, the physician responsible for coordinating his care.
3. The patient has the right to receive from his physician information
necessary to give informed consent prior to the start of any procedure
and/or treatment. Except in emergencies, such information for informed

---

Source: ©1975 by the American Hospital Association, 840 North Lake Shore Drive, Chicago,
Illinois 60611. Reprinted with permission of the American Hospital Association.

consent should include but not necessarily be limited to the specific procedure and/or treatment, the medically significant risks involved, and the probable duration of incapacitation. Where medically significant alternatives for care or treatment exist, or when the patient requests information concerning medical alternatives, the patient has the right to such information. The patient also has the right to know the name of the person responsible for the procedures and/or treatment.

4. The patient has the right to refuse treatment to the extent permitted by law and to be informed of the medical consequences of his action.

5. The patient has the right to every consideration of his privacy concerning his own medical care program. Case discussion, consultation, examination, and treatment are confidential and should be conducted discreetly. Those not directly involved in his care must have the permission of the patient to be present.

6. The patient has the right to expect that all communications and records pertaining to his care should be treated as confidential.

7. The patient has the right to expect that within its capacity a hospital must make reasonable response to the request of a patient for services. The hospital must provide evaluation, service, and/or referral as indicated by the urgency of the case. When medically permissible, a patient may be transferred to another facility only after he has received complete information and explanation concerning the needs for and alternatives to such a transfer. The institution to which the patient is to be transferred must first have accepted the patient for transfer.

8. The patient has the right to obtain information as to any relationship of his hospital to other health care and educational institutions insofar as his care is concerned. The patient has the right to obtain information as to the existence of any professional relationships among individuals, by name, who are treating him.

9. The patient has the right to be advised if the hospital proposes to engage in or perform human experimentation affecting his care or treatment. The patient has the right to refuse to participate in such research projects.

10. The patient has the right to expect reasonable continuity of care. He has the right to know in advance what appointment times and physicians are available and where. The patient has the right to expect that the hospital will provide a mechanism whereby he is informed by his physician or a delegate of the physician of the patient's continuing health care requirements following discharge.

11. The patient has the right to examine and receive an explanation of his bill regardless of source of payment.

12. The patient has the right to know what hospital rules and regulations apply to his conduct as a patient.

No catalog of rights can guarantee for the patient the kind of treatment he has a right to expect. A hospital has many functions to perform, including the prevention and treatment of disease, the education of both health professionals and patients, and the conduct of clinical research. All these activities must be conducted with an overriding concern for the patient, and, above all, the recognition of his dignity as a human being. Success in achieving this recognition assures success in the defense of the rights of the patient.

Appendix 5B

Confidentiality of Patient Health Information: A Position Statement of the American Medical Record Association

The basic research and assembly of this material, which now becomes an AMRA Position Statement, was first prepared as a Report by the Legislative Committee of the Pennsylvania Medical Record Association in 1976-77, as funded by AMRA's Executive Board. For these efforts, AMRA is most grateful.

That Report was then modified and subsequently adopted by the AMRA Executive Board in December 1977.

Preface

The Executive Board of the American Medical Record Association is proud to present this confidentiality document which states our position regarding the appropriate collection, dissemination and protection of an individual's personal health information.

At this time, when legislation is being prepared at the national, state and local levels regarding protection of privacy, confidentiality and freedom of information, it is imperative that our Association and its members, who are responsible for development of ethical practices to safeguard the information entrusted to their care, clearly affirm their position in this regard—to health care providers, third-party payors, government agencies, national and state health officials and legislators.

Source: Reprinted, with permission, from the April, 1978 issue of MEDICAL RECORD NEWS, published by the American Medical Record Association, 875 North Michigan Avenue—(Suite 1850), John Hancock Center, Chicago, IL 60611. Reprinted with permission.

The Executive Board strongly encourages each member to work diligently toward implementation by all health care providers of the letter and spirit of this report, including adoption of policies based on the model included herein by all health care providers.

Table of Contents

VI. Model Policies for Maintenance of Confidentiality of Patient Health Information
    1.0 Data Collection
    2.0 Storage
    3.0 Access

I. Introduction

The American Medical Record Association (AMRA) has traditionally been of service to its members and other health care professionals and agencies by providing guidance in the development of policies and procedures to those concerned with the collection, storage and dissemination of health care information.

AMRA has, since its founding in 1928, been committed to the highest ethical standards for its member practitioners. This position statement reflects a continuing concern in the development of laws, regulations and policies affecting health care information.

AMRA's members are, by training and experience, qualified to provide leadership in information systems which serve the needs of the patient, the institution and the public.

Through this position statement, AMRA establishes the concerns of its members over the abuses of confidentiality of health care information.

II. Philosophy

The primary purposes of the medical record are

a. To document the course of the patient's health care.
b. To provide a medium of communication among health care professionals for current and future patient care.

In order to fulfill these purposes, significant amounts of data must be revealed and recorded. The patient must be assured that the information shared with health care professionals will remain confidential, otherwise the patient may withhold critical information which may affect the quality of the care provided.

Economic issues, social issues, and technological advances have eroded the traditional relationship of confidentiality which exists between the patient and health care professional. Substantiation of payment claims has generated an increasing number of requests for information from patient health records. At the same time, the increase in the amount of computerized health data, the development of large data banks and the advancement of record linkage, pose a threat to the privacy of medical information. The public is generally unaware of this threat and the consequences of a loss of confidentiality in the health care system. Adequate measures to safeguard medical privacy must be established.

AMRA recognizes that patient health information provides a sound data base for a variety of legitimate activities. Through this statement, AMRA reaffirms the patient's right to privacy, including the privacy of the medical record. While the patient does not have the property right to the record, he should have the protected right of information. Further, in keeping with the spirit of informed consent, AMRA supports the right of the patient to have access to his own medical record, unless there are specific contraindications such as: a. Minors, b. Those deemed legally incompetent, c. Specific restriction by attending physician that access could be detrimental to the patient.

Therefore, subject to applicable authorized provisions, release of any individually identifiable medical information for any purpose other than direct patient care, must be done only with the expressed authorization of the patient or his authorized agent.

Further, AMRA recommends greater emphasis on the patient's right to privacy through: a. The establishment of written policies for the collection, storage and dissemination of information, b. Ongoing educational programs for all staff and personnel to enforce these policies.

With respect to this right of privacy, AMRA urges the development and implementation of programs to:

1. Protect the patient from invasion of privacy by protecting against indiscriminate and unauthorized access to confidential health information;
2. Promote appropriate usage and maintenance of confidentiality once health information is disseminated to authorized persons;
3. Educate the patient and the public to: a. Their rights of confidentiality, . . . b. Their right to restrict or limit dissemination of identifiable medical information, c. Their right of access to that information.

III. Current Usage of Patient Health Information

A. Release of Information

Health care facilities receive and respond to numerous requests for information from the medical records in their care. The requests may be written, by telephone or in person, from a broad spectrum of users. The responses are usually written, but in emergencies, may be given by telephone or to the patient or his representative. The health care facilities ordinarily consider the information to be released to fall into two categories:

1. "Confidential" information which requires the patient's written authorization or permission to release.

   Confidential information is provided to users such as insurance companies, credit agencies, attorneys and others who will use it for nonpatient care purposes. The authorizations are obtained from the patient by the insurance company, attorney, etc., at the time the initial agreement is made. Many are worded to permit the collection of information from any future medical records the patient's health care may generate. On some occasions, "confidential" information may be released without the patient's written authorization, but with his implied consent, usually to those who are currently caring for the patient. A record of what information and to whom it was released and a copy of the authorization are usually kept as part of the original medical record.

2. "Non-confidential" information or that information which may be released without the patient's authorization.

Most health care institutions have policies, procedures and systems for the controlled dissemination of information from their medical records to appropriate users.

B. Users and Uses of Health Record Information

The medical record is a compendium of information about an individual patient during the course of treatment of an episode or episodes of illness(es), or while maintaining an individual's state of health.

The record is made up of components, arranged in a logical sequence. The components include the physical and mental history of the current and previous illness, social factors which may contribute to the illness such as job, marital or other personal conflicts, the findings on physical examinations, results of diagnostic tests such as x-rays, electrocardiograms, laboratory values, findings and opinions of consulting specialists, the treatment prescribed, a description of the patient's response to that treatment (or lack of response), diagnoses, operations and the plans for and goals of follow-up care. The primary reason for the collection of this sometimes voluminous and sensitive information is patient care.

The content of the medical record is developed as a result of the interactions of the members of the health care "team" who use it as their communication tool. The "team" is an interdisciplinary group which includes physicians, nurses and numerous allied health personnel.

They inform and advise each other through their entries in the record about their findings, observations, opinions and treatment of the patient. At the conclusion of treatment of the episode of illness the record is sent to the medical record department where it is processed.

Medical record department personnel are responsible to design and implement a system to provide for evaluation, retention and future utilization of patient information. Patient information is used to plan patient care, perform medical research, evaluate patient care and provide information to authorized users.

Current users of medical information and the purposes for which the information is used may be classified as follows:

USERS OF MEDICAL RECORDS

USES OF INFORMATION IN MEDICAL RECORDS

A. Health Care Providers, Institutional and Individual (Primary Users)

1. as a medium of communication among health care providers during the current episode of illness
2. as a reference for treatment of future illnesses
3. for training of physicians and other personnel—to assist students to relate theory with medical practice
4. for prospective and retrospective evaluation of the quality of patient care through review and analysis of patterns of care as documented in the medical record
5. for promotion of effective and efficient use of facilities, equipment, services, personnel and financial resources through statistical analysis of information abstracted from the medical record
6. for documentation of voluntary compliance with standards for accreditation of the institution
7. for research aimed at the improvement of treatment, assessment of disease detection methods, assessment of the effectiveness of medication and other treatments through study of appropriate cases
8. for documentation which demonstrates conformity to government regulations
9. follow-up care of patients with long-term illnesses and assessment of the efficacy of the care given

B. Payors for Services, private insurance plans, government insurance plans and programs (Secondary Users)

1. for substantiation of patient claims for payment of health care services
2. for audits of claims for health care services and professional fees
3. to monitor the quality and equity of care and services rendered to those insured
4. to assess and control the cost of health care services to those insured

C. Social Users

1.	Public Health Agencies	1.	in surveillance of diseases of epidemiologic significance through statistical analysis of information abstracted from medical records
2.	Medical and Social Researchers, institutional and extrainstitutional	1.	for investigations of disease patterns, effects of disease on functions of daily living, including occupational health and safety
3.	Rehabilitation and Social Welfare Programs	1.	in determination of need for specific types of rehabilitation programs through analysis of incidence data
		2.	in development of individual rehabilitation and training plans for participants in programs for the handicapped, retarded and drug and alcohol abusers
4.	Employers	*1.	for administration of employer-provided health insurance plans
		*2.	for determination of employment suitability
		3.	in treatment and analysis of job related injuries and correction of occupational hazards
		4.	to determine disability
5.	Insurance Companies	*1.	in determination of risks in writing insurance
		2.	in determination of liability for claims
6.	Government Agencies: federal, state and local	1.	for allocation of government resources for schools, health care facilities, education institutions, etc. based on vital statistics submitted from medical records
7.	Education Institutions	*1.	for assessment of suitability for admission to selected education programs
		2.	for maintenance of student and employee health programs
8.	Judicial process	1.	in adjudication of civil and criminal matters through use of the medical record as evidence through the legal process
		2.	in judicial process for involuntary admission of mentally ill
9	Law enforcement and investigation	*1.	in criminal investigation
		*2.	for security clearance programs
10.	Credit investigation agencies	*1.	for determination of credit eligibility
11.	Accrediting, Licensing and Certifying Agencies	1.	for demonstration of individual fulfillment of criteria for professional licensing by a state government agency
		2.	to ascertain competence of practitioners
		3.	for determination of compliance with criteria for hospital based education programs
		4.	as documentation of compliance with standards for institutional accreditation
12.	Media: press, radio, TV	1.	for announcements of developments in medical research
		2.	for reporting of health hazards, diseases affecting the public health and newsworthy events

*May in some instances be improper use.

IV. Problem Areas in the Use of Health Information

In a record-generating society, the maintenance of confidentiality is subject to a number of pressures through all stages of collection, storage and retrieval. The result of these pressures is most often the unauthorized access to information, either through routine indiscriminate dissemination or through failure to establish adequate policies and procedures governing individual and organizational access to identifiable data. There are several relevant problem areas which are to some degree interrelated.

A. Ownership of the Health Record and Health Information

The issue of ownership of the patient health record, as distinct from ownership of the information therein, is one which has not been resolved. While the patient may to some extent control access to his record by refusing consent to release of information, in many states he himself has access only through litigation or in accordance with the policy of the individual institution. In the private sector*, the physical document itself is not the patient's property, and in few cases is a full copy made available to him. In addition, many health care providers consider the document and its contents to be their own property, generated by them; by virtue of this "ownership" they feel themselves justified in exercising control over its release to the patient. For the most part, providers and institutions have failed to fully address the issue of ownership and its attendant implications for policy and procedure development. There may be somewhat casual access to the record by almost anyone *except* the patient—by transporters and processors of various levels of training and reliability. Access may also be obtained by unauthorized and in many cases unidentified users, both internal and external to the facility. Another by-product of refusal of patient access has been the recording of inaccurate and inconsistent information with minimal review conducted for relevance.

B. Patient Education

For the most part, patients are unaware of the full range of purposes for which the record is used, or of policies governing the release of information. They are mainly aware of those uses personal to them, such as planning of individual health care, or protection of legal interests in such matters as personal injury suits or applications for life insurance. Less well-known uses are those of medical care evaluation, research (whether internal or external to the institution), planning for facilities, and meeting the require-

---

*as opposed to governmental institutions.

ments of licensing, accrediting, and certifying bodies. Few have any concept of the quantity of information released to third parties, governmental or private.

There is growing emphasis on patient knowledge of self-care as appropriate criteria for patient care audits. This concept must be broadened to include patient knowledge of the record, its contents and its uses. It is the responsibility of the health care providers to act as educators—to focus on the knowledge deficit in the patient population and by correcting it to include the patient as an active contributor to the health care team, to the accuracy of his record, and to the assurance of its appropriate use.

C. *Nature and Extent of Information Collected, Stored and Accessed*

The health information gathered today is substantially different from that gathered in an era preceding the multipart form and word processing. Patient mobility and professional specialization mean that one family physician no longer carries the family health history in his head, with the aid of a few pertinent notes. Multiple providers mean that the record is a major central communication tool. Also, external agency needs and legal requirements affect data collection; social and family histories are now required by both accrediting and governmental agencies, for example. Thus, more and intimate detail of the patient's personal habits, social relationships, emotional and mental status, attitudes and preferences is being collected as part of medical data. This information is generally disclosed willingly by the patient but with the understanding that the confidentiality of the communication will not be breached. Routine processing, storage and retrieval functions are performed on the record as a whole; usually no data are screened or removed at any point. Consequently, a great deal of highly sensitive identifiable information may be retained for decades without review for relevance or propriety.

The sequel to prolonged storage of all information as a unit is often the release of that entire unit. A notable example is that of information released to insurance companies whose attempts to insure payment for no more care than is necessary have led to demands for far more data. These demands, together with facilities' budgetary crises and personnel reductions, have led to the frequent practice of indiscriminate photocopying in order to keep up with the workload. This results in volumes of unedited data released to third parties without restriction of use to a specific need and without requiring destruction of the information or of personal identifiers as quickly as possible. It has, in fact, proven almost impossible to discover what happens to such information; whatever policies for identification, retention and release exist within the agencies have seldom been made known to either the public or the health care providers.

D. Informed Consent

As may be inferred from the preceding paragraphs, the practice of obtaining informed consent is notable chiefly by its absence. There are at least three facets to this particular problem.

First, in "blanket consent", patients or guardians are asked to sign releases which allow facilities to disseminate "any and all" identifiable information to whomever is offering a benefit or service to the patient. The patient is not himself "informed" as to the full extent of the record's content, which segments of it will be open to third party access, or what will happen to the information once it is in the third party's possession. "Blanket consent" does not serve to instill a sense of responsibility in the collectors, storers and users of patient data.

Second, difficulty arises from the common third-party practice of requesting "prospective consent", or consent of release of information prior to treatment. This means that the patient is consenting to the dissemination of that which is not yet collected, a practice which precludes any intelligent decision-making on the part of the patient.

Third, most insurance companies request a form of consent which could be construed as "perpetual consent," since there is no attendant time limit set for validity of the consent. With other requestors, health care institutions vary in the time limits within which they accept patient consent as "current." In some cases health care institutions are adopting more stringent limits, but there is no uniformity of policy in this area.

E. Security Policies and Procedures

Failure to fully acknowledge that the facility owning an information system is directly responsible for its uses has led to practices which do not always support the ethical principles of confidentiality. This applies both to intra- and inter-institutional transactions. In a health facility a large number of persons handle personal information, often at locations remote from any central control area. Partly as a consequence of numbers and inconvenience, close monitoring of their activities is not routine. The categories of persons involved include transporters (e.g. patient escorts, elevator operators, car drivers), handlers (e.g. unit clerks and managers, admissions and billing clerks), internal processors (e.g. key punch operators, chart analysts, file clerks) and external processors (e.g. services for transcription, subpoenas, photocopy, microfilm, data processing, coding, and off-site storage).

The identification of legitimate investigators poses special problems. Law-enforcement officers, for example, sometimes are seen as authority figures and obtain unauthorized information from personnel who are uninformed or somewhat intimidated. Newspaper reporters, credit investigators and a variety of others without any legitimate need-to-know have been known to assume an almost limitless range of identities, including patient relatives, priests, messengers, and physicians, in order to obtain health information.

In an adequate information control system, identification of categories of authorized processors must be followed by clear identification of persons appropriate to perform such functions. Physical, technical and procedural security measures are developed with a degree of refinement dependent to some extent on the adequacies of the personnel control system. None of these controls have been sufficiently expanded to reflect record-keeping practices in today's society.

The emergence of the computer's role in the health care system increases the capacity for information storage and transfer and provides a new range of possibilities for unauthorized access to patient data. The image of giant and possibly unrestrained mechanical data banks has, however, captured a sufficient number of imaginations to result in several studies, publications and legislative proposals designed to assess and minimize the risks associated with automated record-keeping. What has not yet occurred is the translation of those concerns to the manual system. Both manual and computer systems face such risks as: untrained generators, processors or accessors who can inadvertently alter, release or lose information; natural forces such as fire or flood which can destroy any information improperly stored; use of information for purposes not specified at the time of consent to release; and information transferred or sold with malicious intent.

Few data processing policies and procedures are comprehensive, detailed, and applicable to all forms of processing. Operational standards usually are designed in accordance with those of other health-care facilities, whereas the best models are more likely to be found within high-risk industries. Standards devoted to protection of software—the record—rarely approach the caliber of those developed for the testing of expensive hardware. If such deficiencies are corrected, the computer may yet prove the greatest asset to confidentiality rather than the greatest liability.

V. Emergence of Privacy as a Public Issue

In the wake of the Watergate revelations, perhaps no issue has generated more attention than that of privacy. The Privacy Act of 1974 imposed controls on the Federal sector with regard to record-keeping on individuals and specified rights of individuals to gain access to those records maintained by governmental agencies, with the opportunity to correct inaccurate data.

The Privacy Act of 1974 also created the Privacy Protection Study Commission, with a mandate to undertake a study over a three-year period to investigate the feasibility of extending provisions of the Privacy Act to the private sector. The Commission has investigated the record-keeping practices in many areas of the private sector, including medical records, employment and personnel records, education records, records of social agencies, and private investigation firms. The report and recommendations of the Privacy Protection Study Commission were transmitted to President Carter and the Congress on July 12, 1977. This report, *Personal Privacy in an Information Society*, includes a chapter titled "Record Keeping in the Medical-Care Relationship," which summarizes information gathered in hearing testimony and research, and delineates the conclusions and recommendations of the Commission with regard to medical documentation.

The Commission conclusions indicate that medical records now contain more information, are available to more users, are less well controlled and are used for more non-medical purposes than ever before. Further, the Commission concludes that, in many instances, patient authorization to release information may not be consent freely given, when the patient's choice may be to consent or to forego employment, insurance or other benefits. In addition, despite the increasing number of uses and users of a growing volume of patient health information, it is still rare for the patient to exercise his right to direct access, to have the opportunity to review it for completeness, accuracy or timeliness or to control the disclosure of information.

The Commission recommendations have three stated objectives: ". . . (1) to minimize intrusiveness; (2) to maximize fairness; and (3) to create a legitimate, enforceable expectation of confidentiality."[1]

In a separate study, *Computers, Health Records and Citizen Rights*, conducted under the auspices of the Institute for Computer Sciences of the National Bureau of Standards, Alan Westin of the Department of Public Law and Government at Columbia University has stated that "Medical records and health data are being used today in an enormous variety of settings, with computerization present in all of them. Our report has traced such use in doctor's offices, clinics, health centers, and hospitals, in governmental and private facilities; in acute and ambulatory care; in physical medicine and psychiatric treatment; where patients could choose their health care and where they are under various institutional controls (prisons, the army, mental hospitals, etc.). We have seen that beyond primary care lie important uses of personal medical data for service-payment, quality care

---

[1]*Personal Privacy in an Information Society: The Report of the Privacy Protection Study Commission*, July 1977, USGPO, Wash., D.C. 20402 (stock #052-003-00395-3)

review, and all the social processes . . . from credit, employment and licensing to law enforcement, social research, and political life.''[2]

The Westin report is a comprehensive review of the nearly infinite ways that personal health information is used, by both appropriate and unauthorized users, for legitimate, questionable and clearly inappropriate purposes, for transactions in the best interest of the patient, as well as for those which are detrimental to the patient and others.

The medical record practitioner, as "custodian of the records" is increasingly on the horns of a dilemma: how to fulfill the obligations of recordkeeping in providing needed information to serve the patient, the health care facility, and the community, while protecting the patient from unauthorized, inappropriate or unnecessary intrusion into the highly sensitive and personal data of his health record.

Under the watchword of accountability, the long-held tradition of confidentiality of health information has been gradually eroded. Third party payors, both private and governmental, demand more and more personal health information to process a claim, and routinely visit hospitals to review selected patient health records in toto for the purposes of claim verification and audit.

The proposed procedures for Review of Hospital Services for Professional Standards Review Organizations (Federal Register, January 25, 1977, Part II), state in section 101.715 Examination of the operation and records of hospitals, that "(a) Each PSRO is authorized to inspect the operation and records pertinent to the health care services rendered to Title V, XVIII or XIX patients of any hospital in the PSRO area in which services are provided and may require such hospital to provide copies of such records to the PSRO . . ."; further, this section states that, "(b) a PSRO may utilize the records of patients *other than those covered under Titles XVIII, XIX and V*, where access to their records is authorized by the hospital." (emphasis added) Not only have patients who accept benefits under these programs relinquished their rights to privacy of their health records as a condition of acceptance of benefits, but it would now appear that *all* patients, regardless of their payment status, may have their "confidential" health records open to review without the benefit of their knowledge or consent.

The increasing pressures of fiscal accountability, malpractice, risk management, accrediting, licensing and regulatory agencies, public health agencies and third party payors, with their accompanying information requirements, have subjected hospitals, and medical record departments in

---

[2]Westin, Alan F., *Computers, Health Records and Citizen Rights*. U.S. Department of Commerce: National Bureau of Standards Monograph 157, USGPO, Wash., D.C. December 1976.

particular, to demands for patient health information which are staggering. While the work load has increased considerably, employment of sufficient manpower has been prohibited by fiscal constraints facing hospitals. Therefore, medical record departments have made heavy use of photocopy equipment and other document replication media which decrease the effectiveness of control over the types and amount of information released from patient records.

Health care facilities have also turned to automated information handling systems in an attempt to cope with the growing demands for more information in more sophisticated formats. The recipients of this information have turned to such electronic systems as well, in order to process and review the data received, e.g., the massive data systems of Blue Cross/Blue Shield, Medicare, Departments of Welfare, private insurance carriers, and most recently, the PSRO's. The technology that has evolved to manage the "health information explosion" has, in turn, created new problems of data security.

In his conclusion to *Computers, Health Records and Citizen Rights*, Alan Westin states, "As American society redefines and reorganizes its health-care system in the coming decade, it will have to make increased use of computer technology to manage the rivers of data that will be generated . . . If the question is not whether but how such technology will be used in health care, American Society has one nonnegotiable condition for this process: basic citizen rights cannot be made a casualty of technology-assisted health systems. To do so would be to betray the tradition of Hippocrates, and ultimately to dehumanize health care itself."

The health care community has been acutely aware of the insidious erosion of the confidential relationship between the patient and the health care professional through the growing requests for the information shared in this relationship for the purpose of patient care.

The health care community has taken some steps to try to curb this intrusion, and momentum is gathering for more definitive action. In 1973, the American Hospital Association adopted "A Patient's Bill of Rights," which included statements asserting the patient's rights to privacy of his medical care program as well as of all communications and records of his care. In 1974, AMRA adopted a Position Paper on the Confidentiality of Medical Information, recommending the "development and implementation of programs to: (1) protect the patient from invasion of privacy as a result of indiscriminate and unauthorized access to confidential health information and (2) promote appropriate use of medical information once it is disseminated to authorized persons." Also in 1974, at the initiation of the American Psychiatric Association, fifty medical and consumer groups met in Key Biscayne, Florida, to discuss their concerns about the confidentiality of health records. This meeting provided the impetus for the formation of National Commission on Confidentiality of Health Records. In June, 1976 the AMA House of Delegates approved a bill for model state legislation on the confidentiality of health care information.

These are but a few examples of expressions of concern from the health care community. Most of these expressions have been in the form of guidelines or policy statements, without the force of law. A version of the AMA Model bill has been introduced in five state legislatures; however, it has not yet been enacted in any state.

As these guidelines and policy statements have been propounded, the requirements for release of patient health information have continued to grow, both through regulation and through the requirements of private agencies. Integral to the concerns of privacy and confidentiality of patient health information is the issue of patient authorization and the conditions under which a patient consents to release of information from his health record. At this time, it is unusual for a patient to gain direct access to his health record. Without the opportunity to review the contents of his health record, a patient is placed in the untenable position of consenting to the release of information of which the patient has no knowledge. This situation is incompatible with the rationale of informed consent. Further, many patients sign blanket prospective consents to release of medical information as a condition of participation in both private and public health insurance programs. Here, again, the patient is required to consent to the release of information which does not yet exist, and therefore, cannot be considered *informed* consent.

The public has been increasingly subjected to intrusion by a variety of agencies into their personal lives; in recent years, the greatest intrusion into the "medical life" of the individual has been made in the name of accountability. The public has demanded this, too; however, the public at large does not recognize the consequences of these demands nor the price in individual freedom and privacy that is paid to assure that health dollars are spent most appropriately and most effectively. In addition, those who have been pressed to be accountable, have, in some cases, been overzealous in carrying out their charge, and have demanded far more information than necessary to process a claim, to determine eligibility, or to assure quality.

There is now a need for a swing of the pendulum back, for a balance between the needs of society to know and the rights of the individual to be free from unwarranted intrusion into his personal life. AMRA acknowledges the need for patient health information in substantiating health insurance claims, in litigation, and in medical care evaluation. The critical issue is how much information is needed to carry out these functions, under what conditions should the information be gathered and disseminated, who should have access to the information and what criteria should be used to determine legitimacy of purpose.

Many of these questions become moot if the patient is fully informed about the existence of information about his health care, has access to it and can exercise maximum control over its dissemination. In the spirit of this philosophy, AMRA endorses the following model policies for maintenance of confidentiality of health information, and actively supports their implementation.

MODEL POLICIES FOR MAINTENANCE OF CONFIDENTIALITY OF PATIENT HEALTH INFORMATION

General

The health record is the property of the health facility and shall be maintained to serve the patient, the health care providers and the institution in accordance with legal, accrediting and regulatory agency requirements. The *information* contained in the health record belongs to the patient, and the patient is entitled to the protected right of information. All patient care information shall be regarded as confidential and available only to authorized users.

1.0 *Data Collection*

1.1 The types and amount of information gathered and recorded about a patient shall be limited to that information needed for patient care. Supplementary data which is *not* required for patient care but desirable for research, education, etc., may be recorded with the permission of the patient, following explanation of the purpose for which the information is requested.

1.2 All individuals engaged in the collection, handling or dissemination of patient health information shall be specifically informed of their responsibility to protect patient data and of the penalty for violation of this trust. Proven violation of confidentiality of patient information shall be cause for immediate termination of access to further data, and immediate termination of any employer-employee relationship with prejudge for rehire. This policy shall be made known to all employees at the time of employment and each employee shall indicate understanding of this policy through a signed statement at the time of employment, kept with employee's personnel record. An example of statement is attached. Once yearly they will read the policy and again sign a statement of compliance and understanding.

Note: Continued development of State and Federal legislation to impose penalties of fine and / or imprisonment for such violation is recommended.

1.3 The collection of any data relative to a patient, whether by interview, observation or review of documents, shall be conducted in a setting which provides maximum privacy and protects the information from unauthorized individuals.

2.0 *Storage*

2.1 All primary health records shall be housed in physically secure areas under the immediate control of the Director of the Medical Record Department.

2.2 Secondary records, indices or other individually identifiable patient health information maintained by the institution are subject to the stated policies for maintenance of confidentiality of patient health information. A listing of these secondary records with a brief description of content and location shall be maintained in a central location, preferably in the Medical Record Department.

2.3 Primary and secondary health records shall be retained according to legal, accrediting or regulatory agency requirements, then destroyed according to an approved institutional retention schedule unless there is specific need for preservation of these records. The method of destruction shall be specified and the actual destruction witnessed or attested to in writing by the individual(s) responsible for destruction.

2.4 Original health records may not be removed from the premises, except on order of subpoena.

2.5 Access to areas housing health information records shall be limited to Medical Record Department personnel. The sole exception to this policy shall be the individual designated by the Director of Medical Records for access at times when the Department is not staffed. Health records must be available and accessible at all times for patient care.

2.6 When in use within the institution, health records should be kept in secure areas at all times. Health records should not be left unattended in areas accessible to unauthorized individuals.

2.7 If facsimiles of the health record are provided to authorized internal users, the same controls will be applied for return of these facsimiles as for return of the original health record. Wherever possible, internal users will be encouraged to use the original health record rather than to obtain a facsimile.

2.8 When photocopies or other reproductions of the health record are provided to authorized external users, these copies will be accompanied by a statement:

a) prohibiting use of the information for other than the stated purpose.
b) prohibiting disclosure by recipient to any other party.
c) requiring destruction of copies after the stated need has been fulfilled.

3.0 *Access*

3.1 All requests for health records shall be directed to the Medical Record Department.

3.2 Release of information from the health record shall be carried out in accordance with all applicable legal, accrediting, regulatory agency requirements, and in accordance with written institutional policy.

3.3 Health records shall be available for use within the facility for direct patient care by all authorized personnel as specified by the chief executive officer, and documented in a policy manual.

3.4 Direct access to patient health records for routine administrative functions, including billing, shall not be permitted, except where the employees are instructed in policies on confidentiality and subject to penalties arising from violation of these as specified in **1.2**.

3.5 Original health records may not be removed from the premises, except on order of subpoena.

3.6 Subject only to specific contraindications by the attending physician and to any legal constraints such as those governing minors and those adjudicated as incompetent, a patient may have access to his own health record for review upon written request with reasonable notice. A patient may have access to records of his care after discharge and completion of the health record. Photocopies of health record will be provided on written request by the patient and payment of a reasonable fee.

3.7 *All* information contained in the health record is confidential and the release of information will be closely controlled. A properly completed and signed authorization is required for release of all health information except:

a) as required by law
b) for release to another health care provider currently involved in the care of the patient
c) for medical care evaluation
d) for research and education in accordance with conditions specified in Policies **3.11** and **3.12** below.

3.8 In keeping with the tenet of informed consent, a properly completed and signed authorization to release patient information shall include at least the following data:

a) name of institution that is to release the information
b) name of individual or institution that is to receive the information

c) patient's full name, address and date of birth
d) purpose or need for information
e) extent or nature of information to be released, including inclusive dates of treatment

   Note: An authorization specifying "any and all information . . ." shall not be honored

f) specific date, event or condition upon which consent will expire unless revoked earlier
g) statement that consent can be revoked but not retroactive to the release of information made in good faith
h) date that consent is signed

   Note: Date of signature must be *later* than the dates of information to be released

i) signature of patient or legal representative.

3.9 All requests for information from health records shall be directed to the Medical Record Department for processing.

3.10 Information released to authorized individuals/agencies shall be strictly limited to that information required to fulfill the purpose stated on the authorization. Authorizations specifying "any and all information . . ." or other such broadly inclusive statements shall not be honored. Release of information that is not essential to the stated purpose of the request, is specifically prohibited.

3.11 Following authorized release of patient information, the signed authorization will be retained in the health record with notation of what specific information was released, the date of release and the signature of the individual who released the information.

3.12 Health records shall be available to authorized students enrolled in educational programs affiliated with the institution for use within the Medical Record Department. Students must present proper identification and written permission of the instructor with their request. Data compiled in educational studies may *not* include patient identity or other information which could identify the patient.

3.13 Health records shall be made available for research to individuals who have obtained approval for their research projects from the appropriate medical staff committee and administrator or other designated authority. Data compiled as part of research studies may not include patient identity or other information which could identify the patient unless prior authorization from the patient has been obtained. Any research project which would involve contact of the patient by the researcher must have written permission of the patient's attending physician, or in his absence a physician designated by the current chief executive officer of the facility, and consent of the chief executive officer to conduct this study prior to contact. Research projects which involve use of health records shall be conducted in accordance with institutional policies on use of health records for research.

3.14 The names, addresses, dates of admission or discharge of patients shall not be released to the news media or commercial organizations without the express written consent of the patient or his authorized agent.

3.15 All service organizations which process patient-identifiable health information for the institution shall agree in writing to conditions which:

a) mandate the security of the patient information,
b) specify the methods by which the information is handled and transported,
c) limit the number of types of individuals who have access to the information to those directly involved in processing and
d) specify the penalty for any violation of security or confidentiality.

3.16 Requests for health record information received via telephone will require proper identification and verification to assure that the requesting party is entitled to receive such information. A record of the request and information released will be kept.

SAMPLE CONFIDENTIALITY STATEMENT

I understand and agree that in the performance of my duties as an employee of _____ , I must hold medical information in confidence. Further I understand, that intentional or involuntary violation of my employer's confidentiality may result in punitive action including possible fine or imprisonment.

Date	Signature
Date	Signature
Date	Signature
Date	Signature

Appendix 5C

H.R. 668

96TH CONGRESS
1ST SESSION

H. R. 668

To provide for the confidentiality of medical and/or dental records of patients not receiving assistance from the Federal Government, and for other purposes.

IN THE HOUSE OF REPRESENTATIVES

JANUARY 15, 1979

Mr. ROBINSON introduced the following bill; which was referred to the Committee on Interstate and Foreign Commerce

---

A BILL

To provide for the confidentiality of medical and/or dental records of patients not receiving assistance from the Federal Government, and for other purposes.

Be it enacted by the Senate and House of Representatives of the United States of America in Congress assembled, That no officer, employee, or agent of the United States, or any agency, or department thereof, may inspect, acquire, or otherwise require for any reason whatever, any part of medical and/or dental records of patients whose medical and/or dental care was not, or will not be, provided directly by the Federal Government, or was not, or will not be, paid for (in whole or in part) under a Federal program or any other programs receiving Federal financial assistance, unless

I—O

such patient has authorized such disclosure in accordance with section 2.

SEC. 2. A patient may authorize disclosure under section 1 if he furnishes a signed and dated statement in which he—

(1) authorizes such disclosure for a specific period of time;

(2) identifies the patient records which are authorized to be disclosed; and

(3) specifies the purposes for which, and the agencies to which, such records may be disclosed.

SEC. 3. Any person who violates section 1, upon conviction, shall be fined not more than $10,000 or imprisoned for not more than five years, or both.

SEC. 4. In addition to any other remedy contained in this chapter or otherwise available, injunctive relief shall be available to any person aggrieved by a violation or threatened violation of this title.

SEC. 5. Should any other law of the United States grant, or appear to grant, power or authority to any person to violate section 1 of this Act, the provisions thereof shall supersede and pro tanto override and annul such law, except those statutes hereinafter enacted which specifically refer to this title.

SEC. 6. The provisions of this title shall become effective upon the expiration of ninety days following the date of enactment.

Appendix 5D

H.R. 2979

96TH CONGRESS
1ST SESSION

H. R. 2979

To protect the privacy of medical records maintained by medical care facilities, to amend section 552a of title 5, United States Code, and for other purposes.

IN THE HOUSE OF REPRESENTATIVES

MARCH 14, 1979

Mr. PREYER introduced the following bill; which was referred jointly to the Committees on Government Operations, Interstate and Foreign Commerce, and Ways and Means

---

A BILL

To protect the privacy of medical records maintained by medical care facilities, to amend section 552a of title 5, United States Code, and for other purposes.

Be it enacted by the Senate and House of Representatives of the United States of America in Congress assembled,

SHORT TITLE

SECTION 1. This Act may be cited as the "Federal Privacy of Medical Records Act".

TABLE OF CONTENTS

★I—E

TABLE OF CONTENTS—Continued

TITLE I—PRIVACY OF MEDICAL RECORDS

TITLE II—AMENDMENT TO TITLE 5, UNITED STATES CODE

FINDINGS AND PURPOSES

SEC. 2. (a) Congress finds that—

(1) the right to privacy is a personal and fundamental right protected by the Constitution of the United States;

(2) the collection, maintenance, use, and dissemination of medical information can threaten an individual's right to privacy;

(3) the Federal Government is playing an increasingly important role in the provision, payment, and regulation of medical services;

(4) medical information about an individual is routinely made available to public and private organizations for uses not directly related to the provision of medical services to the individual;

(5) in order to prevent unfairness resulting from the misuse of medical information, an individual must be able to exercise more direct control over medical information; and

(6) an individual's right to privacy must be balanced against the legitimate needs of public and private organizations for individually identifiable medical

information in performing their law enforcement, public health, research, fiscal, and other important functions.

(b) The purposes of this Act are—

(1) to establish procedures allowing individuals to inspect medical records relating to them and to make corrections in these records; and

(2) to define the circumstances under which individually identifiable medical information may be disclosed and to whom it may be disclosed.

TITLE I—PRIVACY OF MEDICAL RECORDS
PART A— DEFINITIONS, EFFECT OF STATE LAW, AND RIGHTS OF MINORS AND INCOMPETENTS

DEFINITIONS

SEC. 101. For purposes of this Act:

(1) The term "accounting" means, with respect to a disclosure, the recording, as part of the medical record from which the disclosure was made, of the date, nature, and purpose of the disclosure, of the name and business address of the person to whom the disclosure was made, and of any written certification provided in order to obtain the record.

(2) The term "audit" means [to be supplied].

(3) The term "employee" means, with respect to a facility or person, an individual who is employed by,

responsible to, or performing a function on behalf of, the facility or person.

(4) The term "evaluation" means an assessment of effectiveness, efficiency, or compliance with applicable legal, fiscal, medical, scientific, or other appropriate standards or aspects of performance.

(5) The term "government authority" means any agency or department of the United States, or of any territory or possession thereof, of any State or political subdivision thereof, of the District of Columbia, or of the Commonwealth of Puerto Rico, or any officer, employee, or agent thereof.

(6) The term "health research project" means a biomedical, epidemiologic, or health services research project or a health statistics project.

(7) The term "health services" means [to be supplied].

(8)(A) The term "institutional review board" means an Institutional Review Board established in accordance with regulations of the Secretary under section 474 of the Public Health Service Act.

(B) The term "appropriate institutional review board" means, with respect to a health research project intending to use the medical records maintained by a facility or researcher, (i) the institutional review board for the organization sponsoring the project, (ii) the institutional review board (if any) for the facility or researcher, or (iii) the institutional review board for another medical facility or institution the medical records of which also are intended to be used in the project.

(9) The term "medical care facility" means—

(A) a hospital, skilled nursing facility, or intermediate care facility, or

(B) another entity for which approval by the Secretary is required for participation in or coverage under the program under title XVIII of the Social Security Act or for which certification by a State agency is required for participation in a program under title XIX of such Act, but only with respect to such provisions of this title as the Secretary makes applicable to such an entity by regulation,

which is approved by the Secretary for participation in or coverage under the program under title XVIII of the Social Security Act or certified by a State agency or participation in a program under title XIX of such Act. Such term also includes an entity of the United States which is a hospital, skilled nursing facility, or intermediate care facility.

(10) The term "medical record" means any material that—

(A)(i) contains information relating to the health, examination, care, or treatment of an individual, or (ii) is to be added to such materials under the provisions of this title, and

(B) is in a form enabling the individual to be identified.

(11) The term "Secretary" means the Secretary of Health, Education, and Welfare.

EFFECT ON STATE LAWS

SEC. 102. (a) Except as provided in subsection (b), this title supercedes any State or local laws governing the confidentiality of medical records maintained by medical care facilities to the extent that the records of such facilities are subject to this title.

(b) This title does not supercede—

(1) any restriction on the disclosure of medical records under (A) section 333 of the Comprehensive Alcohol Abuse and Alcoholism Prevention, Treatment and Rehabilitation Act of 1970 or (B) section 408 of the the Drug Abuse Office and Treatment Act of 1972,

(2) any other such restriction of Federal, State, or local law with respect to disclosure of medical records

relating to alcohol or drug abuse, or treatment for such abuse, or

(3) any restriction of Federal, State, or local law on access to or disclosure of medical records relating to psychiatric, psychological, or mental health treatment.

RIGHTS OF MINORS AND INCOMPETENTS

SEC. 103. The rights of (and obligations with respect to) an individual under this title shall be exercised and discharged through—

(1) the parent or guardian of the individual, if the individual is under the age of majority (as determined under the laws of the jurisdiction in which the facility is located); or

(2) an authorized legal representative of the individual, if the individual has been declared to be incompetent by a court of competent jurisdiction.

PART B—RIGHTS OF ACCESS, CORRECTION, AND NOTICE, AND AUTHORIZED DISCLOSURE

INSPECTION OF MEDICAL RECORDS

SEC. 111. (a)(1) Except as provided under subsection (b), a medical care facility shall permit an individual to inspect any medical record that the facility maintains about the individual, and shall permit the individual to have a copy of the record. The individual may, in accordance with section 115, authorize another person to inspect or to have a copy of the record and to accompany the individual during the inspection.

(2) A facility may require a written application for the inspection and copying of a medical record under this section and shall respond to a request for such an inspection or copy within 30 days of the date it receives the request.

(3) A medical care facility may not charge a fee for permitting inspection of a record under this section. The facility may charge a reasonable fee (no greater than the copying fee imposed on third-party payers) for making a copy of such a medical record.

(b) A medical care facility may deny an individual the right to inspect a medical record (or portion thereof) if it determines that the inspection might reasonably be expected to cause sufficient harm to the individual so as to outweigh the desirability of permitting access. If the right to inspect is denied, the facility shall permit an appropriate person (as defined by the Secretary) designated by the individual to inspect the record involved.

(c) The Secretary shall publish recommended criteria by which medical care facilities can determine, pursuant to subsection (b), whether the inspection by an individual of the individual's medical records might reasonably be expected to cause sufficient harm to the individual so as to outweigh the desirability of permitting the inspection.

CORRECTION OF MEDICAL RECORDS

SEC. 112. Not later than 30 days after the date an individual requests in writing that a medical facility correct a medical record that the facility maintains about the individual, the facility shall either—

(1)(A) make the correction requested; (B) inform the individual of the correction that has been made; and (C) upon the request of the individual, inform any person not employed by the facility and to whom the incorrect portion of the record was previously disclosed of the correction that has been made; or

(2) inform the individual of (A) the reasons for its refusal to make the correction, (B) any procedures for further review of the refusal, and (C) the individual's right to file with the facility a concise statement setting forth the individual's reasons for disagreeing with the refusal of the facility.

After an individual has filed a statement of disagreement, the facility, in any subsequent disclosure of the disputed portion of the record, shall include a copy of the individual's statement and may include a concise statement of the facility's reasons for not making the requested correction.

SEC. 113. (a) A medical care facility shall, in accordance with subsection (b), provide an individual with a written notice of record keeping practices describing—

(1) the categories of disclosures from a medical record that the facility may make under part C without the written authorization of the individual;

(2) the individual's rights under this title, including the right to inspect medical records and the right to seek corrections of medical records; and

(3) the procedures established by the facility for the exercise of these rights.

(b) A notice of record keeping practices (described in subsection (a)) shall be provided to an individual—

(1) when the facility first provides services to the individual after the effective date of this title;

(2) when the facility first provides services to the individual more than one year after providing a previous notice; and

(3) when the facility first provides services to the individual after a substantial change has been made in the notice.

(c) The Secretary shall promulgate by regulation a model notice of record keeping practices describing the categories of disclosures and rights of individuals required to be included in notices of record keeping practices under paragraphs (1) and (2) of subsection (a). If a facility's notice of record keeping practices incorporates the model notice promulgated by the Secretary under this subsection, the facility's notice shall be deemed in compliance with the requirements of paragraphs (1) and (2) of subsection (a) for such a notice.

DISCLOSURE OF MEDICAL RECORDS

SEC. 114. A medical care facility—

(1) may not disclose a medical record about an individual other than to the individual (under section 111) unless either (A) the individual has authorized the disclosure under section 115, or (B) the disclosure is permitted under part C without such an authorization;

(2) may not disclose a medical record to any person unless the person is properly identified; and

(3) shall, where practicable, limit disclosure of a medical record to information needed to accomplish the purpose for which the disclosure is made.

AUTHORIZATION FOR DISCLOSURE OF MEDICAL RECORDS

SEC. 115. (a) For purposes of this title, an individual has authorized disclosure to a person of information in a medical record maintained by a medical care facility only if—

(1) the authorization is (A) in writing, (B) dated, and (C) signed by the individual;

(2) the facility is specifically named or generically described in the authorization as authorized to disclose such information;

(3) the person to whom the information is to be disclosed and the purpose for which the person may use the information are specifically named or generically described in the authorization as a person to whom, and a purpose for which, such information may be disclosed; and

(4) the disclosure occurs before the date or event (if any), specified in the authorization, upon which the authorization expires.

(b) An individual may in writing revoke or amend an authorization, in whole or in part, at any time.

(c) A medical care facility that discloses information from a medical record pursuant to this section shall maintain a copy of the authorization as part of the medical record.

PART C—DISCLOSURE OF MEDICAL RECORDS WITHOUT SPECIFIC AUTHORIZATION

EMPLOYEE USE

SEC. 121. A medical care facility may disclose a medical record it maintains about an individual, without the authorization described in section 115(a), if the disclosure is to an employee of the facility who has a need for the medical record in the performance of his duties.

CONSULTATION

SEC. 122. A medical care facility may disclose a medical record it maintains about an individual, without the authorization described in section 115(a), if the disclosure is to a medical care professional who is consulted by the facility in connection with health services provided to the individual.

ADMISSION AND HEALTH STATUS INFORMATION

SEC. 123. A medical care facility may disclose a medical record it maintains about an individual, without the authorization described in section 115(a), if the disclosure only reveals the presence of the individual at the facility or the provision of services to the individual at the facility, his location in the facility, and his general condition, and—

(1) the individual has not objected to the disclosure, and

(2) the information does not reveal specific information about the individual's condition or treatment.

HEALTH RESEARCH

SEC. 124. (a) A medical care facility may disclose a medical record it maintains about an individual, without the authorization described in section 115(a), if—

(1) the disclosure is for use in a health research project (as defined in section 101(6)) which has been determined by an appropriate institutional review board (as defined in section 101(8)(B)) to be of sufficient im-

portance so as to outweigh the intrusion into the privacy of the individual that would result from the disclosure, and

(2) the facility has provided to the person to whom the information is disclosed a copy of the notice (published by the Secretary under subsection (c)) of the requirements of subsection (b).

(b) Any person who obtains a medical record pursuant to subsection (a) shall—

(1) maintain the medical record in compliance with the security standards prescribed by the Secretary pursuant to section 132(b)(1);

(2) remove, where practicable, information enabling individuals to be identified;

(3) not disclose in any public report information contained in the record and enabling individuals to be identified; and

(4) not further use or disclose the information contained in the record and enabling the individuals to be identified, except—

(A) for disclosure to an employee of the person who has a need for the information in performing his duties under the project,

(B) in compelling circumstances affecting the health or safety of any person or involving imminent danger of serious property damage,

(C) for use in another health research project, under the same restrictions on use and disclosure (including approval by an appropriate institutional review board) applicable under this subsection to the original project, and

(D) for disclosure to a properly identified person for the purpose of an audit or evaluation related to the project.

(c) The Secretary shall publish a notice, available for use by medical care facilities, which accurately describes the conditions, described in subsection (b), for the maintenance, use, and further disclosure of information disclosed under this section.

AUDITS AND EVALUATIONS

SEC. 125. (a) A medical care facility may disclose a medical record it maintains about an individual, without the authorization described in section 115(a), if—

(1) the disclosure is for the purpose of an audit or evaluation, and

(2) the facility has provided to the person to whom the information is disclosed a copy of the notice

(published by the Secretary under subsection (c)) of the requirements of subsection (b).

(b) Any person who obtains a medical record pursuant to subsection (a) shall—

(1) maintain the medical record in compliance with the security standards prescribed by the Secretary pursuant to section 132(b)(1);

(2) remove, where practicable, information enabling individuals to be identified;

(3) not disclose in any public report information contained in the record and enabling individuals to be identified; and

(4) not further use or disclose the information contained in the record and enabling the individuals to be identified, except—

(A) for disclosure to an employee of the person who has a need for the information in performing his duties under the audit or evaluation,

(B) for disclosure to the person for whom the audit or evaluation is being carried out,

(C) in compelling circumstances affecting the health or safety of any person or involving imminent danger of serious property damage, and

(D) when required by Federal or State law.

(c) The Secretary shall publish a notice, available for use by medical care facilities, which accurately describes the conditions, described in subsection (b), for the maintenance, use, and further disclosure of information disclosed under this section.

HEALTH AND SAFETY

SEC. 126. (a) A medical care facility may disclose a medical record it maintains about an individual, without the authorization described in section 115(a), if the disclosure is—

    (1) to assist in the identification of a dead person, or

    (2) pursuant to a showing of compelling circumstances (A) affecting the health or safety of any person or (B) involving imminent danger of serious property damage,

and the facility maintains an accounting (as defined in section 101(1)) of the disclosure.

(b) Medical records disclosed by a medical care facility to a governmental authority under this section shall not be further disclosed by the authority except, if not otherwise prohibited by law—

    (1) where necessary to fulfill the purpose for which the record was obtained, or

(2) for the purposes, and subject to the conditions (other than any requirement that an accounting be maintained), specified in sections 124 through 131.

STATUTORILY MANDATED DISCLOSURES

SEC. 127. (a) A medical care facility may disclose a medical record it maintains about an individual, without the authorization described in section 115(a), if the disclosure is to a governmental authority pursuant to a Federal or State law requiring the disclosure of the record to the authority.

(b) Medical records disclosed by a medical care facility to a governmental authority under this section shall not be further disclosed by the authority except, if not otherwise prohibited by law—

(1) where necessary to fulfill the purpose for which the record was obtained, or

(2) for the purposes, and subject to the conditions (other than any requirement that an accounting be maintained), specified in sections 124 through 131.

SECRET SERVICE OR FOREIGN INTELLIGENCE

SEC. 128. (a) A medical care facility may disclose a medical record it maintains about an individual, without the authorization described in section 115(a), if the disclosure is—

(1) to—

(A) the United States Secret Service for the purpose of conducting its protective functions under section 3056 of title 18, United States Code (relating to Secret Service powers), under section 202 of title 3, United States Code (relating to the Executive Protective Service), or under Public Law 90-331 (relating to Secret Service protection of Presidential and Vice Presidential candidates), or

(B) an authority of the United States authorized to conduct foreign counter- or positive-intelligence activities for the purpose of conducting such activities, and

(2) the government authority seeking the disclosure provides the facility with a written certification, signed by a supervisory official of a rank designated by the head of the government authority, that the record is being sought for a legitimate Secret Service or foreign intelligence purpose.

(b) No medical care facility, or employee of the facility, shall disclose to any person that a government authority has sought or obtained access to a medical record under this section.

(c) Medical records disclosed by a medical care facility to a governmental authority under this section shall not be further disclosed by the authority except, if not otherwise prohibited by law where necessary to fulfill the purpose for which the record was obtained.

LAW ENFORCEMENT FUNCTIONS

SEC. 129. (a) A medical care facility may disclose a medical record it maintains about an individual, without the authorization described in section 115(a), if the disclosure is to a government authority, and is—

(1)(A) for use in an investigation or prosecution (directed at any person other than the individual) of fraud, abuse, or waste in a program or project funded or operated by a government authority, or (B) to assist in the identification or location of a suspect or fugitive in a legitimate law enforcement inquiry;

(2) the government authority seeking the disclosure provides the facility with a written certification, signed by a supervisory official of a rank designated by the head of the government authority, that the record is being sought for a legitimate purpose under this section; and

(3) the facility maintains an accounting (as defined in section 101(1)) of the disclosure.

(b) Medical records disclosed by a medical care facility to a governmental authority under this section shall not be further disclosed by the authority except, if not otherwise prohibited by law—

(1) where necessary to fulfill the purpose for which the record was obtained, or

(2) for the purposes, and subject to the conditions (other than any requirement that an accounting be maintained), specified in sections 124 through 131.

JUDICIAL AND ADMINISTRATIVE PROCEEDINGS

SEC. 130. (a) A medical care facility may disclose a medical record it maintains about an individual, without the authorization described in section 115(a), if the disclosure is not otherwise prohibited by law, is made pursuant to the Federal Rules of Civil or Criminal Procedure or comparable rules of other courts or administrative agencies in connection with litigation or proceedings to which the individual is a party.

(b) Medical records disclosed by a medical care facility to a governmental authority under this section shall not be further disclosed by the authority except, if not otherwise prohibited by law—

(1) where necessary to fulfill the purpose for which the record was obtained, or

(2) for the purposes, and subject to the conditions (other than any requirement that an accounting be maintained), specified in sections 124 through 131.

SUBPOENAS, SUMMONS, AND SEARCH WARRANTS

SEC. 131. (a) A medical care facility may disclose a medical record it maintains about an individual, without the authorization described in section 115(a), if—

(1) the disclosure is pursuant to an administrative, judicial, or grand jury summons or subpoena or pursuant to a search warrant;

(2) the facility is provided a written certification by the person seeking the record that the person has complied with the access provisions of section 141; and

(3) the facility maintains a copy of the summons, subpoena, or search warrant as part of the medical record.

(b) Medical records about an individual disclosed by a medical care facility under this section pursuant to a subpoena issued under the authority of a Federal grand jury—

(1) shall be returned and actually presented to the grand jury;

(2) shall be used only for the purpose of considering whether to issue an indictment or presentment by that grand jury, or of prosecuting a crime for which that indictment or presentment is issued, or for a purpose authorized by rule 6(e) of the Federal Rules of Criminal Procedure;

(3) shall be destroyed or returned to the medical care facility if not used for one of the purposes specified in paragraph (2); and

(4) shall not be maintained, or a description of the contents of such records shall not be maintained, by any government authority other than in the sealed records of the grand jury, unless such record has been used in the prosecution of a crime for which the grand jury issued an indictment or presentment or for a purpose authorized by rule 6(e) of the Federal Rules of Criminal Procedure.

(c) Medical records disclosed by a medical care facility to a governmental authority under this section shall not be further disclosed by the authority except, if not otherwise prohibited by law—

(1) where necessary to fulfill the purpose for which the record was obtained, or

(2) for the purposes, and subject to the conditions (other than any requirement that an accounting be maintained), specified in sections 124 through 131.

OTHER PROVISIONS RELATING TO DISCLOSURES WITHOUT
SPECIFIC AUTHORIZATION

SEC. 132. (a) Nothing in this part shall be construed as requiring a medical care facility to disclose information not otherwise required to be disclosed by law.

(b)(1) The Secretary shall prescribe security standards with respect to the use and maintenance by researchers, auditors, and evaluators of identifiable medical record information disclosed by facilities under sections 124 and 125. The standards shall establish appropriate administrative, technical, and physical safeguards for insuring the security and confidentiality of these records. The Secretary may prescribe different standards for researchers, auditors, and evaluators, and may vary the standards according to the sensitivity of the information disclosed.

(2) The Secretary shall publish guidelines on how medical care facilities can fulfill the accounting requirement of sections 126 and 129, including suggestions for such methods and procedures as will meet this requirement inexpensively and with minimal disruption to the medical treatment process and to standard record keeping practices.

(c) The Secretary shall prepare a notice, for use under section 141(a)(2), detailing the rights of an individual who wishes to challenge, under section 142, the disclosure of the individual's medical record under such section.

PART D—GOVERNMENT ACCESS, CHALLENGE RIGHTS, AND REPORTING

ACCESS PROCEDURES

SEC. 141. (a) A government authority may obtain a medical record about an individual from a medical care facility pursuant to an administrative, judicial, or grand jury summons or subpoena under section 131, if not otherwise prohibited by law, only if—

(1) there is reasonable cause to believe that the record will produce information relevant to a legitimate law enforcement inquiry being conducted by the government authority;

(2) except as provided in subsection (c), a copy of the summons or subpoena has been served upon the individual or mailed to his last known address on or before the date on which the summons or subpoena was served on the medical care facility, together with a notice (published by the Secretary under section 132(c)) of the individual's right of challenge under section 142; and

(3)(A) 14 days have passed from the date of service or mailing and within such time period the individual has not initiated a challenge in accordance with section 142, or

(B) it is ordered by a court under section 142.

(b) A government authority may obtain a medical record about an individual from a medical care facility pursuant to a search warrant if, not later than 30 days after the date the search warrant was served on the medical care facility, it serves the individual with, or mails to the last known address of the individual, a copy of the search warrant together with the notice (published by the Secretary under section 132(c)) of the individual's right of challenge under section 142.

(c)(1) A government authority may apply to an appropriate court to delay (for an initial period of not longer than 90 days) serving a copy of a summons or subpoena and a notice otherwise required under subsection (a)(2) with respect to a law enforcement inquiry. The government authority may apply to the court for extensions of the delay.

(2) An application for a delay, or extension of a delay, under this subsection shall state, with reasonable specificity, the reasons why the delay or extension is being sought.

(3) If the court finds that—

(A) the inquiry being conducted is within the lawful jurisdiction of the government authority seeking the medical records;

(B) there is reasonable cause to believe that the records being sought will produce information relevant to the inquiry;

(C) the government authority's need for the record in the inquiry outweighs the individual's privacy interest; and

(D) there is reasonable cause to believe that receipt of a notice by the individual will result in—

(i) endangering the life or physical safety of any person;

(ii) flight from prosecution;

(iii) destruction of or tampering with evidence;

(iv) intimidation of potential witnesses; or

(v) jeopardy (with a comparable degree of seriousness to the circumstances described in clauses (i) through (iv)) to an investigation or official proceeding or undue delay in trial or ongoing official proceeding,

the court shall enter an ex parte order delaying, or extending the delay of, the notice and an order prohibiting the medical care facility from revealing the request for, or the disclosure of, the records.

(3) Upon the expiration of a period of delay of notice under this subsection, the government authority shall serve, with the service of the summons or subpoena and the notice, a copy of any applications filed and approved under this subsection.

CHALLENGE PROCEDURES

SEC. 142. (a) Within 14 days of the date of service or mailing of a summons or subpoena of a government authority seeking a medical record about an individual from a medical care facility under section 131, the individual may file in the appropriate United States district court or state court a motion to quash the the subpoena or summons, with a copy served upon the government authority (specified in the notice which the individual received under section 131(a)) by delivery or registered or certified mail.

(b)(1) Upon receipt of such a motion, the government authority may file with the appropriate court such affidavits and other sworn documents as sustain the validity of the summons or subpoena. The individual may file, within five days of the date of the authority's filing, affidavits and sworn documents in response to the authority's filing.

(c) If the court is unable to determine the motion on the basis of the initial filings, the court may conduct additional proceedings as it deems appropriate. All such proceedings shall be completed, and the motion decided, within ten calendar days of date of the government authority's filing.

(d)(1) A court may only deny an individual's timely motion under subsection (a) if it finds that there is reasonable cause to believe that the law enforcement inquiry is legitimate and that the records sought are relevant to that inquiry, and the court shall sustain the motion if it finds that the individual's privacy interest outweighs the government authority's need for the record.

(2) The court may assess against a Federal government authority reasonable attorney fees and other litigation costs

reasonably incurred in the case of any motion brought under subsection (a) against the authority and in which the individual has substantially prevailed.

(e) A court ruling enforcing process under this section shall not be deemed a final order and no interlocutory appeal may be taken therefrom by the individual. An appeal of a ruling enforcing the process under this section may be taken by the individual (1) within such period of time as provided by law as part of any appeal from a final order in any legal proceeding initiated against him arising out of or based upon the medical record, or (2) within 30 days after a notification that no legal proceeding is contemplated against him. The government authority obtaining the medical record shall promptly notify an individual when a determination has been made that no legal proceeding against him is contemplated. After 180 days from the date of the enforcement of the process, if the government authority obtaining the record has not initiated such a proceeding, a supervisory official of the government authority shall certify to the appropriate court that no such determination has been made. The court may require that such certifications be made at reasonable intervals thereafter, until either notification to the individual has occurred or a legal proceeding is initiated as described in clause (1).

(f) The challenge procedures of this section constitute the sole judicial remedy available to an individual to prevent disclosure of a medical record pursuant to a judicial or administrative summons or subpoena.

(g) Nothing in this section shall enlarge or restrict any rights of a medical care facility to challenge requests for a medical record made by a government authority under existing law. Nothing in this section shall entitle an individual to assert the rights of a medical care facility.

REPORTING REQUIREMENTS

SEC. 143. In April of each year (beginning with the year after the year in which this Act is enacted), each Federal government authority that requests access to medical records from a medical care facility pursuant to sections 126 through 131, shall submit a report to the Speaker of the House of Representatives and the President of the Senate, for referral to the appropriate committees of Congress, which report shall include the number of (1) requests for medical records made under each of such sections, (2) delays of notice sought under section 141(c), (3) successful and unsuccessful challenges made under section 142, in the proceeding calendar year, and such other information as the authority deems appropriate.

PART E—ENFORCEMENT

COMPLIANCE AS A CONDITION FOR PARTICIPATION IN
MEDICARE AND MEDICAID PROGRAMS

SEC. 151. (a) A medical care facility may not participate and may not continue to participate in the program
under title XVIII of the Social Security Act unless the facility provides adequate assurances, and evidence from time to
time, to the Secretary of its substantial compliance with the
provisions of parts B and C of this title.

(b)(1) Except as provided in paragraph (2), a medical
care facility may not participate and may not continue to
participate in the program of a State under title XIX of the
Social Security Act unless the facility provides adequate assurances, and evidence from time to time, to an appropriate
State agency (as determined under regulations of the Secretary) of its substantial compliance with the provisions of parts
B and C of this title.

(2) A medical care facility is not required to provide the
assurances and evidence otherwise required under paragraph
(1) if it has provided the assurances and evidence required
under subsection (a).

CRIMINAL PENALTY FOR OBTAINING A MEDICAL RECORD
THROUGH FALSE PRETENSES

SEC. 152. Any person who, under false or fraudulent
pretenses or with a false or fraudulent certification required

under this Act, requests or obtains a medical record about an individual from a medical care facility or an authorization from an individual to disclose such a record shall be fined not more than $10,000, or imprisoned for not more than one year, or both.

CIVIL SUITS

SEC. 153. (a) Any person aggrieved as a result of—

(1) a violation by a medical care facility, government authority, researcher, auditor, or evaluator of any provision of part B or C of this title, or

(2) the commission by a person of an act which constitutes a crime under section 152,

may bring a civil action in any appropriate United States district court, without regard to the amount in controversy, or in any other court of competent jurisdiction, against the medical care facility, government authority, researcher, auditor, evaluator, or other person, respectively.

(b) If the court determines in such an action that a violation or commission has occurred, the aggrieved person may—

(1) recover the sum of—

(A) actual damages sustained as a result of the violation or commission or $1,000, whichever is greater, and

(B) the costs of the action together with reasonable attorney fees as determined by the court; and

(2) obtain such other relief, including punitive damages and equitable relief, as the court determines to be appropriate.

TITLE II—AMENDMENT TO TITLE 5, UNITED STATES CODE

AMENDMENT TO TITLE 5, UNITED STATES CODE

SEC. 201. Section 552a of title 5, United States Code, is amended by adding at the end the following new subsection:

"(r) Any medical record contained in a system of records maintained by a medical care facility subject to title I of the Federal Privacy of Medical Records Act shall not be subject to the provisions of subsections (b) through (d), (e)(3), (e)(11), (f)(3), and (g) through (k) of this section, if the maintenance and disclosure of the medical record are subject to the provisions of such title.".

TITLE III—EFFECTIVE DATE AND REGULATIONS

EFFECTIVE DATE AND PROMULGATION OF REGULATIONS

SEC. 301. This Act and the amendments made by this Act shall take effect on the first day of the first calendar quarter beginning more than 180 days after the date of the enactment of this Act.

PROMULGATION OF REGULATIONS

SEC. 302. The Secretary shall first establish final regulations to carry out the amendments made by this Act not later than the first day of the second month that begins before the effective date of such amendments (as specified under section 301).

Appendix 5E

S. 503

96TH CONGRESS
1ST SESSION

S. 503

To amend the Privacy Act of 1974 to provide for the confidentiality of medical records, and for other purposes.

IN THE SENATE OF THE UNITED STATES

MARCH 1 (legislative day, FEBRUARY 22), 1979

Mr. JAVITS (for himself, Mr. RIBICOFF, Mr. COHEN, Mr. LEVIN, Mr. MATHIAS, and Mr. SASSER) introduced the following bill; which was read twice and referred jointly by unanimous consent to the Committees on Governmental Affairs and the Judiciary, with instructions that if and when ordered reported by one committee, the other has not to exceed 30 days

---

A BILL

To amend the Privacy Act of 1974 to provide for the confidentiality of medical records, and for other purposes.

Be it enacted by the Senate and House of Representatives of the United States of America in Congress assembled, That this Act may be cited as the "Privacy Act Amendments of 1979".

AMENDMENTS TO THE PRIVACY ACT

SEC. 2. The Privacy Act of 1974 is amended by—

II—E

(1) inserting the heading "TITLE I—GENERAL PRIVACY PROVISIONS" immediately above section 2;

(2) striking out "this Act" each place it appears in sections 8 and 9 and inserting "this title"; and

(3) inserting at the end the following new title:

"TITLE II—CONFIDENTIALITY OF MEDICAL RECORDS

"FINDS AND PURPOSES

"SEC. 201. (a) The Congress finds that—

"(1) the right to privacy is a personal and fundamental right;

"(2) due to rapidly changing technology, record-keepers are able to compile and disseminate detailed and highly personal information about individuals;

"(3) the collection, maintenance, use, and dissemination of confidential information about individuals by governmental and private sector organizations may threaten the individual's right to privacy;

"(4) as evidenced by the testimony of the Privacy Protection Study Commission before the Committee on Governmental Affairs of the Senate, existing statutory protection of confidential information between patients and health care service providers is inadequate;

"(5) as evidenced by the report of the Privacy Protection Study Commission—

"(A) in addition to the service provider, the number of people who have access to individually identifiable medical information is very large, although the patient is often denied access to such information, and

"(B) there is a need for the extension of statutory privacy protection to the relationship between patients and service providers; and

"(6) it is essential that patients have the right to exercise more direct control over confidential information relating to their own health care, particularly in light of the availability of such information to third parties and its effect on the individual's ability to obtain employment, insurance, medical care, and other important societal benefits.

"(b) It is the purpose of this title to—

"(1) clearly define the circumstances under which confidential health care information in individually identifiable form may be disclosed, and to whom it may be disclosed;

"(2) provide procedures by which the patient may have access to his own health care information and may take steps to assure the fairness and objectivity of those records; and

"(3) carefully balance the legitimate need of certain governmental and private sector organizations to have access to confidential information with the individual's expectation of, and right to, the confidentiality and privacy of such information.

"DEFINITIONS

"SEC. 202. For purposes of this title, the term—

"(1) 'confidential information' means data or information in any recorded medium created or maintained by a service provider that—

"(A) reveals or contains the fact that an individual is or has been a patient; or

"(B) relates to the health (including dental and mental health) history, diagnosis, condition, treatment, or evaluation of a patient;

"(2) 'patient or former patient' means an individual who consults with, or is examined, interviewed, treated, or is otherwise served by, a service provider with regard to a health condition (medical, mental, or emotional) or social deprivation or dysfunction;

"(3) 'patient identifier' means—

"(A) the patient's name, or other descriptive data from which it could be reasonably anticipated that a person—

"(i) could identify such patient, or

"(ii) be led to other data from which such patient might be identified; or

"(B) a code, number, or other means used to identify the patient in relation to confidential information regarding him;

"(4) 'person' means any individual, court, corporation, association, partnership, State or local government or agency or part thereof, or the Federal Government or agency or part thereof;

"(5) 'Secretary' means the Secretary of Health, Education, and Welfare;

"(6) 'service provider' means—

"(A) a hospital, skilled nursing facility, intermediate care facility, or ambulatory care facility as defined in title XVIII or XIX of the Social Security Act, which has been approved by the Secretary for participation under such title XVIII or certified by a State agency for participation under a State plan approved under such title XIX;

"(B) any entity (other than an individual physician) not described in subparagraph (A)

which has been approved by the Secretary for participation under such title XVIII or certified by a State agency for participation under such State plan, but only with respect to the provisions of this title which the Secretary by regulation makes applicable to such entity; and

"(C) a health maintenance organization, medical group, or individual practice association, as defined in title XIII of the Public Health Service Act, which has received a Federal grant, loan guarantee, or contract pursuant to such title, but only with respect to the provisions of this title which the Secretary by regulation makes applicable to such entity;

"(7) 'individuals employed by or affiliated with a service provider' includes—

"(A) persons engaged in good faith in training programs with a service provider, or clinical supervisors employed by the service provider, and

"(B) persons employed by the service provider who are involved in financial auditing or preparation of bills, or who are otherwise engaged in the collection of payments of charges for services to patients;

"(8) 'bona fide medical emergency' means any situation in which the health or safety of the patient or any other individual is in immediate danger;

"(9) 'qualified personnel' means persons whose training and experience are appropriate to the nature and level of the work in which they are engaged; and

"(10) 'law enforcement inquiry' means a lawful investigation or official proceeding inquiring into a violation of, or failure to comply with, any criminal or civil statute or any regulation, rule, or order issued pursuant thereto.

"PATIENT ACCESS TO INFORMATION

"SEC. 203. (a) Except as provided in subsection (c), a service provider shall, within thirty days of a written or oral request by a patient, allow the patient access to his complete health care record, for purposes of inspection and copying. The service provider may not impose a charge for permitting such an inspection, and may not impose more than a reasonable charge (in any event no greater than the charge imposed on third persons) for providing such a copy.

"(b) The service provider shall, in accordance with regulations promulgated by the Secretary, establish procedures which—

"(1) allow a patient or former patient to contest the accuracy or completeness of confidential information pertaining to that individual;

"(2) allow confidential information to be corrected upon request of the patient or former patient when the service provider concurs in the proposed correction;

"(3) allow a patient or former patient who believes that the service provider maintains inaccurate or incomplete confidential information concerning him to add a statement to the record stating what he believes to be an accurate or complete version of that information if the service provider does not so concur.

A statement added under paragraph (3) shall become a permanent part of the service provider's medical record system, and shall be disclosed to any person receiving the disputed information.

"(c) If a service provider determines that disclosure of a patient's or former patient's records to that individual would be detrimental to that individual, the service provider may refuse to disclose such information. Upon such refusal, the service provider shall advise the patient or former patient that he may appoint another individual of his own choice to be his authorized representative. The service provider shall provide access to the confidential information to the authorized representative for purposes of exercising the patient's rights under subsections (a) and (b) if the authorized representative complies with the procedures specified in section 205(a).

"(d) If a patient or former patient is under twelve years of age, or as a consequence of physical or mental incompetence has been placed under guardianship, his parents, guardian or duly appointed legal representative may exercise all the rights set forth in subsections (a) and (b) on behalf of that individual.

"CONFIDENTIAL INFORMATION

"SEC. 204. Except as provided by this title a service provider shall not, without the authorization, as provided in section 205(a), of the patient or former patient to whom the confidential information pertains—

"(1) disclose or transmit any confidential information together with a patient identifier to any person,

"(2) disclose or transmit a patient identifier to any person, or

"(3) disclose or transmit confidential information if the person disclosing or transmitting such confidential information has reason to believe that the recipient may have a patient identifier for such information.

"AUTHORIZATION OF DISCLOSURE

"SEC. 205. (a) A patient or former patient who is twelve years of age, or older, and not physically or mentally incompetent, may authorize the disclosure of his confidential information. Such authorization shall—

"(1) be in writing and signed by the patient or former patient;

"(2) designate the nature and content of the information to be disclosed, who may disclose such information, and to whom such information may be disclosed;

"(3) designate the use of the disclosed information; and

"(4) designate the expiration date, which shall not exceed one year from the date the authorization was signed.

"(b) If a patient or former patient is under twelve years of age, or incompetent as a consequence of physical or mental disability, the patient's parents, guardian, or legal representative may authorize the disclosure of the confidential information in accordance with the authorization requirements of subsection (a).

"(c) The service provider shall retain a copy of each authorization form, and shall keep a permanent record of each disclosure made pursuant to such authorization, including the nature of the data disclosed and to whom it was disclosed. The authorization form and disclosure records shall be treated as part of the confidential information to which authorization under this section applies.

"(d) A patient or former patient may withdraw such authorization at any time by written notice to the service provider. After receipt of such written notice, or after the expiration of the authorization under subsection (a), the service provider shall not release any additional confidential information concerning such patient or former patient.

"DISCLOSURE WITHOUT AUTHORIZATION

"SEC. 206. (a) Except as provided in subsection (b), no disclosure of confidential information shall be made without authorization.

"(b) Disclosure of confidential information without authorization may be made—

"(1) to individuals employed by or affiliated with a service provider and described in section 202(7)(A), if the performance of their duties requires that they have access to such information;

"(2) to individuals employed by or affiliated with a service provider and described in section 202(7)(B) to the extent that the information is essential to financial auditing or preparation of bills and submission of claims for payment of charges for services to a patient;

"(3) subject to the provisions of subsections (e) and (f), for purposes of audit and evaluation, whether or not such audit or evaluation is required by law;

"(4) subject to the provisions of subsections (d) and (e), to Federal, State, and local public health officials, if the service provider is required by law to report specific conditions to such officials;

"(5) subject to the provisions of subsections (e) and (h), to Federal, State, or local law enforcement officials, if the service provider is required by law to report to such officials concerning specified items of confidential information that indicate that the patient may have been involved in, or a victim of, a violation of law;

"(6) to the parent, guardian, or legal custodian of a patient—

"(A) less than twelve years of age, or

"(B) physically or mentally incompetent,

if the service provider determines that such disclosure is appropriate under the circumstances;

"(7) to medical or law enforcement personnel to the extent necessary to meet a bona fide medical emergency;

"(8) subject to the provisions of subsection (h), to the immediate family or any other individual with whom the patient is known to have a responsible relationship, if the patient is incapable of giving authorization due to a bona fide medical emergency, except that the service provider shall notify the patient at the earliest opportunity that the disclosure was made, and to whom it was made;

"(9) subject to the provisions of subsections (g) and (h), to qualified personnel for use in a biomedical, epidemiologic, or health services research project, or a health statistics project, if the research plan is first submitted to, and approved by, an appropriate institutional review board and the director of the service provider or his designee; or

"(10) pursuant to an administrative summons, judicial subpoena, search warrant, or formal written request as provided in sections 207, 208, and 209.

"(c) Individuals receiving confidential information under paragraphs (1) and (2) of subsection (b) shall not disclose such information, except as authorized by this title.

"(d) The Secretary shall promulgate regulations to assure that disclosures of confidential information made pursuant to subsection (b)(4) are made under conditions that adequately protect the confidential information from unauthorized disclosure.

"(e) Any organization or agency to which information is disclosed under subsections (b) (3), (4), and (5) shall not disclose such information except to the extent required by Federal law, and shall destroy any patient identifiers in such information and the records containing such information at the earliest opportunity consistent with the requirements of Federal law.

"(f) In the case of a disclosure of confidential information without authorization pursuant to subsection (b)(3), for purposes of an audit or evaluation not specifically required by statute, the Secretary shall, by regulation, establish procedures to assure that adequate safeguards, including a program for removal or destruction of patient identifiers, are established by the user or recipient of confidential information to protect such information from unauthorized disclosure.

"(g) Qualified personnel granted access to confidential information under subsection (b)(9) may not identify, directly or indirectly, any individual patient in any report of such research project, or otherwise disclose the identity of a patient in any other manner.

"(h) If confidential information is disclosed under subsection (b), the service provider shall retain a record of each such disclosure.

"(i) A service provider shall not release confidential information or patient identifiers to a Federal, State, or local governmental authority until such authority certifies in writing that it has complied, or will comply, with the applicable provisions of this title.

"ADMINISTRATIVE SUMMONS OR JUDICIAL SUBPOENA

"SEC. 207. (a) For purposes of section 206(b)(10), a Government authority may obtain confidential information pursuant to an administrative summons or judicial subpoena only if—

"(1) there is reason to believe that the information sought is relevant to a legitimate law enforcement inquiry;

"(2) a copy of the subpoena or summons has been served upon the subject of the confidential information or mailed to his last known address on or before the date on which the subpoena or summons was served on the service provider together with the following notice which shall state with reasonable specificity the nature of the law enforcement inquiry:

"'Information concerning your health care held by the health care provider named in the attached subpoena or summons are being sought by this (agency or department or authority) in accordance with title II of the Privacy Act of 1974 for the following purpose:

"'If you desire that such records or information not be made available, you must:

"'1. Fill out the accompanying motion paper and sworn statement or write one of your own, stating that you are the patient or former patient whose confidential information is being requested by the Government and either giving the reasons you believe that the confidential information is not relevant to the legitimate law enforcement inquiry stated in this notice or any other legal basis for objecting to the release of the confidential information.

"'2. File the motion and statement by mailing or delivering them to the clerk of any one of the following [   ] courts:

"'3. Serve the Government authority requesting the confidential information with a copy of your motion and statement by mailing or delivering them to

"'4. Be prepared to come to court and present your position in further detail.

"'5. You do not need to have a lawyer, although you may wish to employ one to represent you and protect your rights.

If you do not follow the above procedures, upon the expiration of ten days from the date of service of this notice or fourteen days from the date of mailing of this notice, information requested therein will be made available. This information may be transferred to other Government authorities for legitimate law enforcement inquiries, in which event you will be notified after the transfer.'; and

"(3) ten days have expired from the date of service of the notice or fourteen days have expired from the date of mailing the notice to the patient or former patient and within such time period the patient or former patient has not filed a sworn statement and motion to quash in an appropriate court, or the patient or former patient has complied with the provisions of this section.

"(b) Upon application of the Government authority, the notice to the patient or former patient required under subsection (a), may be delayed by order of an appropriate court if the presiding judge or magistrate finds that—

"(1) the investigation being conducted is within the lawful jurisdiction of the Government authority seeking the confidential information;

"(2) there is reason to believe that the confidential information being sought is relevant to a legitimate law enforcement inquiry; and

"(3) there is reason to believe that such notice will result in—

"(A) endangering the life or physical safety of any person;

"(B) flight from prosecution;

"(C) destruction of or tampering with evidence;

"(D) intimidation of potential witnesses; or

"(E) otherwise seriously jeopardizing an investigation or official proceeding or unduly delaying a trial or ongoing official proceeding to the same extent as the circumstances in the preceding subparagraphs.

An application for delay must be made with reasonable specificity.

"(c) (1) If the court makes the findings required in paragraphs (1), (2), and (3) of subsection (b), it shall enter an ex parte order, granting the requested delay for a period not to exceed ninety days and issuing an order prohibiting the service provider from disclosing that confidential information has been obtained or that a request for confidential information has been made, except that, if the court finds that there is reason to believe that such notice may endanger the lives or physical safety of a patient or former patient or group of patients, or any person or group of persons associated with a patient or former patient, the court may specify that the delay be indefinite.

"(2) Upon expiration of the period of delay of notification under paragraph (1), the patient or former patient shall be served with, or mailed, a copy of the process or request, together with the following notice which shall state with reasonable specificity the nature of the law enforcement inquiry:

" 'Information concerning your health care held by the health care provider named in the attached process or request was supplied to or requested by the Government authority named in the process or request on (date). Notification was withheld pursuant to a determination by the (title of court so ordering) under title II of the Privacy Act of 1974 that such notice might (state reason). The purpose of the investigation or official proceeding was   .'.

"(d) If access to confidential information is obtained pursuant to section 210(b) (emergency access), the Government authority shall, unless a court has authorized delay of notice pursuant to subsection (b), as soon as practicable after such records are obtained, serve upon the patient or former patient, or mail by registered or certified mail to his last known address, a copy of the request of the service provider together with the following notice which shall state with reasonable specificity the nature of the law enforcement inquiry:

" 'Information concerning your health care held by the health care provider named in the attached request were obtained by (agency or department) under title II of the Privacy

Act of 1974 on (date) for the following purpose: . Emergency access to such records
were obtained on the grounds that (state grounds).'.

"(e) Any memorandum, affidavit, or other paper filed in
connection with a request for delay in notification shall be
preserved by the court. Upon petition by the person to whom
such confidential information pertains, the court may order
disclosure of such papers to the petitioner unless the court
makes the findings required in subsection (b).

"(f) For purposes of section 206(b)(10), and in accordance with the notice provided under subsection (a)(3), within
ten days of service or within fourteen days of mailing of a
subpoena or summons, a patient, or former patient may file a
motion to quash an administrative summons or judicial subpoena, with copies served upon the Government authority. A
motion to quash an administrative summons or judicial subpoena shall be filed in the appropriate court. Such motion
shall contain an affidavit or sworn statement—

"(1) stating that the applicant is a patient or
former patient of the health care entity from which
confidential information pertaining to him has been
sought; and

"(2) stating the applicant's reasons for believing
that the confidential information sought is not relevant
to the legitimate law enforcement inquiry stated by the

Government authority in its notice, or that there has not been substantial compliance with the provisions of this title.

Service shall be made under this section upon a Government authority by delivering or mailing by registered or certified mail a copy of the papers to the person, office, or department specified in the notice which the patient or former patient received pursuant to this title. For purposes of this section, 'delivery' has the meaning stated in rule 5(b) of the Federal Rules of Civil Procedure.

"(g) If the court finds that the patient or former patient has complied with subsection (f), it shall order the Government authority to file a sworn response, which may be filed in camera if the Government includes in its response the reasons which make in camera review appropriate. If the court is unable to determine the motion on the basis of the parties' initial allegations and response, the court may conduct such additional proceedings as it deems appropriate. All such proceedings shall be completed and the motion decided within seven calendar days of the filing of the Government's response.

"(h)(1) If, after the proceedings under subsection (g), the court finds that—

"(A) the applicant is not the patient or former patient to whom the confidential information sought by the Government authority pertains, or

"(B) there is a demonstrable reason to believe that the law enforcement inquiry is legitimate and a reasonable belief that the information sought is relevant to that inquiry,

the court shall deny the motion, and, in the case of an administrative summons or court order other than a search warrant, order such process enforced.

"(2) If the court finds, after the proceedings under subsection (g), that the applicant is the patient or former patient to whom the confidential information sought by the Government authority pertains, and that—

"(A) there is not a demonstrable reason to believe that the law enforcement inquiry is legitimate and a reason to believe that the confidential information sought is relevant to that inquiry, or

"(B) there has not been substantial compliance with the provisions of this title,

the court shall order the process quashed.

"(i) A court ruling denying a motion under this section shall not be deemed a final order and no interlocutory appeal may be taken therefrom. An appeal of a ruling denying a motion under this section may be taken by the patient or former patient—

"(1) within such period of time as provided by law as part of any appeal from a final order in any legal proceeding initiated against him arising out of or based upon the confidential information, or

"(2) within thirty days after a notification that no legal proceeding is contemplated against him.

The Government authority obtaining the confidential information shall promptly notify a patient or former patient when a determination has been made that no legal proceeding against him is contemplated. After one hundred and eighty days from the denial of the motion, if the Government authority obtaining the confidential information has not initiated such a proceeding, a supervisory official of the Government authority shall certify to the appropriate court that no such determination has been made. The court may require that such certifications be made, at reasonable intervals thereafter, until notification to the patient or former patient that a legal proceeding has been initiated.

"(j) The challenge procedures of this title constitute the sole judicial remedy available to a patient or former patient to oppose disclosure of confidential information pursuant to this title.

"(k) Nothing in this title shall enlarge or restrict any rights of a service provider to challenge requests for confidential information made by a Government authority under existing law. Nothing in this title shall entitle a patient or former patient to assert the rights of a service provider.

"SEARCH WARRANTS

"SEC. 208. (a) A Government authority may obtain confidential information if it obtains a search warrant pursuant to the Federal Rules of Criminal Procedure in the case of Federal courts or comparable rules in the case of other courts.

"(b) No later than ninety days after the Government authority serves the search warrant, it shall mail to the patient's or former patient's last known address a copy of the search warrant together with the following notice:

" 'Information concerning your health care held by the health care provider named in the attached search warrant were obtained by this (agency or department) on (date) for the following purpose: . You may have rights under title II of the Privacy Act of 1974.'.

"(c) Upon application of the Government authority, a court may grant a delay in the mailing of the notice required in subsection (b), which delay shall not exceed one hundred and eighty days following the service of the warrant, if the court makes the findings required in section 207(b). If the court so finds, it shall enter an ex parte order granting the requested delay and an order prohibiting the service provider from disclosing that confidential information has been obtained or that a search warrant for such confidential information has been executed. Additional delays of up to ninety days may be granted by the court upon application, but only in accordance with this subsection. Upon expiration of the period of delay of notification of the patient or former patient, the following notice shall be mailed to the patient or former patient along with a copy of the search warrant:

" 'Information concerning your health care held by the health care provider named in the attached search warrant were obtained by this (agency or department) on (date). Notification was delayed beyond the statutory ninety–day delay period pursuant to a determination by the court that such notice would seriously jeopardize an investigation concerning   . You may have rights under title II of the Privacy Act of 1974.'.

"FORMAL WRITTEN REQUEST

"SEC. 209. A Government authority may request confidential information under section 206(b)(10) pursuant to a formal written request only if—

"(1) no administrative summons or subpoena authority reasonably appears to be available to that Government authority to obtain confidential information for the purpose for which such information is sought;

"(2) the request is authorized by regulations promulgated by the head of the agency or department;

"(3) there is reason to believe that the information sought is relevant to a legitimate law enforcement inquiry; and

"(4)(A) a copy of the request has been served upon the customer or mailed to his last known address on or before the date on which the request was made to the service provider together with the following notice which shall state with reasonable specificity the nature of the law enforcement inquiry:

" 'Information concerning your health care held by the service provider named in the attached request are being sought by this (agency or department) in accordance with title II of the Privacy Act of 1974 for the following purpose:

" 'If you desire that such information not be made available, you must:

" '1. Fill out the accompanying motion paper and sworn statement or write one of your own, stating that you are the patient whose information is being requested by the Government and either giving the reasons you believe that the information is not relevant to the legitimate law enforcement inquiry stated in this notice or any other legal basis for objecting to the release of the information.

" '2. File the motion and statement by mailing or delivering them to the clerk of any one of the following United States District Courts:

" '3. Serve the Government authority requesting the information by mailing or delivering a copy of your motion and statement to

" '4. Be prepared to come to court and present your position in further detail.

" '5. You do not need to have a lawyer, although you may wish to employ one to represent you and protect your rights.

If you do not follow the above procedures, upon the expiration of ten days from the date of service or fourteen days from the date of mailing of this notice, the information requested therein may be made available. This information may be transferred to other Government authorities for legitimate law enforcement inquiries, in which event you will be notified after the transfer.'; and

"(B) ten days have expired from the date of service or fourteen days from the date of mailing of the notice by the customer and within such time period the customer has not filed a sworn statement and an application to enjoin the Government authority in an appropriate court, or the patient challenge provisions of section 207 have been complied with.

"EXCEPTIONS

"SEC. 210. (a) Nothing in this title prohibits the disclosure of any confidential information which is not identified with or identifiable as being derived from the health care records of a particular patient or former patient.

"(b) Nothing in this title shall apply when confidential information is sought by a Government authority under the Federal Rules of Civil or Criminal Procedure or comparable rules of other courts in connection with litigation to which the Government authority and the patient or former patient are parties.

"(c) Nothing in this title shall apply when confidential information is sought by a Government authority pursuant to an administratiave subpena issued by an administrative law judge in an adjudicatory proceeding subject to section 554 of title 5, United States Code, and to which the Government authority and the patient or former patient are parties.

"(d)(1) Nothing in this title (except sections 206(i) and 216) shall apply when confidential information is sought by a Government authority in connection with a lawful proceeding, investigation, examination, or inspection directed at the service provider in possession of such information or at a legal entity which is not a patient or former patient.

"(2) If confidential information is sought pursuant to this subsection, the Government authority shall submit to the service provider the certificate required by section 206(i).

"(3) Confidential information obtained pursuant to this subsection may be used only for the purpose for which they were originally obtained, and may be transferred to another agency or department only when the transfer is to facilitate a lawful proceeding, investigation, examination, or inspection directed at the service provider in possession of such information, or at a legal entity which is not a patient or former patient.

"(e) Nothing in this title (except section 218) shall apply to any subpoena or court order issued in connection with proceedings before a grand jury.

"(f) This title shall not apply when confidential information is sought by the General Accounting Office pursuant to an authorized proceeding, investigation, examination or audit directed at a government authority.

"SPECIAL PROCEDURES

"SEC. 211. (a)(1) Nothing in this title (except sections 216 and 219) shall apply to the production and disclosure of confidential information pursuant to requests from—

"(A) a Government authority authorized to conduct foreign counterintelligence or foreign positive-intelligence activities for purposes of conducting such activities; or

"(B) the Secret Service for the purpose of conducting its protective functions under section 3056 of title 18, United States Code, the joint resolution entitled 'Joint Resolution to authorize the United States Secret Service to furnish protection to major presidential or vice presidential candidates', approved June 6, 1968 (Public Law 90–331; 82 Stat. 170) or section 202 of title 3, United States Code.

"(2) In the instances specified in paragraph (1), the Government authority shall submit to the service provider the certificate required in section 206(i) signed by a supervisory official of a rank designated by the head of the Government authority.

"(3) No service provider, or officer, employee, or agent of such service provider, shall disclose to any person that a Government authority described in paragraph (1) has sought or obtained access to the confidential information of a patient or former patient.

"(4) A Government authority specified in paragraph (1) shall compile an annual tabulation of the occasions in which this subsection was applicable.

"(b)(1) Nothing in this title shall prohibit a Government authority from obtaining confidential information from a service provider if the Government authority determines that delay in obtaining access to such records would create imminent danger of—

> "(A) physical injury to any person;
>
> "(B) serious property damage; or
>
> "(C) flight to avoid prosecution.

"(2) In the instance specified in paragraph (1), the Government shall submit to the service provider the certificate required in section 206(i) signed by a supervisory official of a rank designated by the head of the Government authority.

"(3) Within five days of obtaining access to confidential information under this subsection, the Government authority shall file with the appropriate court a signed, sworn statement of a supervisory official of a rank designated by the head of the Government authority setting forth the grounds for the emergency access. The Government authority shall thereafter comply with the notice provisions of section 207(d).

"(4) The Government authority specified in paragraph (1) shall compile an annual tabulation of the occasions in which this section was used.

"DUTY OF SERVICE PROVIDER

"SEC. 212. Upon receipt of a request for confidential information made by a Government authority under section 206(b)(10), the service provider shall, unless otherwise provided by law, proceed to assemble the confidential information requested and be prepared to deliver the confidential information to the Government authority as provided in this title.

"NOTIFICATION OF DISCLOSURES

"SEC. 213. A service provider shall notify a patient or former patient, in such form and manner as the Secretary may require, of the disclosures of confidential information concerning that patient or former patient that may be made without his authorization, and of the right of access, and any other patient protection, provided in this title. The service provider shall make such notification, unless it cannot reasonably do so under the circumstances—

"(1) when it first records any confidential information concerning that patient; and

"(2) when it first provides services after the effective date of this title.

"USE OF INFORMATION

"SEC. 214. Confidential information originally obtained pursuant to this title by a Government authority shall not be transferred to another authority unless the transferring authority certifies in writing that there is reason to believe that the information is relevant to a legitimate law enforcement inquiry within the jurisdiction of the receiving authority.

"WARNING REQUIRED

"SEC. 215. (a) All written disclosures of confidential information shall bear the following statement: 'The protection of the confidentiality of information contained herein is required by Federal law. This material shall not be disclosed to anyone without authorization as provided by law, and violations are punishable under the law.' A copy of the authorization form specifying to whom, and for what specific use, such information may be disclosed, or a statement setting forth any other statutory authorization for disclosure, shall accompany all such written disclosures.

"(b) Service providers shall insure that all persons in their employ or under their supervision are aware of their duty to maintain the confidentiality of information protected by this title, and of the existence of penalties and civil liabilities for violation of this title.

"(3) shall be destroyed or returned to the service provider if not used for one of the purposes specified in paragraph (2); and

"(4) shall not be maintained, or a description of the contents of such records shall not be maintained by any Government authority other than in the sealed records of the grand jury, unless such record has been used in the prosecution of a crime for which the grand jury issued an indictment or presentment or for a purpose authorized by rule 6(e) of the Federal Rules of Criminal Procedure.

"REPORTING REQUIREMENTS

"SEC. 219. (a) In April of each year, the Director of the Administrative Office of the United States Courts shall send to the appropriate committees of Congress a report concerning the number of applications for delays of notice and the number of patient challenges made pursuant to section 207 during the preceding calendar year. Such report shall include the identity of the Government authority requesting a delay of notice; the number of notice delays sought and the number granted under each subparagraph of section 207(b)(3); the number of notice delay extensions sought and the number granted; and the number of patient challenges made and the number that were successful.

"(b) In April of each year, each Government authority that requests access to confidential information of any patient or former patient from a service provider pursuant to section 206(b)(10), 207, 208, 209, or 211, shall send to the appropriate committees of Congress a report describing requests made during the preceding calendar year. Such report shall include the number of requests for records made pursuant to each section of this title listed in the preceding sentence and any other related information deemed relevant or useful by the Government authority.

"PREEMPTION

"SEC. 220. No State or political subdivision of a State may establish or continue in effect any law or regulation that is less stringent than the provisions of this title.

"EFFECTIVE DATE

"SEC. 221. This title shall take effect one hundred and eighty days after enactment, and shall apply to all information maintained by service providers regardless of whether that information was first maintained prior to the effective date of this title.

"SAVING PROVISION

"SEC. 222. Nothing in this title shall be construed as in any way affecting, modifying, repealing or suspending the provisions of the Drug Abuse Office and Treatment Act, the Comprehensive Alcohol Abuse and Alcoholism Prevention,

Treatment and Rehabilitation Act, section 303(a) of the
Public Health Service Act, or section 502(c) of the Controlled Substances Act.".

O

Chapter 6

Organizations and Professionals Who Influence Medical Records

CHAPTER OBJECTIVES

1. Identify the organizational components of the American Medical Record Association
2. Differentiate between the education and role of a medical record technician and a medical record administrator
3. Identify the professional activities of medical and allied health practitioners that directly interface with medical record development and use
4. Identify medical staff functions that impact the role and function of the medical record professional
5. Identify 4 characteristics of a medical record professional
6. Relate the American Medical Record Association's Code of Ethics to the managerial responsibilities of an administrative medical record professional

THE AMERICAN MEDICAL RECORD ASSOCIATION

The American Medical Record Association (AMRA) was founded in 1928. Grace Whiting Myers was the first president of the association. Many events, occurrences, and people were instrumental in the development of the organization that eventually became known as the American Medical Record Association. Some of these events have already been discussed, particularly in Chapter 1. Now let's take a more detailed look at some of the historic precursors of the AMRA.

For many centuries hospitals had been organized as places where patients could receive treatment. A particularly meaningful hospital in any discussion of the AMRA is St. Bartholomew's Hospital in London. This medieval institution, started in 1137, is still in existence today. What is even more interesting is that it still has some of the records of patients treated there during its earliest times. This gives us some insight into the importance placed on documentation, even in that early stage of hospital history. St. Bartholomew's went so far as to develop bylaws and organizational departments, one of which was analogous to the medical record department of today.

Another hospital of historic interest to us is the Pennsylvania Hospital, started in 1752 through the efforts of Benjamin Franklin. Its earliest records are analogous to the modern master patient index, with a little bit of the disease and operation index thrown in. The indexes from the Pennsylvania Hospital have been retained and are still available for viewing. More detailed records were kept starting in 1803, and these records include pen-and-ink illustrations.

Massachusetts General Hospital was opened in 1821 and has the distinction of having retained its complete file of records from the day it opened, including catalogues of these records. This famous hospital, still very active in treatment of patients, has taken a leadership role in medical record administration, in the computerization of functions of medical recordkeeping as well as in the operation of a school of medical record administration.

We can see from the study of these three hospitals that documentation of patient care had a high priority from very early times. Using these three in addition to other teaching hospitals in the United States as a starting point, we start to see an increasing emphasis on documentation of records during the twentieth century in the United States. Teaching hospitals were the prime developers of useful medical records. At its annual meeting in 1902 the AHA focused some of its attention on medical records. Two items given attention at that meeting were the lack of uniformity in the methods of compiling medical data and the lack of individuals designated as responsible for the development of records. Physicians tended to avoid involvement with medical records, probably as a result of working with poor records. Because there were no models, there was little encouragement for and interest in developing good records. Also, there was no coordinated effort to bring about good records. In 1905 the AMA, at its annual meeting, discussed the value and necessity of medical records.

In 1913 the ACS was founded. As we discussed in Chapter 1, the ACS was the originator of hospital standardization. The standardization it proposed at that time (and eventually developed to a very fine degree) was not total standardization of all methods and activities involved in the provision of health care through hospitals but was really a standardization of the most common functions inherent in serving patients. It selected particular functions that could be standardized without jeopardizing unique services on the part of individual hospitals. One of the areas in which it set standards was documentation of patient care.

At the direction of the ACS and its director of hospital activities, Dr. Malcolm T. MacEachern, a meeting was called in October 1928. All individuals who were involved in medical recordkeeping were invited to this meeting. Grace Whiting Myers, librarian emeritus of Massachusetts General Hospital, was asked to chair the original meeting and to direct preparation of the program, plan exhibits, and organize committees. It was at this meeting that the newly formed association took as its main objective "to elevate the standards of clinical records in hospitals, dispensaries, and other distinctly medical institutions." At the end of the first year there were 58 charter members of the AMRA. In 1979 the membership of this group totaled more than 23,000. Today's AMRA is a nonprofit organization with headquarters in Chicago, Illinois. Figure 6-1 shows the components of the association.

The stated purpose of AMRA is to promote the art and science of medical record administration and to improve the quality of comprehensive health information services for the welfare of the public. The AMRA has clearly stated its goals.

1. Provide leadership in all areas affecting the health record profession.
2. Provide leadership in promoting the appropriate use of health record information in the best interests of the public.
3. Promote unity and a sense of common purpose among health record practitioners in all settings.
4. Provide appropriate communication channels to meet the needs of the members.
5. Represent the health record profession in its dealings with government and other national groups and international organizations.
6. Delineate and promote on an on-going basis the appropriate roles, functions, and qualifications of health record personnel.
7. Promote and evaluate educational activities that enable the health record practitioner to achieve and maintain professional and technical competence.
8. Develop and update standards for health record practice and credentialing of practitioners.
9. Maintain and encourage adherence to a stated code of ethics.
10. Promote and conduct research programs relating to the health record field.

Figure 6-1 Organizational Components of the American Medical Record Association

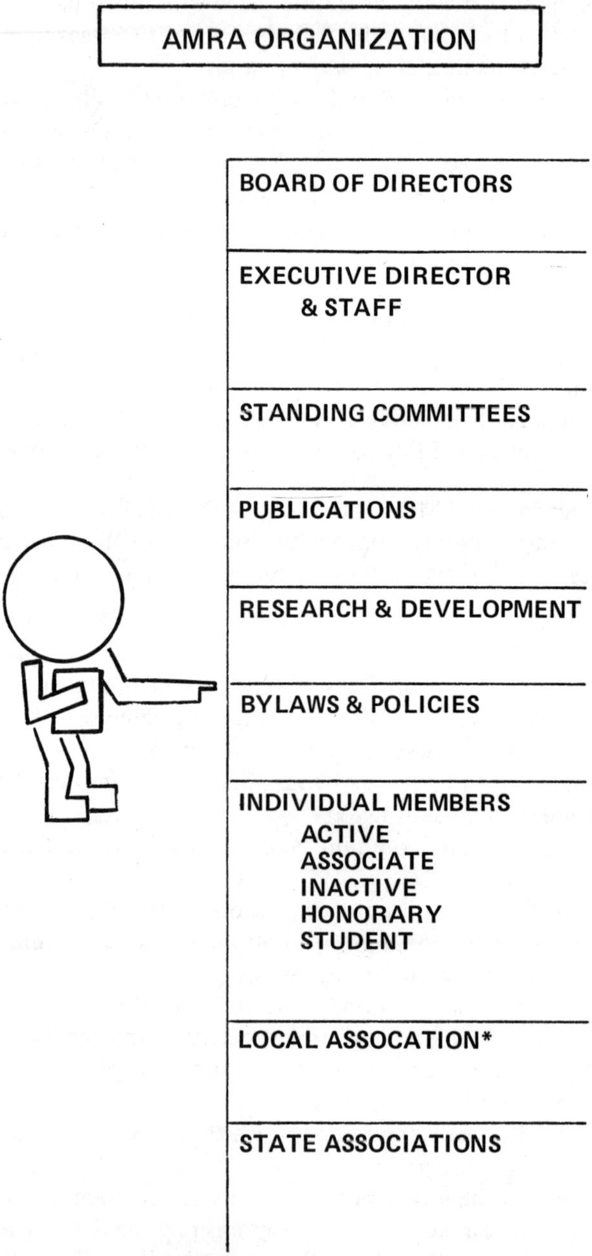

*Not formally part of the AMRA structure.

Objectives of the Association as Approved in 1978

To carry out its objectives, AMRA continues to establish and develop standards of competency, encourages and develops educational programs, promotes the professional growth of its members, and continuously addresses itself to greater professional effectiveness in the development and use of records for patient care and secondary uses. Membership in the AMRA is open to anyone who is interested in the association and its purposes.

There are five categories of membership. *Active members* are medical record technicians and medical record administrators actively working in the profession. *Associate members* are other individuals engaged in medical record work or related fields. This category of membership includes individuals who are nonregistered or nonaccredited record professionals. *Inactive members* are those individuals who are no longer employed in the field. *Honorary membership* is awarded to individuals whose special qualifications are publicly recognized by the AMRA House of Delegates. *Student members* are those individuals who are enrolled in approved programs for medical record administrators or medical record technicians. Individual members are represented most effectively through component state associations. Individual state associations are organized as integral components of the national association, as national bylaws provide for one association to be organized for each state in the union. Members belong concurrently to both the national association and the association of the state where they work. Determination of the state association to which the member belongs is based on the place of employment, and a member may not belong to more than one state association at a time. Student members may belong to the association of the state where they attend school. For those members who are no longer employed, their place of residence is used in determining the state association with which they are affiliated.

The House of Delegates of the AMRA is the official legislative body, and delegates to the national association are elected by component state associations. Local and regional medical record groups are not official components of the AMRA, but they are an important part of state associations. Because members reside in one small geographic area, local associations provide a continuing opportunity for association members to meet and share the benefits of organizational communication at the local level.

The number of delegates is determined by the number of active members in the state association. Each state can have a maximum of ten delegates and a minimum of two. The House of Delegates convenes once a year at the annual meeting of the association.

The executive board was renamed by action of the 1978 House of Delegates. Now titled the Board of Directors, it is a ten-member board elected by the active membership. The major purpose of the board of directors is to act for the association between annual meetings and to manage the business and professional activities and determine the direction of the association. It fulfills these important functions by direct action through association committees that it creates and directs. There are currently seven standing committees of the association. They are:

1. *The Education and Registration Committee.* Its duties include establishing and maintaining standards for accreditation and registration, establishing policies for the correspondence education program, and determining eligibility of candidates for the qualifying examinations.
2. *The Record and Research Development Committee.* This committee is responsible for the review of new concepts of potential significance in the art and science of medical record administration. It recommends a course of action to be taken in the areas of innovative and developing research topics.
3. *Planning and Bylaws Committee.* This committee serves as an advisory body to the board of directors for long- and short-range planning and formulation of policy and bylaw amendments.
4. *Professional Publications Committee.* This committee attempts to stimulate and encourage the development of publications on medical record administration. It serves the needs of both continuing education and formal education programs.
5. *The Nominating Committee.* The Nominating Committee prepares a ballot of candidates for the offices of president-elect and members of the board of directors. Each candidate is requested to prepare a statement of philosophy that is published and mailed with the ballots.
6. *The Program Committee.* The function of this group is to develop the general theme that will be carried out at each annual meeting. It has the responsibility to select specific topics and schedule speakers for each annual program.
7. *Item Writing Committee.* This committee is charged with the maintenance and continual updating of the bank of questions used for the National Qualifying Examinations. Both the record-administration and record-technician examinations are made up from items compiled and retained in the data bank.

The board employs an executive director who is responsible for carrying out the directions, policies, and everyday activities of the national office. The board gets its direction and derives its authority from the membership through bylaws and policies established by the House of Delegates. The board currently meets at least four times a year.

The executive director, under the direction of the board of directors, is the chief administrative officer of the association. The executive director acts as the agent of the board in all spheres of association activity and is responsible for the administration of all association programs. This individual is also responsible for the performance of the executive office staff. The duties of the executive director are determined by the board of directors, but the executive director selects and supervises the national office staff and professional personnel. Departments within the executive office include the academic division, professional services division, correspondence education division, continuing education division, and administrative services division.

One of the benefits of membership in the AMRA is communication with others whose professional interests are similar to one's own. Individual members' interests are represented before related health professional associations, educational institutions, accrediting agencies, and various levels of government. Because the association endeavors to maintain liaison with many other health associations, members benefit from this relationship in the form of information sharing provided through such publications as *Medical Record News*, a journal published six times a year, or *Counterpoint*, a newsletter published six times a year. Component state association membership provides an opportunity to attend meetings and share information through state bulletins or newsletters in which ideas and activities of professional associates are published. Salary surveys, group insurance, and retirement plans are all benefits available to members of the AMRA. Individual members have an opportunity to influence the direction of the association through active participation at the state level. Delegates, who are selected from active members in the state associations, have a direct impact on the bylaws and the policies that determine the course of action the association takes. Membership on committees or on the board of directors is the highest level of AMRA direction that a member can achieve and active members who actively participate enhance their opportunity to be appointed to a national committee or nominated for election to the board of directors.

Today there are two levels of recognized professionals in medical record administration. In October 1971 the AMRA House of Delegates changed the title of Medical Record Librarian to Medical Record Administrator. This name change was the result of a problem stemming from confusion created by the original title: Medical Record Librarian. For years, health professionals and laypersons alike were unable to determine what individual was responsible for the development of medical records. By changing the word librarian to administrator, the AMRA gave notice to all interested parties that the job responsibilities and educational backgrounds of those who practiced the administration and development of medical records would henceforth be identified by the established title Medical Record Administrator. The title Medical Record Technician identifies professional individuals who are active participants in the development of medical record systems.

These titles reflect the focus of the profession but can also be used, with slight modification, to reflect the educational and professional achievements of the practitioners. A Registered Record Administrator is one who has completed a baccalaureate degree program in medical record administration and has successfully completed a national registry examination. Other avenues to registration include completion of a baccalaureate degree, certain prerequisite courses, and a program of study in medical record administration, usually known as a certificate program.

An Accredited Record Technician (ART) is a high school graduate who has completed either a school program or an AMRA-sponsored correspondence course in medical record technology and successfully completed a national accreditation examination.

Individuals who work with medical records but have not successfully completed these examinations are usually known as medical record practitioners. Only those individuals who have passed the examination are entitled to use the professional designations indicated above, which are distinct from position or job titles. Registered record administrators may have job titles that vary greatly, depending on where they work. This is also true of accredited record technicians. Some job titles that either of these individuals may have are: Director of Medical Records, Assistant Professor, Consultant, Research Associate, Department Head, Systems Manager, Information Manager, Records Manager, and so on.

The registration examination was first established in 1932 and the accreditation examination in 1951. Figure 6-2 displays the educational avenues available to individuals who wish to become either record technicians or record administrators or to record technicians who wish to become record administrators.

The educational programs of the AMRA are accredited through the Committee on Allied Health Education and Accreditation. This group is composed of representative health profession associations. The original sponsor of accreditation for medical record programs was the AMA.

Medical stenographers and those who work as transcribers and clerks in medical record departments or with medical record development in its many applications are not currently included in the educational programs of the AMRA. Some of these individuals do have professional associations with which they are affiliated, and some are members of the AMRA.

To get a better understanding of the professional performance of the administrator and technician, the following excerpts from the "Essentials of Accredited Educational Programs of AMRA" are reproduced.

Figure 6-2 Educational Path to Registered Record Administrator

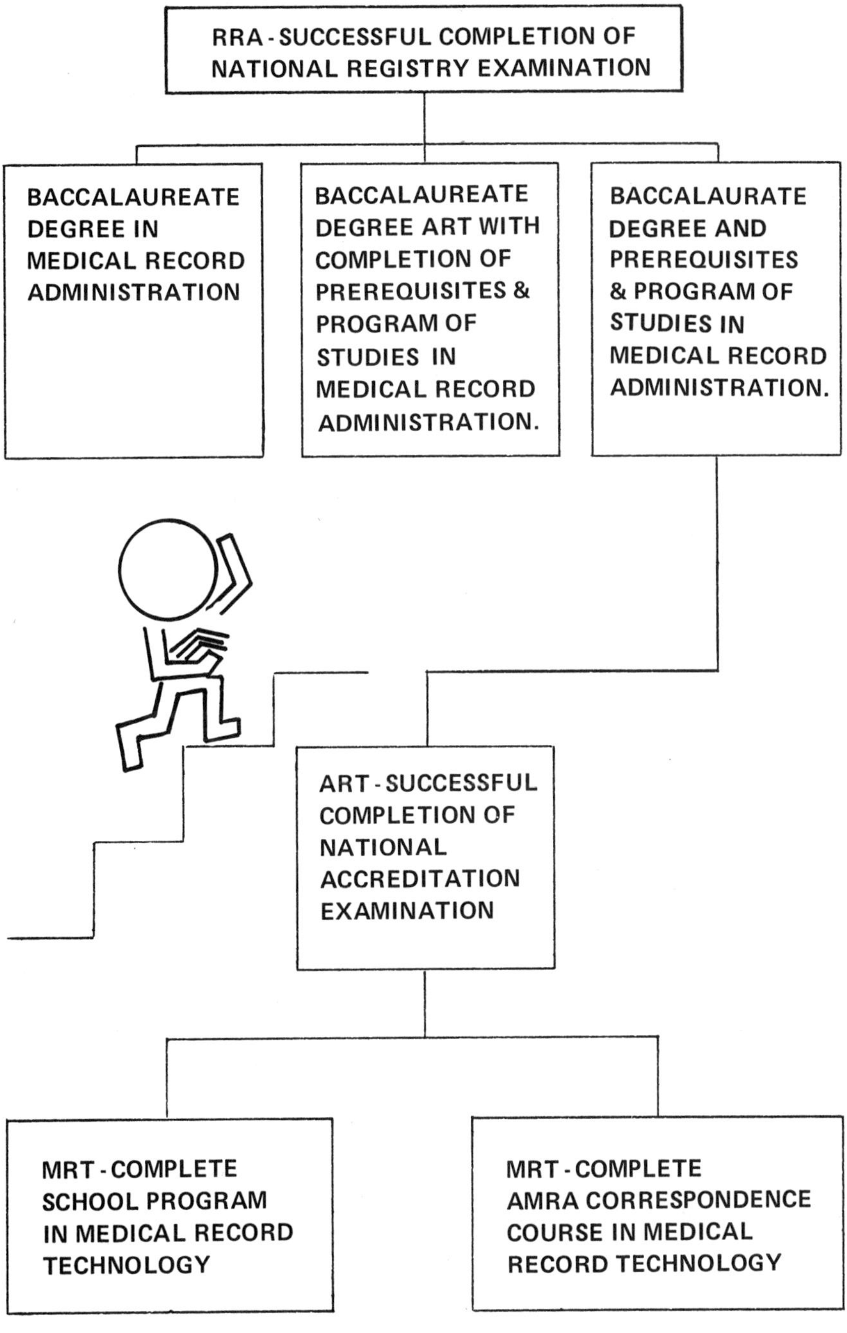

Medical Record Administrator*

The medical record administrator is the professional responsible for the management of health information systems consistent with the medical, administrative, ethical, and legal requirements of the health care delivery system.

The common functions of the medical record administrator include, but are not limited to, the following:

1. Plan and develop a system of medical records to attain the institutional goals and meet standards of accrediting and regulatory agencies.
2. Develop, analyze, and technically evaluate medical records and indexes.
3. Assist the medical staff in evaluating the quality of patient care and in developing criteria and methods for such evaluation.
4. Participate in committee functions relative to medical records and patient information systems.
5. Collect and analyze patient and institutional data for health care and health related programs.
6. Develop in-service education materials and offer instructional programs for health care personnel.
7. Design health information systems appropriate for varying sizes and types of health care facilities.
8. Design and direct a health record abstracting system for regional health data systems.
9. Engage in basic and applied research in the health care field.
10. Provide consultant services to various types of health care facilities, health data systems, health related organizations, and governmental agencies.
11. Direct a total health record program for an individual health care facility or a system of health care institutions.
12. Design facilities in which medical record services may be offered efficiently.
13. Prepare and manage departmental budgets.
14. Select and order equipment and supplies.
15. Participate in development of institutional policies and procedures.
16. Initiate, conduct, or participate in research and development of systems, services, and equipment.

---

*Reprinted with permission of the American Medical Record Association.

17. Coordinate and integrate the efforts of the medical record department with those of other departments to achieve institutional goals.
18. Manage the human resources of the medical information service.
19. Evaluate the organization and operation of medical record services in relation to established standards and new technology and make appropriate revisions.
20. Evaluate and improve the systems, forms, procedures, methods, and motions used in accomplishing departmental work.
21. Select and utilize management tools appropriate for achieving specified objectives in the health care setting.
22. Develop and implement policies and procedures for processing medico-legal documents, insurance and correspondence requests in accordance with professional ethics and in conformity with federal, state, and local statutes.

Medical Record Technician

The medical record technician possesses the technical skills necessary to maintain components of health information systems consistent with the medical, administrative, ethical, legal, accreditation, and regulatory requirements of the health care delivery system.

The functions of the medical record technician include, but are not limited to, the following:

1. Technically analyze and evaluate health records according to standards established by current law, regulations, and accrediting agencies.
2. Compile and utilize various types of administrative and health statistics, e.g., patient census, daily discharge analysis, monthly patient data reports, and vital statistics.
3. Code symptoms, diseases, operations, procedures, and other therapies according to recognized classification systems.
4. Release health information (medico-legal, insurance, and correspondence requests) in accordance with professional ethics and in conformity with institutional policy and legal provisions.
5. Maintain and utilize a variety of health record indexes, storage, and retrieval systems.

6. Perform patient registration activities.
7. Transcribe medical reports.
8. Complete and/or verify discharge data abstracts.
9. Prepare health data input for computer processing, storage, and retrieval.
10. Maintain specialized registries, such as cancer, trauma, stroke.
11. Abstract and retrieve health information used for evaluating and planning in health care and health related programs.
12. Participate in committee functions relative to health records and patient information systems.
13. Provide data to the health care facility staff in patient care evaluation, utilization review, planning, and research activities.
14. Supervise one or more health record service activities such as: transcription, word processing, filing, coding and indexing, statistics, and correspondence.
    This function may include:
    — Planning and assigning work loads
    — Communicating work priorities to appropriate personnel
    — Assisting in planning and implementing short- and long-range departmental objectives
    — Assisting personnel under their supervision in their work
    — Preparing appropriate reports on activities in units under their supervision
    — Assisting in in-service education and the training of personnel
    — Assisting in evaluating and improving the systems, forms, procedures, methods, and motions used in accomplishing work in units under their supervision
    — Assisting in the preparation of departmental budgets
    — Assisting in research and selection of systems, services, supplies, and equipment.

Employment Opportunities

Employment opportunities for record administrators and record technicians include:

- Hospitals
- Skilled nursing facilities
- Clinics
- X-ray departments
- Mental health centers
and

- Special areas, such as:

Ambulatory cardiac units	Insurance companies
Veterinary hospitals	Community health centers
Medical schools	Home health care agencies
Government agencies	Commercial companies
Prison systems	Pharmaceutical firms

This partial listing of places where record administrators and record technicians are employed is not intended to be an exhaustive list. These facilities, agencies, and institutions represent employment achieved by graduates with whom the authors are acquainted. Another role is that of a consultant. The AMRA publishes guidelines for consultants and part-time supervisors in medical records, and their guidelines provide information that is useful to those who need the services of a record consultant yet are not familiar with functions that record consultants perform.

Another group responsible for developing health information is those individuals who provide technical and clerical assistance needed to pull the data together in a composite, useful form. These individuals may be typists or clerks whose responsibility requires abstracting, coding, indexing, filing, transcribing, analyzing, keypunching, or computer-terminal typing. To fully participate in developing health information, clerical and technical personnel must have training in the confidentiality of the information and its uses, in medical terminology, and in determining accuracy and completeness. For the clerical staff to participate in developing and managing health information, it is necessary that they have a leader who can explain, teach, and motivate. For them to achieve job effectiveness they must believe that their work is an integral part of a system that is vital to patient care.

Leadership skills must be demonstrated by the medical record administrator. These skills are needed because the medical record administrator is a liaison between those who perform the daily routine functions of health data management and the more sophisticated users of the data. The medical record administrator is also a liaison between those who enter data on the original medical document and the clerical staff. Leadership skills are required in almost any employment position that a medical record administrator chooses. We emphasize leadership skills because almost any employment position for a medical record administrator requires that the individual work closely with clerical, administrative, and medical staff. Most medical record administrators find themselves in a middle management position when employed in a hospital. As such, they must be an information source for all other departments regarding the resources available in the medical record department. The medical record administrator works very closely with the medical staff in many secondary functions of patient care (see Fig. 6-3). Some of these secondary functions of patient care are:

Figure 6-3 Medical Record Department Relationship with Medical Staff
Committees

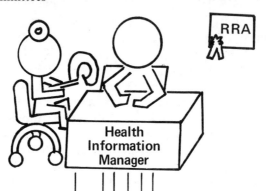

UTILIZATION REVIEW

Prospective, concurrent and
retrospecitve review of
appropriateness of admission
and services. Works with
fiscal intermediary for
reimbursement of services.
Assists medical staff in
committee work, design of
UR plan, appeals & surveys.

MEDICAL AUDIT

Assists in Topic selection, in
criteria development and
clarification. Performs initial
screening, reports results and
variances. Makes recommendations. Performs re-audit. Provides data displays, trend
analysis, and suggests topics
to consider.

TISSUE COMMITTEE

Quantitative analysis of records.
Reports variances in pathological
findings against diagnosis. Reports
inappropriate removal of tissues.

SPECIAL TASK FORCE

Special assignments - ie Research
Committee, Tumor Registry.

PHARMACY ADVISORY

Screens records — Reports all
adverse reactions to drugs, IV.'s,
blood utilization. Reports
inappropriate use of drugs
were documented - ie administration of antibiotics to resistant
organism.

INFECTIONS CONTROL

Does qualitative analysis of
records. Reports all hospital
acquired infections, reportable disease, trend analysis,
special studies upon request.
Morbidity statistics tabulated
for entire facility.

- Utilization review
- Evaluation of care
- Review of medical staff bylaws
- Review of departmental procedures and documents that relate to accrediting and licensing
- Coordination of medical staff policies related to completing and documenting patient records

The importance of the leadership function can be understood by looking at Figure 6-4. This describes the essential task facing health information professionals who represent health information to a variety of users. While doing so, they communicate on a management level with representatives of all those users so that there is a smoothly functioning system that shares the information with those who need it when they need it.

Insert Figure 6-4

By studying the figure, one can see that an essential role of the record professional is to provide direction to others in the collection of data, methodology of data management, and the many uses of data. In its 1979 manual the Joint Commission on Accreditation of Hospitals (JCAH) describes what medical record professionals should be qualified for and what they should be able to do in the hospital setting. This description is included as Appendix 6A.

Figure 6-5 shows some sample organizational charts representing medical record professionals in various departments. These are given to demonstrate some of the organizational components where record administrators and technicians work and interact in various types of facilities. These are samples only and we realize that there are various roles in a variety of settings. Many ARTs serve in departmental management capacities without the services of a medical record administrative consultant.

HEALTH AND MEDICAL INFORMATION ORGANIZATIONS

There are several professional associations whose purpose and function is compatible with record professionals' education and professional background and direction. We have already discussed the AMRA. Other associations that have a historic relationship with medical record professionals have also been discussed: the ACS, the AHA, and the AMA.

Two other groups of contemporary origin that are excellent associations for medical record professionals are the Association for Health Records (AHR) and the Society for Computer Medicine (SCM). The AHR was founded in 1969 as a multidisciplinary forum for the exchange of information among all persons in the field of medical and health information. This

Figure 6-4 Alternative Titles for Health Information Managers

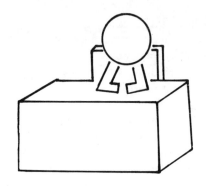

HEALTH INFORMATION PROFESSIONAL
MEDICAL RECORD ADMINISTRATOR
HEALTH DATA ANALYST
HEALTH DATA BANK ADMINISTRATOR

RECOGNIZES WHAT DATA
MUST BE COLLECTED IN
ANY GIVEN APPLICATION

PLAN METHODS AND
CREATE FORMATS FOR
EFFECTIVE COLLECTION
OF THE DATA

recognize emerging role of
individual patient in directing
personal health care program
AND WORK WITH options for
making health information
available to meet that
objective

management of the impact of technology
on manual, paper record systems and
identify appropriate and effective
strategies for implementation of
technology.
RECOGNIZE THE USE OF DATA
PATIENT medical statistics, medical
research and seek ways of displaying it

management of dynamic information
linkage throughout the health care
environment - foster inter-agency
cooperation

release of information scope
and character-establish policies
of responsible confidentiality

Figure 6-5 Examples of Various Roles of Medical Record Personnel

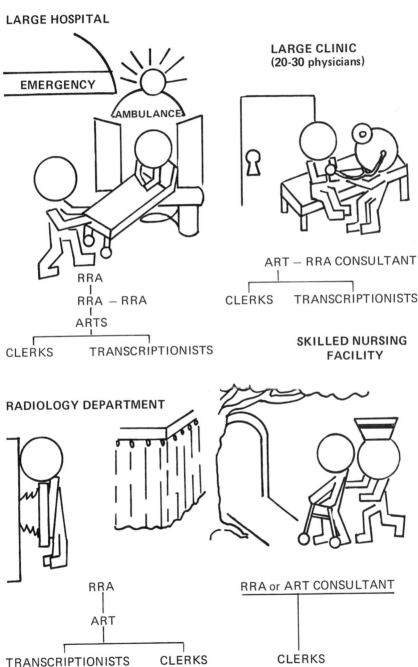

LARGE HOSPITAL

EMERGENCY

AMBULANCE

RRA
|
RRA — RRA
|
ARTS
CLERKS   TRANSCRIPTIONISTS

LARGE CLINIC
(20-30 physicians)

ART — RRA CONSULTANT
|
CLERKS   TRANSCRIPTIONISTS

SKILLED NURSING
FACILITY

RADIOLOGY DEPARTMENT

RRA
|
ART
TRANSCRIPTIONISTS   CLERKS

RRA or ART CONSULTANT
|
CLERKS

group has dedicated itself to problems in the medical and health record field, with particular interest in the shortage of qualified medical record personnel. The AHR was formed to meet the growing needs of individuals with a variety of backgrounds but with a common interest in medical and health records. It was organized so that these individuals could meet and share ideas about such things as:

- Computers
- Standardization
- Hospital information systems
- Telecommunications
- Health data banks
- Health care information systems
- Federal legislation directed at health information
- Comprehensive health planning
- Integrated health care
- Education and credentials
- Progressive care
- Community health centers
- Industrial health records

It was founded with the following goals:

1. The AHR shall recognize as its primary function the encouraging of the free interchange of ideas concerning medical and health records.
2. The AHR shall encourage, sponsor, develop, and support whenever possible, a broad and very educational program for its members and for others concerned with medical and health records.
3. The AHR shall work toward establishing graduated standards of proficiency within the field of medical and health records.

The primary method chosen by the AHR to share information and foster its purposes is an annual interdisciplinary conference on health records that addresses current topics. Its membership includes such individuals and professions as:

- Physicians
- Health record analysts
- Hospital administrators
- Nurses
- Statisticians
- Laboratory administrators
- Insurance executives
- Actuaries

- Biostatisticians
- Nosologists
- Medical record administrators
- Medical record technicians
- Computer programmers
- Systems analysts
- Optometrists
- Health planners
- Microfilm specialists
- Medical record researchers
- Medical record educators
- Medical information specialists

Membership is open to all persons engaged or interested in the field of health records. All members have the right to vote and to hold office. The AHR is headquartered in Ann Arbor, Michigan.

The SCM was organized in 1970. Its original members were physicians; its current membership includes a vast array of health and related professionals who work with computerized health information. It has promoted the use of computers in medicine through its annual meeting, clinics and training sessions, newsletter, and published proceedings of its annual conference. The annual conference and the proceedings that describe papers presented is one of the most excellent sources of current state-of-the-art descriptive information available concerning computerized health information. The thrust of this group and its publications is promotion of currently existing technology, not theoretical proposals. Medical record professionals have been warmly received into membership in this well-organized and sophisticated group of computer-medicine technologists. The society has its main office in Arlington, Virginia.

Since membership is still rather small—approximately 400 members—there is only one standing committee in SCM. Other committees are appointed as needed, based on the decision of the current president or the president and the board. The society is currently considering expanding its organization to include additional committees and to improve the scope and the direction of the organization, thereby assuring its members of more opportunity to participate in the plans, policies, and products of the group.

Among others who influence medical records are The American Society of Allied Health Professions, and governing bodies, boards of trustees, and administrative staffs of facilities, institutions, or agencies that are involved in developing health information. In any health care facility it is the board of trustees, the governing body, or any other group, whatever the title, that makes up the highest level of organizational administration that bears the full legal and moral responsibility for the professional services provided by the facility. Individuals at this highest level of responsibility usually are selected from prominent members of the community, representing business, the professions, and other areas of civic responsibility. These individuals are selected to represent the best interests of the facility and the members of the community. They offer their services without remuneration and cannot be employees of the organization. To carry out the specific functional activity of the organization, an administrator is hired who works under the direction of the board of trustees. The administrative officer of the health care facility is responsible to the board for carrying out established policies in conjunction with the board and the administration. These policies are usually based on economic and human needs. The administrator is responsible for all members of the staff. Included in this responsibility is direction of the medical staff in all except specifically medical decisions. Under the direction of the administrator, the health care facility is organized into departments. These departments carry out specialized activities necessary to an organization that provides full-service, contemporary health care. Hospital departments with which the medical record administrator has a management relationship are listed below.

Accounting
Admitting
Anesthesia
Dietary
Emergency
Housekeeping
Maintenance
Medical education
Medical illustrations
Medical library
Medical staff
Medical staff committees
Nursing
Outpatient
Pathology
Personnel
Pharmacy
Physical medicine and rehabilitation
Public information
Purchasing
Radiology
Respiratory therapy
Social services
Teleprocessing

The medical record administrator in the role of director of the medical record department generally reports directly to a member of the administrative staff, such as the administrator in a small facility or an assistant administrator in a large facility. Medical record administrators serve in a line capacity; that is, they are responsible to administrators for directing and developing medical record departments. Decisions that are made are carried out with the concurrence of the appropriate administrator. Medical record administrators may serve in staff or consultative positions to other departments as well as be equally responsible with them to specific administrators.

Some policies might be established by a governing body of a hospital and jointly carried out by the administration and the medical record department; for example, policies on the retention and release of information, policies on the completion of the record, and policies on medical staff duties regarding dictation and completion of medical records. In home health care agencies, neighborhood health centers, or other ambulatory care facilities, the essential elements described here also apply. One particular difference might be a heavy representation of consumers on the board of governors or the board of trustees of an ambulatory care facility. Many of these facilities have sprung from a grassroots need and, therefore, are highly represented at the board level by those who initiated the development of the facility. Members of the medical profession often serve as members of the boards of trustees of ambulatory care facilities and, in some instances, of hospitals. No members of the medical profession serve on such boards, however, if they are in any way employed by the facility.

MEDICAL STAFF AND PHYSICIAN COMPONENTS

The medical staff in a hospital is organized and functions to provide optimum patient care through efficient use of physicians' education and their skill in using the facilities of the institution. We have seen that the governing board is the highest level of administrative responsibility in a hospital or other health care facility. Working directly under the board of trustees is the administrator. Also responsible to the board of trustees is that group of individuals who are the primary providers of care—the medical staff. The medical staff has overall responsibility for the quality of all medical care provided to patients and for the ethical conduct and professional practices of individual physicians. It is accountable to the governing body, just as the administrator is. The medical staff can be on a line relationship to the governing body or may work on a line to the administrator. In many organizations the medical staff serves in a staff or advisory capacity to the administrator with line authority only to and from the governing body. The medical staff must consist of qualified members whose aim is to achieve the optimal level of professional performance. It achieves this through selection of individuals for appointment to the medical staff and special delineation of clinical privileges for each individual member. The medical staff addresses itself to periodic reappraisal of each member. Unlike other functioning units of the hospital, the medical staff is composed so that it is, in itself, an independently organized body. It achieves its identity and organizational uniqueness through establishing bylaws, rules, and regulations that provide a framework for self-government and a means of accountability to the governing body. The medical staff must address itself to qualifications of individuals who will serve on the staff. Privileges of individual members of the medical staff must be delineated and a mechanism for appointing, reappointing, and appraising the qualifications of the individual members of the medical staff must be established.

Typical categories of medical staff are: active, associate, courtesy, consulting, honorary, provisional, and temporary. Let's take a closer look at these.

Active medical staff includes physicians and dentists who are responsible for the greatest amount of medical practice within the hospital and who perform all significant staff, organizational, and administrative functions.

Associate medical staff consists of physicians or dentists who are being considered for advancement to the medical staff. Included in this is a definition of the period of time to be served in associate medical staff as outlined in the bylaws. At the end of this period the member is considered for advancement through a mechanism established by staff bylaws.

Courtesy medical staff is a group of physicians or dentists who have privileges to admit and treat patients only occasionally. The number of patients who may be admitted by these members is defined by medical staff bylaws along with any exceptions related to bed availability. If a physician or dentist finds the need to regularly increase the number of patients admitted to a particular facility, then that individual seeks admission to associate or other staff membership status. Courtesy staff members are usually active or associate staff members in other hospitals, where they do the majority of their practice and participate in quality care evaluation studies.

Consulting medical staff is a group established for those medical or dental practitioners of recognized professional ability who, on an on-call or regularly scheduled basis, provide consulting services to other members of the staff.

Honorary staff are those individuals who are recognized for their noteworthy contributions to patient care, their outstanding professional reputation, and/or their long service to the hospital. If honorary status is to be established automatically at a certain age, this is defined in the medical staff bylaws.

Provisional staff includes all initial appointments to the medical staff except honorary and consulting. The initial provisional period should be the same for all new members of the medical staff. All characteristics of this group are defined in the bylaws. Each newly appointed medical staff member is usually assigned to a department or service where his or her performance and clinical competence are observed by a chairman, chief of the department, or some other physician or dentist assigned to perform the review function. If at the end of the provisional period individuals have not satisfied the requirements for staff eligibility, provisional status is usually automatically terminated and they are given written notice of such termination and of any rights that they have under the procedures specified in the medical staff bylaws to contest this decision.

Temporary staff are physicians or dentists who have been granted temporary privileges for a limited period of time by the chief medical staff officer or on the recommendation of the chief of a particular department.

Temporary status is given to physicians or dentists who for some reason have a temporary need to provide patient care in a hospital where they do not usually work. Temporary privileges may be given for a stated period or for a period spanning the time needed for the specialized care of a specific patient. Where there is no urgency, physicians or dentists are asked to sign acknowledgments of having received and read the current medical staff bylaws, rules, and regulations, and agreements that specify that they will be bound by all the terms relating to the temporary clinical privileges.

In the case of any kind of emergency in the hospital, any physician or dentist member of the medical staff is permitted to do everything possible to save the patient's life or to save a patient from serious harm. An emergency, in this case, is defined as any condition in which serious permanent harm or aggravation of injury or disease could result to a patient, or in which the life of a patient is in immediate danger and any delay in treatment could add to that danger. In assisting in emergency care, of course, the physician or dentist can perform only to the degree permitted by the license of that individual physician or dentist, regardless of departmental or staff status or clinical privileges. In providing emergency care, therefore, the professional is obligated to summon all available consultative help.

To have an effective organization the medical staff must provide effective self-regulation. The duties, qualifications, and method of selecting officers of the medical staff should be defined in medical staff bylaws, rules, and regulations. Important to the medical record administrator are such organization components of the medical staff as departments and committees. The executive committee of the medical staff is empowered to act for the staff in the intervals between medical staff meetings. This committee usually performs the following functions:

- Serves as a liaison between medical staff and hospital administration
- Receives and acts upon reports and recommendations from medical staff committees, departments, services, and assigned activity groups
- Implements the approved policies of the medical staff
- Recommends to the governing body all matters relating to appointments and reappointments, staff categorization, department service assignments, clinical privileges, and (except where there is such a function of the medical staff) corrective action
- Accounts to the governing body for the quality of the overall medical care rendered to the patient by the medical staff
- Initiates and pursues corrective action when warranted in accordance with medical staff bylaw provisions
- Informs the medical staff of accrediting programs and the accreditation status of the hospital

- Assures that all medical staff members are actively involved in the accreditation process, including participation in any surveys or final critique session

In a hospital where duties and functions are too complex to be handled by the staff as a whole, the medical staff will be organized in departments. Department chairmen of the medical staff should be chosen for their experience and administrative ability. As will all other organizational components of the medical staff, methods of selection, terms of office, and responsibilities of department chairmen should be specified in the bylaws. Usual duties of department chairman should include:

- Accountability to the executive committee for all professional and medical staff administrative activities within departments
- Continuing surveillance of the professional performance of medical staff members who exercise privileges in the department, submitting regular reports on each member, at least at the time of reappointment/reappraisal
- Recommending to the medical staff the criteria for granting privileges in the department
- Conducting concurrent and retrospective patient care evaluation studies to determine the quality of care being given within the department
- Assuring participation of department members in continuing education programs and required meetings
- Appointing committees as needed to conduct department functions
- Participating in department budgetary planning and assisting in preparation of all required reports

The 1979 JCAH *Manual for Hospitals* has an excellent section describing medical staff bylaws, which is reproduced as Appendix 6B. We have already pointed out that this manual is updated annually; therefore, this particular section could be updated in the next year's edition. However, it should be pointed out that the JCAH does not make whimsical or radical changes over a short period of time. This section will probably retain essentially the same information for the next several years.

There are six major medical staff committees that are traditionally found in hospitals. These committees are found in all accredited hospitals because they encompass functions recommended by the JCAH. In hospitals that are not accredited, however, and in many ambulatory care facilities and other health-care-providing facilities, similar committees exist.

Medical Staff Committees

The major committees of the medical staff are:

- The Medical Record Committee
- The Tissue Committee
- The Infection Committee
- The Pharmacy Advisory Committee
- The Utilization Review Committee
- The Medical Audit Committee

As can be seen by the following committee descriptions, the medical record administrator has an integral role in the committees of the medical staff.

The Medical Record Committee

The primary purpose of the medical record committee is to see that accurate and complete medical records are developed and retained for every patient treated. Records are reviewed for their timely completion, clinical pertinence, and overall adequacy for use in patient care, patient care evaluation studies, and in some circumstances medico-legal documentation. The medical record committee review insures that records reflect the condition and progress of the patient, including results of all tests and therapy given. Some other functions that may come under the consideration of the medical record committee are decisions on the format of the complete medical record, forms to be used in the record, and methods of retaining and retrieving medical data. Members of the medical record committee include members of the medical staff and the medical record administrator.

The Tissue Committee

Its prime responsibility is the review of surgical procedures, both those in which a specimen or human tissue was removed and those in which no specimen or human tissue was removed. The committee reviews documented indications for surgery and attempts to evaluate the relationship between the preoperative and the postoperative diagnoses. It is also concerned with the pathologic diagnoses of any specimens or tissue removed during surgery. Members of the tissue committee include members of the medical staff, the clinical laboratory, and the medical record administrator.

The Infection Committee

Its prime responsibility is distinguishing hospital from nonhospital-acquired infections, control of infection, and the coordination of all other activities regarding infection control, including the reporting, evaluating, and maintaining of records of infections among patients and personnel. This committee is responsible for written policies regarding specific requirements for isolation and for the prevention, surveillance, and control procedures regarding sterilization and disinfection practices in all departments of the hospital. Members of this committee include members of the medical staff, administration, the nursing staff, a microbiologist (if one is part of the clinical laboratory) or other laboratory representative, and often the medical record administrator.

The Pharmacy Committee

Its primary responsibility is the development of policies and practices relating to the selection and distribution of drugs, including policies regarding safety and effective use of pharmaceuticals. This group also serves the medical staff in an advisory capacity on matters pertaining to drugs and develops and reviews periodically the formulary that is a drug list for the entire hospital. Members of this committee include a pharmacist, physicians, and nurses.

The Utilization Review Committee

Its primary purpose is the review of all aspects of care to assure high-quality patient care through the effective use of equipment, personnel, materials, and the facility as a whole. This committee utilizes medical records for most of its deliberations. The committee is always concerned that the need for care is well documented, including justification for admitting patients to the inpatient facility. The utilization review committee must have a written plan that describes the methods it will use for evaluating appropriateness and medical necessity of admissions, continued stays, supportive services, and the provision for discharge planning. This plan must specify the time frame in which the reviews will be conducted and outline the specifications for both concurrent and retrospective reviews. Concurrent review is an evaluation of individual patients during their hospitalization, and retrospective review is a review of patients after they have been discharged. Members of the utilization review committee include members of the medical staff, administration, and the medical record administrator or record technician.

The Medical Audit Committee

This committee, with its more contemporary title of Patient Care Evaluation Committee, has as its prime responsibility an evaluation of the quality of patient care provided to patients by the medical and other professional staffs. Criteria against which standards can be applied and care measured must be established or adapted by the medical and other professional staffs. The criteria must be explicit and measurable and must reflect components of care to enable verification that patients are receiving current technologic and professional services. Members of this committee include physicians, nursing personnel, and medical record professionals.

The JCAH includes specific functions in its recommendations for Patient Care Evaluation. They are tissue review, pharmacy and therapeutics review, medical record review, blood utilization review, antibiotic usage review, and other functions, such as infection control, internal and external disaster plans, and hospital safety.

ALLIED HEALTH PROFESSIONALS AND NURSES

This important group of individuals who provide direct and indirect patient care also influence medical records in many important ways. Central services, housekeeping, and dietetic services, for instance, must have written policies and procedures covering such important patient care factors as requirements for sterilization of equipment, selection of supplies, and maintenance of cleaning schedules. In the case of dietetic services, entries of dietetic histories and other patient care factors are necessary in the medical records of patients who must receive special dietary services. Anesthesia services must evaluate all categories of anesthesia care, and these evaluations must be documented. This pertains to care rendered by all anesthesia personnel, including anesthesiologists, nurse anesthetists, and anesthesiology residents.

The nursing service must have established policies that deal with the assigning of nursing staff to patients, policies regarding medication errors and reactions, and a written plan that reflects the staffing patterns and characteristics of patient assignment. The nursing service is also responsible for audit of its professional staff. A retrospective audit program of the nursing department must include:

1. Development of outcome audit criteria
2. Measurement of nursing practice against the criteria
3. Analysis of the results and identification of deficiencies
4. Provision for corrective action
5. Follow up to determine effectiveness of action taken as previously recommended
6. Submission of reports to appropriate individuals, as previously recommended

The pharmaceutical service must have written records that describe periodic inspections by pharmacist or supervised designee of all drug storage and medication centers throughout the hospital. The pharmacy must also have policies that describe (1) designation of personnel who are allowed to administer medication and (2) specifications developed for the procurement of all drugs, chemicals, and biologicals. In the absence of the pharmacist, only prepackaged drugs should be allowed to be removed from the pharmacy. The director of the pharmaceutical services should participate in all aspects of the hospital's patient care evaluation program that relate to drug utilization and effectiveness.

The physical medicine and rehabilitation department must have written guidelines that relate to:

1. Activities and duties of personnel
2. Discussion with patients/family of the treatment goals and capabilities of the physical medicine and rehabilitation service
3. Staff participation and plans for patient discharge and follow-up care
4. Provision of written after-care instructions for the patient
5. Coordination of care between physical medicine and physical medicine rehabilitation unit and the rehabilitation aspects of nursing

There should be specific reference to any speech therapy unit of this department. There should be an established provision for the reception of patients receiving physical medicine services. There should be an ongoing program of evaluation of this particular unit of the hospital.

Safety and sanitation personnel are another necessary part of the hospital team. There must be a qualified individual designated as safety director and officer, and there must be written policies and procedures approved by the governing body of the administration, the medical and nursing staffs, and all departments and services to assure the safety and sanitation of all areas of the hospital.

The items listed above are a partial description of the many facets of the various departments that must function in any type of health care facility so that care will be adequate. Many other duties are carried out in these departments.

PROFESSIONAL ATTITUDE DEVELOPMENT

The medical record professional must work in an atmosphere of growth and development. New technology and other advances will continually be added to the environment of the contemporary professional. To interact effectively with others in the health profession and to continue to develop a professional perspective on the medical record profession, it will be necessary for the active medical record professional to:

- Maintain a curiosity about new methods
- Abide by an ethical code that provides a framework in which to act
- Foster a personal attitude of responsibility about continuing education

The medical record profession is a rather young profession in comparison with some other medical and health professions. What is a professional? What are some of the elements that define and describe professionals? A professional is one who renders a personal service. The desire to provide this service often arises out of interest in the community or individuals in the community rather than out of self-interest. A professional possesses a specialized body of knowledge attained through higher education. Successful assimilation of this body of knowledge can be demonstrated through successful completion of examinations or other evaluation methods. A professional observes ethical principles and maintains high standards. The standards, formulated through the knowledge and direction of a group of individuals, must be continually updated to reflect current information and technologic advances. A professional must participate in continuing education to maintain a level of knowledge and skills compatible with current needs and technology. Professionals also participate in the education process through teaching others. Educating those they work and come in contact with is one mark of a professional. The professional is capable of performing in an independent mode. There is no reliance on others for basic judgments and professional directions. This also means that professionals rely heavily on intellectual and cognitive resources in the performance of their work. If physical resources are utilized, they are secondary to the cerebral tools of judgment, decision making, innovation, identifying relationships, and application of moral and ethical principles.

It is not easy to evaluate a professional, and for those unfamiliar with the profession's objectives, educational level, and competencies, it is useful to be aware of the ethics of the profession.

Using the foregoing comments as a guideline to identify characteristics that describe a professional, let's apply them to the medical record profession by citing some examples.

We discussed the role of the medical record administrator or technician as a patient advocate, particularly in sponsoring policies that provide speedy retrieval of accurate records for patient care and also in promoting the patient-carried personal health record. These two activities demonstrate the professional quality of service to others. They also point out the aspect of professionalism through education of others. The ability to function independently is demonstrated by the role many record professionals take in consulting and education. Educational excellence based on a defined body of knowledge is seen through the successful completion of the registration and accreditation examination as well as the curricula and publications of medical record schools and publications and the research of medical record professionals. To maintain active registration or accreditation, medical record professionals participate in continuing education and must achieve set levels of continuing education credit for continued credentialing.

The code of ethics of the American Medical Record Association is printed here in its entirety for those who are interested in this important professional guideline.

Code of Ethics for the Practice
of Medical Record Administration*

The medical record practitioner is concerned with the development, use, and maintenance of medical and health records for medical care, preventive medicine, quality assurance, professional education, administrative practices and study purposes with due consideration of patients' right to privacy. The American Medical Record Association believes that it is in the best interests of the medical record profession and the public which it serves that the principles of personal and professional accountability be reexamined and redefined to provide members of the Association, as well as medical record practitioners who are credentialed by the Association, with definitive and binding guidelines of conduct. To achieve this goal, the American Medical Record Association has adopted the following Code of Ethics:

1. Conduct yourself in the practice of this profession so as to bring honor and dignity to yourself, the medical record profession, and the Association.
2. Place service before material gain and strive at all times to provide services consistent with the need for quality health care and treatment to all who are ill and injured.
3. Preserve and secure the medical and health records, the information contained therein, and the appropriate secondary records in your custody in accordance with professional management practices, employer's policies, and existing legal provisions.

*Reprinted with permission of the American Medical Record Association.

4. Uphold the doctrine of confidentiality and the individual's right to privacy in the disclosure of personally identifiable medical and social information.
5. Recognize the source of the authority and powers delegated to you and conscientiously discharge the duties and responsibilities thus entrusted.
6. Refuse to participate in or conceal unethical practices or procedures in your relationship with other individuals or organizations.
7. Disclose to no one but proper authorities any evidence of conduct or practice revealed in medical reports or observed that indicates possible violation of established rules and regulations of the employer or professional practice.
8. Safeguard the public and the profession by reporting to the ethics committee any breach of this code of ethics by fellow members of the profession.
9. Preserve the confidential nature of professional determinations made by official committees of health and health-service organizations.
10. Accept compensation only in accordance with services actually performed or negotiated with the health institution.
11. Cooperate with other health professions and organizations to promote the quality of health programs and the advancement of medical care, ensuring respect and consideration for the responsibility and the dignity of medical and other health professions.
12. Strive to increase the profession's body of systematic knowledge and individual competency through continued self-improvement and application of current advancements in the conduct of medical record practices.
13. Participate in developing and strengthening professional manpower and appropriately represent the profession in public.
14. Discharge honorably the responsibilities of any Association position to which appointed or elected.
15. Represent truthfully and accurately professional credentials, education, and experience in any official transaction or notice, including other positions and duality of interests.

Sources of Information

A vitally important aspect of the medical record professional's management of time is that which pursues new information. In the area of published information we will describe several sources considered essential for active professionals who seek continuing sources of new methods, research, concepts, and federal regulations.

The Federal Register

The *Federal Register* is a publication that makes regulations and legal notices issued by federal agencies available to the public. It is published five days a week, every week of the year. It contains notices of proposed legislation as well as approved legislation. The volumes devoted to the Department of Health, Education, and Welfare are those that pertain most particularly to medical records and should be consulted often by those who need to know what is being proposed regarding health information and what has been legislated that affects health information.

MEDLARS

The Medical Literature Analysis and Retrieval System (MEDLARS) is a computer-based system derived from journals indexed for *Index Medicus*, *Index to Dental Literature*, and the *International Nursing Index*. It contains more than 1.8 million citations to almost 3,000 medical- and health-related scientific journals going back as far as 1964. A computer printout provides author, title, and bibliographic notations under subject headings derived from medical descriptor terms. The computer base for this system is located in the National Library of Medicine in Bethesda, Maryland. More than 400 medical schools and hospital libraries in the United States have access to the MEDLARS system. A backup system of 11 regional medical libraries in the United States provides MEDLARS searches for health scientists in hospitals that do not have computer terminals. These federally designated regional medical libraries also provide consultative services and interlibrary loan privileges to other medical libraries within their region. These 11 regional medical libraries are listed below:

- The Francis A. Countway Library of Medicine, Boston, Massachusetts
- New York Academy of Medicine Library, New York, New York
- College of Physicians Library, Philadelphia, Pennsylvania
- National Library of Medicine, Bethesda, Maryland
- Wayne State Medical Library, Detroit, Michigan
- Emory University Medical Library, Atlanta, Georgia
- John Crerar Library, Chicago, Illinois
- University of Nebraska Medical Library, Omaha, Nebraska
- University of Texas Medical Library, Dallas, Texas
- Health Science Library, University of Washington, Seattle, Washington
- Center for Health Sciences Library, Los Angeles, California

The location of medical libraries providing MEDLARS services is available from the National Library of Medicine. Since the use of automated information retrieval systems has been expanding at an extremely rapid rate, it is important for the researcher to keep abreast of the innovations and changes that are occurring in this field. The costs and services connected to the MEDLARS system vary throughout the country.

MEDLINE

MEDLARS on Line (MEDLINE) is a shortened form of the MEDLARS system. It contains more than 400,000 citations selected from 1,200 major journals indexed for *Index Medicus*. The MEDLINE system is usually programmed to include journal citations for the past two years. If a researcher in September 1979 uses the MEDLINE system, journal articles from 1977 to about 1979 (considering a five-month lag from publisher to inclusion in MEDLINE) would be available on computer tape.

Current Research

Current research not included in computer retrieval systems or annual reviews can be found in the most recently published periodicals. Most university and medical libraries have reading rooms where current scientific journals are placed on open shelves. A perusal of newly published journals sometimes is helpful in gaining an overview of a topic and frequently an up-to-date bibliography of related literature. Current journals will also be helpful in locating individuals engaged in ongoing research. It is very useful to request from researchers current reprints of articles, unpublished research, and conference papers. A charge for copying costs should be expected. In general, most scholars will be flattered to receive requests by individuals genuinely interested in their work and they will readily respond. The standard format in requesting reprints is to list the bibliographic notation, i.e., journal, volume, and date.

Research Grants Index

This source is published annually by the U.S. Department of HEW, PHS, NIH and Division of Research Grants, Bethesda, Maryland 20014, ". . . as a source of information on health research currently . . . supported by the health agencies of DHEW. . . ." Thus, scientists and administrators of science programs may find this publication useful in identifying current research activities in areas relating to their own endeavors.

REFERENCES

Accreditation Manual for Hospitals. Chicago, Ill.: Joint Commission on Accreditation for Hospitals, 1979.

Huffman, Edna K. *Medical Record Management*. Berwyn, Ill.: Physicians' Record Co., 1972.

Essentials of an Accredited Educational Programs of AMRA. Chicago, Ill.: American Medical Association, 1975.

Appendix 6A

1979 JCAH Manual for Hospitals: Standards for Medical Record Services

Standard IV—The medical record department shall be provided with adequate direction, staffing, and facilities to perform all required functions.

INTERPRETATION

A qualified medical record individual, responsible to the chief executive officer or his designee, should be employed on at least a part-time basis, consonant with the needs of the hospital and medical staff. This individual shall be either a registered record administrator or an accredited record technician, based upon successful completion of examination requirements of the American Medical Record Association. Where highly developed organization, management, and departmental evaluative skills are needed, a registered record administrator or a person with documented equivalent training and/or experience should be employed. When employment of a registered or accredited individual is impossible, the hospital must secure the consultative assistance of a qualified registered record administrator or accredited record technician. The consultant's primary responsibility should be to evaluate the ability and efficiency of the medical record personnel and the quality of the services being provided by the medical record department, and to assist in correcting any deficiencies found. Consultative assistance should not be used as a supplement to or substitute for medical record department personnel's performance of routine duties. The consultant should visit not less than quarterly and should render written reports of the findings and recommended actions to the chief executive officer.

When a qualified registered record administrator or a qualified accredited record technician is available only on a consultative basis, individuals who are charged with medical record supervisory responsibility, but are not registered or accredited, must demonstrate their current competence. In addition to supervisory ability, competence must be demonstrated by a working knowledge of all medical record department activities, including preparation of medical records, filing and record storage, indexing, coding, statistical reporting, and security and confidentiality of records; orientation, on-the-job training, and in-service education of medical record departmental personnel; the application of automated data processing to medical records where indicated; and the role of the medical record department in medical staff or departmental committee functions, such as those related to patient care evaluation studies and utilization review. Supervisory personnel who do not possess the recommended medical record credentials should participate at least in an approved preparatory correspondence course for medical record personnel leading to eligibility for accredited status.

Other personnel should be employed as needed in order to perform effectively the functions assigned to the medical record department, including support of the hospital's patient care evaluation programs.

Medical record personnel should be involved in education programs related to their activities, including orientation, on-the-job training, and regular in-service educational programs At least supervisory and management personnel should participate in outside workshops, professional association or other organizational meetings, and pertinent correspondence courses. Educational achievement should be documented for each individual.

The medical record department should be provided with sufficient space and equipment to enable personnel to function in an effective manner and to maintain medical records on all patients so that they are easily accessible. Microfilmed records must be accessible, and equipment for reviewing them convenient, for medical staff use.

The length of time that medical records are to be retained is dependent upon the need for their use in continuing patient care and for legal, research, or educational purposes. Whatever filing and storage system is used, it must provide for easy retrievability of records. Retrievability of pertinent information shall be assured by the use of an acceptable coding system for disease and operation classifications, and by the use of an indexing system to facilitate the acquisition of medical statistical information. The latest revision, or adaptation thereof, of *International Classification of Diseases*, which includes an operative procedure classification, is recommended.

Basic medical statistical information should be readily obtainable through the medical record department, the type and amount to be determined by hospital and medical staff needs. If the hospital participates in an automated medical record data processing system, the data should be available to both the hospital and medical staffs for use in patient care evaluation programs.

The types of data collected and systems of collection within the hospital require internal quality control measures to assess the proficiency of personnel responsible for abstracting and coding medical record information. Verification checks for accuracy, consistency, and uniformity of data recorded and coded for indexes, statistical record systems, and patient care evaluation programs should be a regular part of the medical record abstracting process.

Standard V—The role of medical record personnel in the hospital patient care evaluation programs and in committee functions shall be defined.

INTERPRETATION

The degree of participation of medical record personnel in patient care evaluation activities and in committee functions is related to the size of, and the services provided by, the facility; the capabilities of the departmental personnel; and the requirements of the professional staffs.

The role of medical record personnel in such activities may include, but is not limited to:

- supervision of data gathering, with documentation of the reliability of data produced at all levels;
- training of clerical personnel engaged in locating the most useful sources of required information;
- determination of the incidence of various relevant review topics for the use of committees and individuals, the topic selection being a medical staff responsibility;
- screening of medical records for compliance with established criteria and designated exceptions or equivalents, the establishment of clinical criteria being a medical staff responsibility;
- participation in the selection and design of all forms used in the medical record or for data display, and participation in the determination of the sequence and format of the contents of the medical record;
- suggesting to the professional staffs methods of improving the primary source data that will facilitate data retrieval, analysis, tabulation, and display;

- performing ongoing informational surveillance of practice indicators or monitors for medical staff review; and
- ensuring a mechanism to protect the privacy of patients and physicians whose records are involved in quality-of-care review activities.

When an automated data processing system is used for comparative study purposes, personnel involved with the above medical record administrative functions shall be sufficiently knowledgeable about the system to meet the medical staff requirements.

Appendix 6B

1979 JCAH Manual for Hospitals: Medical Staff

Standard III—The medical staff shall develop and adopt bylaws, rules and regulations to establish a framework of self-government and a means of accountability to the governing body.

INTERPRETATION

To accomplish effectively its functions and responsibilities, the medical staff must develop and adopt bylaws, rules and regulations that create an atmosphere and framework within which each staff member can act with a reasonable degree of freedom and confidence. Such bylaws, rules and regulations shall be subject to the approval of the governing body. The medical staff shall regulate itself by these bylaws, rules and regulations, which shall reflect current staff practices, shall be enforced, and shall be reviewed annually and revised as necessary. The bylaws shall at least provide for:

- the qualifications and procedures for staff membership, including application, appointment and reappointment, periodic appraisal, and provisional status. Qualifications shall be specifically related to proper licensure, training/experience, and documented current competence.
- the method of performing the credentials review function.
- the mechanism for delineation and retention of privileges, and reduction or withdrawal of privileges. This includes the privileges of nonphysician and nondentist practitioners who require medical staff processing because of the patient services to be rendered.
- a request for a statement by the applicant releasing from civil liability those reviewing or providing information relative to credentialing, staff membership, and privileges.
- the establishment of a mechanism for corrective action and automatic and summary suspension.

- the establishment of fair hearing and appellate review mechanisms, when requested by the practitioner in connection with medical staff recommendations for denial of staff appointments, as well as the denial of reappointments, or the curtailment, suspension, or revocation of privileges. It is recognized that the mechanism for individuals applying for initial medical staff appointment or privileges may differ from that which is applicable to medical staff members. These mechanisms should specify the following: the period of time beyond which the right to request a hearing is waived; the right to introduce witnesses or evidence; the role, if any, of legal counsel, and the fixed periods of time in which each action shall be completed, including final action by the governing body. Where a grievance mechanism is established by law, as in the case of employed medical staff members in a governmental facility, this mechanism shall be deemed to be acceptable.
- the organizational structure of the medical staff, including departmentalization/nondepartmentalization; selection, qualifications, responsibilities, and terms of office of staff officers and department/service chairmen; and designation of the committees and/or functions. When committees are established, their responsibilities, composition, and interval of meeting shall be stated.
- the establishment of requirements regarding the frequency of, and attendance at, general staff and departmental/service meetings of the medical staff.
- the establishment of mechanisms to ensure effective communication with the governing body, particularly with reference to the quality of patient care in the hospital. Representatives of the medical staff should participate in any hospital deliberations that affect the discharge of the medical staff responsibilities. Where a joint conference committee exists, the medical staff must select its representatives to this committee.
- the establishment of continuing education requirements.
- a requirement for an ethical pledge from each practitioner, including, but not limited to:

  - refraining from fee splitting or other inducements relating to patient referral,
  - providing for continuous care of his patients,
  - refraining from delegating the responsibility for diagnosis or care of hospitalized patients to a medical or dental practitioner who is not qualified to undertake this responsibility and who is not adequately supervised,
  - seeking consultation whenever necessary, and
  - refraining from providing "ghost" surgical or medical services.

- the mechanism for termination of employment of a physician or dentists in a medico-administrative position.
- the mechanism for adopting, amending, repealing, or otherwise revising the medical staff bylaws, rules and regulations.
- other requirements as specified elsewhere in this *Manual.*

Where there is a medical staff policy that permits patient care orders to be written by the house staff, the policy must not be extended to prohibit orders from being written by the patient's private physician or dentist without his agreement. Further, the staff member's declination to participate in this practice shall not in itself be a basis for sanctions relating to staff membership or the holding of clinical privileges, or to the loss of other medical staff prerogatives. This principle should be made clear in the medical staff bylaws, rules and regulations.

Medical staff rules and regulations shall specifically relate to the role of the medical staff in the care of inpatients, outpatients, emergency patients, and home care patients. The rules and regulations may be general in nature, applicable to the whole staff, such as those relating to medical record delinquency and deficiencies, or may be department-/service-specific. The mechanism for providing emergency care shall be defined. The rules and regulations of each department/service shall not conflict with each other or with the bylaws, rules and regulations of the medical staff or bylaws of the governing body.

The rules and regulations shall include the following medical record requirements:

- The use of symbols and abbreviations only when they have been approved by the medical staff and there is an explanatory legend;
- The specific identity of categories of personnel who are qualified to accept and transcribe verbal orders, regardless of the mode of transmission of the orders;
- The period of time following admission of the patient in which a history and physical examination must be entered in the medical record;
- The specific time period in which medical records must be completed following patient discharge; and
- The entries in medical records that must be dated and authenticated by the responsible practitioner.

Medical staff bylaws, rules and regulations that are centrally established for a number of hospitals related by ownership, such as in governmental or corporation hospital systems, shall be acceptable if equivalent in intent and properly enforced.

Chapter 7

Keeping the Medical Record Where It Can Be Located and Used

CHAPTER OBJECTIVES

1. Recognize the significance of retention/retrieval as a unified concept
2. Identify 4 major systems used in retention/retrieval of patient data
3. Differentiate between numbering and filing systems
4. Relate the retention of master patient index data elements to the retrieval of individual patient records
5. Relate the rate of readmission to the selection of appropriate data elements for the master patient index
6. Identify the major use of computer output microfiche in medical record retention/retrieval
7. Recognize the relationship of retention/retrieval systems to the quantity and type of data under consideration

RETENTION/RETRIEVAL SYSTEMS

The role of the record administrator in the retention/retrieval of data is very much a planning and management role. A systems approach to retention leads one directly to retrieval, and the medical record administrator cannot plan a retention system without directing attention to retrieval and vice versa. Because it is impossible to separate the two functions, retention and retrieval, we have written them with a / to indicate the importance of linking these two words. The management focus starts at the outset of systems design to plan all of the component activities, procedures, and other elements necessary to retain/retrieve information. We need to stop for a moment and take a look at what retention is. *Retention* is, in its very simplest definition, keeping something so that it may be used in the future. Retention for the medical record administrator's purposes, then, is the planning, implementation, and control of a system that safeguards the physical and information characteristics of medical or health data for future retrieval. The record administrator, knowing that the data are going to be used, needs to plan a record system that will allow easy, quick, accurate retrieval. This is very much a management function. Data must be preserved in a useful medium so that, among other functions, they can be studied, copied, abstracted, and summarized.

Four Phases of Data Development

In retention/retrieval, we look at four phases of what takes place in data development. The design phase was examined in detail in our description of the variety and source of data entries in Chapter 2. There is an implementation phase to develop the design within specific forms and formats as outlined in Chapter 4. There is also an evaluation phase. For example, when a new form is designed, you probably won't order a gross; you'll get a six-month supply and then consider them carefully to refine them. That's evaluation. The product of the evaluation is then established for retrieval. The retrieval phase, analogous to feedback, reflects the closing of the loop in problem solving.

When one develops or controls data retrieval/retention, all four phases must be involved. To understand data retrieval better, let's continue our exploration of data retention. In determining the proper selection of retention methods, equipment, material, procedures, personnel qualifications, etc., some of the things that one must determine are:

- Storage medium for data: paper records, computer tape, punch cards, microfiche, microfilm
- Storage medium and retention schedules of indexes, registers, and other types of information
- Content and distribution of medical record summaries
- Development and distribution of information that committees use in their study of diseases, facilities planning, etc.
- Development and distribution of data that federal, local, and state agencies use for research and funding

- Development of data that agencies use in accrediting and licensing facilities
- Development and distribution for evaluation of care

These elements, then, are some of the considerations in planning a data retention/retrieval program. Initial deliberations on the totality of elements in data retrieval and retention constitute a planning function. Once the program is established and becomes operational, there are coordination, leading, and controlling to provide continuous support for the system. Let's take a more thorough look at the management steps in the data retrieval stage.

Management Role in the Retrieval Phase

The health information manager must be prepared to establish the data retrieval phase as a subsystem within the department. This subsystem, ideally, will provide a coordinated approach to all data retrieval within the department, ranging from individual patient information to collective health information. Establishing this subsystem will require the following steps.

Step 1—Organize the data; give prime consideration to the sequence, accuracy, and completeness of the data.

Step 2—Review policies on data retention/retrieval.

Step 3—Relate policies to specific requests for data.

Step 4—Initiate the transfer of data from original documents.

Step 5—Transmit data requested; this may include copying, summarizing, listing, commenting on data requested, and so on.

Step 6—Audit data retrieval; maintain a check and balance system to verify accuracy, completeness, timeliness, appropriateness of records, reports, and so forth.

Establishing Objectives

As in any other system, we must first set some *objectives*. What is the outcome we want? The design of all the records that describe or recount data will then meet the objectives we have established for our retention/retrieval system. Two sample objectives are:

- During the next fiscal year, perform at least eight medical audits on topics to be selected by the medical staff.
- Establish a regular program of record retention to include definitions and schedule of retention for the following types of data: master

patient index, medical audit reports, register of reports sent out of the facility, death records, and emergency reports.

The need to design a retention/retrieval system that will foster accomplishment of these and other related objectives should be obvious. The idea of setting an objective and coordinating all other activities—staffing of personnel, selection of equipment, etc.—that must support the objectives brings us to an important consideration: data that have not been included in a systems design. To work with data that have not been developed according to planned objectives is difficult. It is important to take steps to bring data into a system approach. Regardless of the current condition of the records, the seeming lack of coordination in data flow, and problems of data control, a retention/retrieval system can be developed if the steps described here are followed.

In establishing objectives for a data retention/retrieval program, there are three primary factors that must be taken into consideration to establish a useful system: activity or usage of the data, the space available for the data, and the laws regarding retention.

Activity of Records: In designing a system, it is necessary to prepare some type of *activity list* or other report that will give feedback on how many times the records are used. It is necessary to determine how many requests for information are being received and what type of information is requested. The kind of information requested depends to some extent on the type of health care facility. Many requests for information can be answered by consulting indexes, registers, file cards, or various reports. It is not necessary to use the complete record as a source to adequately answer many inquiries. Larger, more sophisticated departments are designed to satisfy requests without the necessity of pulling the complete record to do so. In a teaching hospital, records usually have a much higher activity rate than records in a community hospital or a long-term care facility. Neighborhood health centers, mental health centers, and other types of ambulatory care facilities may have varying rates of activity, depending on the stability of the patient population, the kinds of research studies in progress, or the kinds of administrative uses for records. For instance, in a facility where old records are seldom used and there are no sanctions that prevent discarding the information, it is probably most effective to establish a regular cycle to destroy old records. Destruction of records is usually based on one of the following conditions: lack of space, information so poorly recorded or maintained that it is no longer legible, and records no longer active.

Space Available for Storage: Retention of records depends a great deal on current and future space allocations. The selection of paper, microfilm, or microfiche is determined to some extent by the amount of storage space allocated to the records. If space is to be reduced, there should be a plan to accommodate alternative methods of storage or destruction as outlined in a predetermined *destruction program*. Regardless of whether storage space is being expanded or reduced, new records continually enter the system. One easily applied rule of thumb is to retire old records at the same rate that new records enter the system. A chief consideration in allocating space for record activity is tying the activity level of the record to space considerations. In some facilities, records may become inactive when they are only three to four years old. Patients may no longer live in the community or receive treatment in the facility, or there may be various other reasons why the records have become inactive. There may be space in the facility for only five years of active records. How one ties together space and the activity of the file, then, becomes a key element in determining space allocation.

Legal Requirements for Retention: Laws vary from state to state, but it is generally accepted that records of juveniles, pediatric cases, or newborns —in other words, all minor patients—must be retained until the patient reaches *majority*, which is age 21 in most states. The medical record administrator is the patient's advocate in this case and should be primarily concerned with the needs of patients. Consideration of the patient, verification of legal statutes, and determination of organizational objectives all come into play regarding retention. The patient, upon reaching majority, can elect to ask and receive information from the records. To become familiar with the legal requirements in a state, it is necessary to determine what the statute of limitations is for various business and medical documents. This requires familiarity with the legal codes and all types of information contained in medical records. Once again, in planning a retention system, one must consider data as a system of parts, rather than thinking only of the medical record as a whole. Registers, indexes, consent forms, forms for the release of information from the institution, medical records, and the various departmental diagnostic and therapeutic reports are all data that must be considered individually when determining the statute of limitations for retention purposes.

Developing the System

Now let us turn our attention to the record administrator in the role of a systems developer. Some of the considerations and questions that must be raised in developing a retention system are the following:

- Who organizes the system and determines what is to be retained?
- What is to be retained?

- Why is it retained?
- Where is it to be retained?
- How long will it be retained?
- How is it to be processed?
- How is it to be retrieved?
- How is it to be controlled?
- What will the destruction schedule and procedures include?
- Will the system fulfill its needs?
- What is the cost in relationship to all of these activities?
- How much supervision does it take?

Answers to the questions will reveal that there is more than one type of document included in the retention function. Documents and data to include when using the guideline questions are: master patient, disease, operation, reason for visit, procedure, and physician or provider indexes; number register; admission and discharge lists; census reports; discharge analysis reports; memos; budgets; administrative reports; committee reports; and all other data reports utilized by the institution, facility, or agency in its operations. Not all data fit into such concise units as those just listed. So, the *guideline questions* are also used to address such functional aspects of the data as content or subject of the information. For instance, laboratory data, vital statistics, cancer research, nutrition studies, and audit reports are all subjects that are addressed by the guideline questions when determining retention policies, methods, and procedures. When approached from the aspect of subject or content, retention becomes a more interesting aspect of record administration than first impressions might reveal. For instance, someone may come to the medical record administrator and ask what is being fed diabetics during their hospital stay. Other questions for the medical record administrator might be what kind of lab tests are being run on pediatric patients who are treated for otitis media or what the average age is of people treated in the institution during January 1978. Considering the possibility of being asked to answer questions such as these at the outset of a retention/retrieval program will help determine the choice of particular components, such as filing equipment, media for records, paper vs. microfiche or computer tape, personnel positions and procedures, material and equipment, and all other elements that are necessary for an effective retention/retrieval system.

Other questions to be considered at the outset of developing a retention/ retrieval program, questions that will help define objectives specifically, are those dealing with such things as cost of personnel and equipment for data retention. What specific kinds of requests for information are received? Is it necessary to pull the complete medical record to give information to inquirers or is there an index somewhere that can be used as a source of reply? (If there is, it will save time and money.) What are the agencies that request information and what do they usually request? For instance, some agencies that request information do so on a regular basis. It is true that occasionally they change the data elements of the information requested, creating a continuing source of annoyance to record administrators who do not have flexible data retrieval systems. Are there instances when one can refuse to give information and, if so, are the reasons for refusal justified? All of these questions and their answers make a strong case for the necessity of a retention/retrieval system that is continually evaluated and updated to reflect current needs and costs. Graduates can become discouraged if they go to work in a facility that does not have a retention/retrieval system. Beset by such reasons as "this is the way we have always done it," or worse still, by the fact that there is no authority vested in one person to establish and maintain a retention/retrieval system, those new to the profession can become convinced that such a system is not possible. If one is able to use a systems approach through objective reasoning based on cost and effective service, it is likely that money and time will be allocated for the medical record administrator to develop and maintain a functional system, even in an organization that has never had a retention/retrieval program. One only has to think of the primary purpose of data retention to recognize that it is eminently possible for any administrator to understand that a record retention/retrieval system is essential. The primary reason for keeping data is patient or client care.

To effectively provide patient care there has to be a sound retention/retrieval program. For there to be any medical research and education, there must be a functioning and useful retention/retrieval program. For administrative purposes and legal protection of the facility, there must be a system that provides accurate, complete, and useful data upon request. None of the foregoing can be accomplished unless there is an established retention/retrieval program for which one individual has full organizational authority. This is, of course, one of the medical record administrator's prime responsibilities.

Systems to Retrieve Data

In Chapter 2 we described four major types of data: identification, financial, medical or treatment, and social. These are still excellent sign-posts for us to consider in assessing data. Using these four categories of data elements leads us to look at all possible elements of data retrieval. Figure 7-1 describes the life cycle of a patient record. Categorized as major sources of data are:

Figure 7-1 Life Cycle of the Patient Record

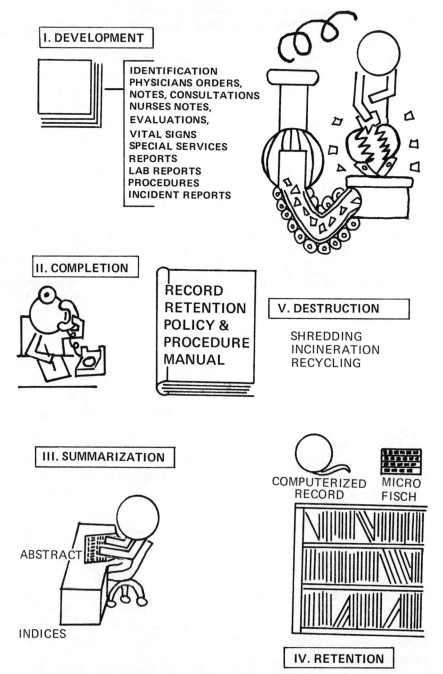

- Patients/clients
- Nurses' notes and evaluations, procedure reports, lab reports, incident reports, vital signs records, diagnostic and other indices
- Physicians and other direct care providers
- Indirect providers and users
- Scheduling and appointments functions

These sources may be thought of as entry gates to all the data developed, preserved, and available for retrieval.

These sources of data retrieval will be discussed in detail later on in this chapter. It must always be remembered that in retrieving data, consideration must be given to confidentiality, timeliness, and cost. Confidentiality must be preserved, and this responsibility lies with the record administrator or other person responsible for reporting the information. Speed of retrieval is an essential concern, for it has an impact on the efficiency of patient care provision and information reporting. Cost is the overriding element of both of the above considerations and in itself is a base line for the other two because without accurate cost projection and control of planned expenditures, the system will not function at all. The cost of a retention/retrieval program must be predicated on the importance of preserving the data in a useful, accessible manner. Objectives that specifically identify these and other needs of retention/retrieval systems must be directly linked to particular cost benefits. For instance, a rather simple-sounding objective, such as "Data will be retained in a retrievable format for ten years after the patient's last treatment episode," will directly influence such cost items as:

- Forms and formats for original entries
- Media for data entries (paper, mag tapes, fiche, etc.)
- Personnel positions, salaries, benefits, and educational programs
- Filing and storage equipment
- Office furniture and furnishings
- Supplies and materials
- Transcription equipment
- Teleprocessing equipment
- Overhead

What one process can be considered as the most effective in locating data? *Indexing* is the process that provides the master key to this initial step in retrieval. Indexing may be described as an organized listing of data pertaining to one subject or source of information. The most important index in a health information retention/retrieval program is the master patient index.

Master Patient Index

The master patient index is the vehicle used to locate records. As in other methods described in this text, the master patient index is used whether the data are in a hospital medical record department, a physician's or dentist's office, a mental health facility, or even in secondary data locations, such as insurance companies and health planning agencies. This index, known by various titles in some of the places described above, is simply a condensed listing that provides information to help locate major documents or data elements. That is, this index is a simplified, condensed version of data from original documents. It is filed separately from original documents. Data in the master index are used to locate original documents or reproduce elements of data from original documents when the whole documents are not needed. Very few health care facilities can have an effective data retention/retrieval system without utilization of a master patient index. (One exception that the authors are familiar with is a clinic that simply uses original documents filed by terminal digit on open shelves. The color-coded, terminal-digit-numbered file folders serve as their own index. The most common elements reproduced on a master patient index card are the patient's full name, full address, telephone number, birthdate, record identification number, admission and discharge dates, and name of the attending physician or other health care provider. Data elements for this index are optional, however, and vary according to the needs of the facility. Once again, in planning a retention/retrieval program one will have to ask questions and receive answers regarding the use of data. It is important that data elements in this index be individually accessible when only those data are required. This avoids pulling the complete record in those instances when only a limited number of data elements are sufficient to satisfy the inquiry.

The Soundex System: A common method used in maintaining the patient index is the *Soundex system*. This is a product of the Remington-Rand Office Systems Division of Sperry Rand Corporation that was designed to facilitate filing in geographic areas where there is a preponderance of vowels in last names (for example, Spanish surnames). However, it has received widespread recognition and use. The Soundex system is a phonetic filing system. Primarily, the Soundex system uses a combination letter and number code to identify names. Listed below are the letters and their number equivalents:

Letter	Number Equivalent
B, F, P, V	1
C, G, J, K, Q, S, X, Z	2
D, T	3
L	4
M, N	5
R	6

Letters that have no number equivalent are not coded. Those letters are A, E, I, O, U, W, H, and Y.

There are ten rules that make this system work.

1. The first letter of the surname is the "initial" letter, and it is never coded. It indicates the section of the file to which the name belongs. (The surname ADAMS will go to the "A" file and BROWN will go to the "B" file.) The remainder of the surname is then coded to three digits.

Example:

Anderson is coded   A-536

The first letter of this name is A. As it is the "initial" letter, it is never coded but merely designated just as it is. The next letter is N, and in the above table it has a numerical equivalent of 5. The next letter is D, and it has an equivalent of 3. The next letter is E, which is a vowel and is never coded. Therefore, you go to the next letter, which is R—the equivalent for that is 6. You now have three digits and that is as far as you have to go. No code contains more than three digits.

Other examples:

Blanchard is coded   B-452

Carter is coded   C-636

2. When there are insufficient letters in the surname to give you a three-digit code, add one zero, two zeros, or three zeros.

Examples:

Smith is coded   S-530

Moore is coded   M-600

Lee is coded   L-000

If a surname has double letters, consider them as though they were a single letter for coding purposes.

Examples:

Abbott is coded   A-130

Farrell is coded   F-640

3. If the name has any combination of two or more letters with the same numerical equivalent, code as a single letter.

Examples:

Jackson is coded   J-250

Biggs is coded   B-200

Herschel is coded   H-624

Rakoczy is coded   R-220

Todt is coded   T-300

Henman is coded   H-550

If one or more letters immediately following the "initial" letter are its numerical equivalent, do not code them but continue through the name until you come to the first letter that you are able to code. This rule applies to any letter that immediately follows the "initial" letter and its equivalent. Examples are often found in names beginning with the letters C, G, L, and P, but most often in names beginning with the letter S. Please note in examples below that the letters in parentheses are similar or equivalent to the first or "initial" letter and, therefore, are not coded.

    Examples:

        Lloyd is coded L(l)oyd   L-300
        Pfeffer is coded P(f)effer   P-160
        Scott is coded S(c)ott   S-300
        Skow is coded S(d)ow   S-000
        Scklaren is coded S(ck)laren   S-465
        Schmidt is coded S(ch)midt   S-530
        Czerny is coded C(z)erny   C-650

4. The vowels A, E, I, O, U, and Y are used as separators. Codable letters, when separated by these vowels, are coded individually.

    Examples:

        Borealis is coded   B-642
        Danilos is coded   D-542
        Hagemann is coded   H-255
        Staten is coded   S-335
        Lyles is coded   S-420

5. The letters W and H, when either or both appear within the name, are to be considered as having no bearing whatsoever on the code. They should be thought of as nonexistent and can be crossed out mentally. The letters W and H are never used as separators and should be remembered as letters only when appearing in a name.

    Examples:

        Withers is coded Wit(h)ers   W-362
        Church is coded C(h)urc(h)   C-620
        Vawter is coded Va(w)ter   V-360
        Shaw is coded S(h)aw   S-000
        Rawll is coded Ra(w)ll   R-400
        Paschka is coded Pasc(h)ka   P-200

6. Foreign and other prefixes such as DI, LA, DE, LE, LOS, LAS, VON, VAN, MC, and MAC, etc., are actually a part of the surname, even if spaced separately. For coding purposes, consider the different parts of the name as though all in one.

Examples:
Di Bello as though Dibello   D-140
De Los Santos as though Delossantos   D-425
Dela Cruz as though Delacruz   D-426
Le Droit as though Ledroit   L-363
L'Oise as though Loise   L-200
D'Aubugny as though Daubugny   D-125
Von Suppe as though Vonsuppe   V-521
Van Den Berg as though Vandenberg   V-535
Vander Meer as though Vandermeer   V-536
O'Farrell as though Ofarrell   O-164
McDonald as though Mcdonald   M-235
Mac Murray as though Macmurray   M-235

7. Compound names are treated as though they are a single name. If there is a hyphen between two names, consider it as all one name for coding purposes. Compound names are most common in Spanish-speaking countries. Frequently a resident of these countries will assume both his father's surname and his mother's maiden name in that order and may or may not hyphenate the two names. Occasionally the second part of the compound name will be abbreviated to just one initial, but this initial must be included in the coding of the entire name. Care should be used to differentiate between a true compound surname and a middle name.
Examples:
Mary Smith-Williams is coded Smithwilliams   S-534
J. A. Bulwer-Lytton is coded Bulwerlytton   B-464
Juan Gomez-Garcia is coded Gomezgarcia   G-526
Juan Jose GARCIA GOMEZ is coded Garciagomez   G-622
Maria Torres F.   All are coded   T-621
Maria Torres Fernandez   These are variations of ways in
Maria Torres-Fernandez   which the same surname may
Maria TORRES FERNANDEZ   be reported.
Enrique Luis Camacho is coded Camacho   C-520
In the last example LUIS is a middle name and is not part of the compound name.

8. Abbreviations of Saint (St.) are coded as though spelled out. Occasionally the French or Spanish abbreviation of SAINTE (Ste.) or SANTA (Sta.) is used. Always be sure that this is coded together with the given name that follows it.

Examples:
   St. John is coded Saintjohn   S-532
   Ste. Marie is coded Saintemarie   S-535
   Sta. Lucia is coded Santalucia   S-534

American Indian names are treated thus: If the reported name includes a given name and a tribal name, code the full tribal name as though it were a compound name.

Examples:
   Jim *Running Deer* is coded Runningdeer   R-552
   Mary *Big White Eagle* is coded Bigwhiteagle   B-232

If no given name appears with the tribal name, consider the tribal name as the only name and code it as a whole.

Example:
   Red Stone Face is coded Redstoneface   R-323
   Chief Black Rain Cloud is coded Blackraincloud   B-323

9. Disregard all titles appearing before or after the surname.
   Examples:
   (Mr.) Smith, John H.
   (Miss) Brown, Mary Jane
   Williams, (Rev.) James Edward
   Paul Johnson, (Sr.)
   Murphy, (Jr.) Charles A.

10. Chinese names are coded thus: If a sequence of two, three, or four names appears, choose the final one for coding.
   Examples:
   Tai Yat Low; code only Low   L-000
   Harry Yat Bun Sing; code only Sing   S-520

If a sequence of names appears and the first one has been underscored or marked with an asterisk, that name is indicated as the family name or surname and is to be coded. A given name or names may follow the family name without punctuation, and care should be taken to code only the family name. Sometimes the family name is printed in capitals and the balance of the name in lowercase letters. Occasionally the given names will be connected by a hyphen.

Examples:
   Wu King Lee; code only Wu   W-000
   Soong Mei Ling; code only Soong   S-520
   Chiang Kai-Shek; code only Chiang   C-520

The Soundex system is especially useful in large organizations that file a heavy volume of information by name. Because many names sound alike but have different spellings, there is a great chance for misfiling in a straight alphabetic system. The phonetic character of Soundex reduces the chance of error by bringing similar sounding names together in one file location. Therefore, the person who is responsible for filing and finding the cards has the advantage of many names filed together in one location, particularly those names that have similar sounds. If there is an error in the spelling of the name, cards of individuals who have similar sounding names will all be filed in one general location. This reduces the filing and finding search that goes on in cases of misspelling or other filing errors. It eliminates the file clerk having to take time to search out misfiles. It is said that this system detects duplication in files and disposes of 96 percent of all transposition of letters.

Alphabetic Filing: The other obvious way to keep a master patient index is through straight alphabetic filing. This, of course, is a very common system and one that requires very little training to learn. The alphabetic system has the advantage of being familiar, easy to teach, and accessible to any user of the file. However, the disadvantage of the alphabetic system is its high error rate. In a large patient population, as in any large card file, there is a tremendous risk of duplication of errors, such as loss or misfile of cards. However, there are rules to make alphabetic filing as easy and accurate as possible.

1. File each name in this sequence: Last name, first name or initial, and middle name or initial. (Arrange units in alphabetic order throughout. When the last names are exactly alike, use the first names to distinguish. When the first names are also the same, use the middle name or initial to differentiate.)

When the full names of two or more individuals are identical, go next to the name of the city, then state, then street name, and finally the numeric order of the house numbers.

A last name with a first name but no middle initial precedes the same name with an initial. Or a last name, when used alone, precedes the same last name with a first name or initial. That is, *nothing* comes before *something*.

Brown
Brown, H
Brown, Harold
Brown, Harold E.
Brown, Harold Edward

2. Treat as part of the last name such prefixes as De, Du, La, Los, Mac, Mc, San, Van, etc., and file exactly as spelled. An exception is sometimes made for M', Mc, and Mac. Theoretically they should be indexed as if beginning with Mac, but this is not generally known. They are sometimes

filed together as a block at the beginning of the M section. When this is done, follow the practice consistently.

de Bonneval, Albert	*Mac's Grouped*
DeByle, Jacqueline	or
Larue, Charles	MacAdam, James
LaRue, Walter	MacNish, Janie
Lefevre, Iris	McAdam, Cora
MacAdam, James	
Macnee, Tom	Macnee, Tom
MacNish, Janie	Mazure, Carole
McAdam, Cora	Meade, Sarah
Van Dam, Bud	
Van der Haas, Kaye	
Van der Schalie, Elaine	
Van Liere, Sharon	

3. Treat hyphenated last names as one complete unit. In computer applications, the hyphen occasionally is not recognized and the name may appear without it.

Cuyler-Curtis, Hazel
Cuylerton, Paul

4. When surnames and forenames are distinguishable (i.e., in either anglicized or foreign names), the names are filed according to usual rules; otherwise, they are filed as written. Modification, accents, diacritics, or other markings are disregarded.

Mohammed Ali
Samuel B. K. Chang
Albwar ur-Sol Siderer

5. File abbreviations as though spelled in full *when the meaning is known*:

Geo. Hayden   File as Hayden, George
but Bud Lofton   File as Lofton, Bud

6. The legal name of a married woman includes her own first name. If the husband's first name is known, her name *may be* cross-referenced to his. *Mrs.* is put into parentheses at the end of the name.

Logan, Lois E. (Mrs.)
Cross-reference: Logan, Richard G. (Mrs.)
                           Filed Logan, Lois E.

In alphabetic filing, certain letters of the alphabet expand more than others. In working with a large master patient index it is helpful to be familiar with a *letter distribution classification* prepared by the Department of the Navy and the Social Security Administration. That classification is shown as Exhibit 7-1.

Exhibit 7-1 Classification Division Frequencies in Name Files[1]

Letter Category	Navy Frequency* (%)	SSA Frequency† (%)	Letter Category	Navy Frequency (%)	SSA Frequency (%)
A	3.15	(3.051)	F	3.58	(3.622)
A-Ak	.72		F-Fd	.54	
Al	.72		Fe-Fh	.43	
Am-Aq	.84		Fi-Fk	.57	
Ar-Az	.87		Fl-Fq	1.07	
B	9.46	(9.357)	Fr-Fz	.97	
B-Bd	2.06		G	4.92	(5.103)
Be-Bh	1.61		G-Gd	1.04	
Bi-Bk	.43		Ge-Gh	.37	
Bl-Bn	.46		Gi-Gn	.85	
Bo-Bq	1.11		Go-Gq	.86	
Br-Bt	2.30		Gr-Gz	1.80	
Bu-Bz	1.49		H	7.74	(7.440)
C	7.40	(7.267)	H-Hd	2.91	
C-Cg	2.07		He-Hh	1.27	
Ch-Ck	1.04		Hi-Hn	.79	
Cl-Cn	.68		Ho-Ht	1.77	
Co-Cq	2.33		Hu-Hz	1.00	
Cr-Ct	.78		I	.39	(.387)
Cu-Cz	.50		J	2.84	(2.954)
D	5.17	(4.783)	J-Jd	.68	
D-Dd	1.31		Je-Jn	.39	
De-Dh	1.24		Jo-Jz	1.77	
Di-Du	.63		K	3.91	(3.938)
Do-Dt	1.17		K-Kd	.52	
Du-Dz	.82		Ke-Kh	1.03	
E	1.94	(1.888)	Ki-Kn	1.25	
E-Ek	.71		Ko-Kq	.46	
El-Em	.45		Kr-Kz	.65	
En-Ez	.78		L	4.69	(4.664)
L-Ld	1.46		Ri-Rn	.90	
Le-Lh	1.26		Ro-Rt	1.84	
Li-Ln	.62		Ru-Rz	.64	
Lo-Lt	.79		S	10.03	(10.194)
Lu-Lz	.56		S-Sb	1.04	
M	9.57	(9.448)	Sc-Sd	1.31	
M-Mb	2.73		Se-Sg	.52	
Mc-Md	2.30		Sh	1.09	
Me-Mh	.74		Si-Sl	1.03	
Mi-Mn	1.30		Sm	1.21	
Mo-Mt	1.65		Sn-So	.50	
Mu-Mz	.85		Sp-Ss	.54	

Exhibit 7-1 Continued

Letter Category	Navy Frequency* (%)	SSA Frequency† (%)	Letter Category	Navy Frequency (%)	SSA Frequency (%)
N	1.72	(1.785)	St	1.97	
N-Nd		.24	Su-Sz		.82
Ne-Nh		.67	T	3.31	(3.450)
Ni-Nz		.81	T-Tg		.93
O	1.43	(1.436)	Th-Tn		1.11
O-Ok		.47	To-Tq		.41
Ol-Oz		.96	Tr-Tz		.86
P	4.90	(4.887)	U		.22	(.238)
P-Pd		1.32	V	1.09	(1.279)
Pe-Pg		1.79	W	6.26	(6.287)
Ph		.26	W-Wd		1.61
Pi-Pn		.62	We-Wg		1.00
Po-Pq		.77	Wh		.68
Pr-Pz		.74	Wi-Wn		1.96
Q	.18	(.175)	Wo-Wz		1.01
R	5.14	(5.257)	X	(‡)	(.003)
R-Rd		.74	Y		.49	(.555)
Re-Rh		1.02	Z		.47	(.552)

Better File Operations, Navy Management Office, Department of the Navy, Washington 25, D.C. (1957), pp. 27-28.

†Social Security Administration distribution of last names by initial letter. The SSA has also published a list of some 1,500 most common names arranged alphabetically by size.

‡Less than 0.005.

From this table, we see that S and M are likely to be the largest sections in an alphabetic name file, and X, Q, and U the smallest. Sizes of sections may vary according to geographic location and concentrations of names of certain nationalities; but for the most part, the distributions shown here can safely be used for planning an alphabetic name file anywhere in the United States. Provision for expanding a large file can be projected according to this information. That is, more expansion can be anticipated in the C or H sections than in the E, N, or O sections.

Source: Irene Place and Estelle C. Popham, *Filing and Records Management* (Englewood Cliffs, N.J.: Prentice Hall, 1966), pp. 54-55. Reprinted with permission.

Computer Output Microfiche: The third method for maintaining the master patient index is *computer output microfilm*, the process of translating computer information into a miniature image on film. This process is generated through computer-created magnetic tape that contains master patient information. These tapes are read on a tape drive and captured by a computer output microfilm recorder. When the film is developed, duplicates are prepared from the original. Microfilm formats can take the form of roll film or 4″ by 6″ *microfiche film cards*, each containing up to 208 pages of computer output. The microimage can be enlarged, read on a microfilm viewer, and, if necessary, printed on paper. This makes storage easy because the original physical size of the data is greatly reduced.

Small skilled nursing facilities (less than 100 beds), residential facilities for the mentally ill or developmentally disabled, and small intermediate care facilities can often store records alphabetically and maintain effective retrievability. With infrequent use of the record and/or long-term stay of the patients, alphabetic filing may be the most efficient method to use. When the number of people who need access to the record or when patient volume expands, medical record departments are established. At this point, other means of storage come into consideration and we turn to numbering.

Numbering

For the medical record department to function efficiently, it is necessary to have an organized method for storing medical records. This is true in clinics, physicians' offices, ambulatory care facilities, or any other type of facility that compiles and retrieves health records.

Because of the potentially large number of medical records that can quickly accumulate in any setting where patient care is offered, the most efficient method of filing the actual documents is through a numbering system. The *numbering system* is basically an identifying factor used to label the record and facilitate its being filed in a systematic manner for easy retention and retrieval. There are three *major* types of numbering systems.

1. *Serial numbering* is that system of numbering in which the patient is assigned a new number each time treatment is received. In other words, each time the patient enters the system or is admitted for treatment, a new number is assigned to the record. This number is then entered on the master patient index and on each new record as it is prepared. Consequences of the serial numbering system are:

   — The patients will have many numbers assigned to their names.
   — There must be a continual updating of the record and the master patient index.

2. *Unit numbering* is a system in which one number is assigned to a patient's record. That patient's record retains that one number forever. Regardless of the number of times that the patient enters or leaves the system, that one number is retained and entered on the master patient index to identify the patient's record.
3. *Serial unit numbering* is a system in which the patient is assigned a new number each time he or she enters the system. All previous records are brought forward and reassigned the new number.

Family numbering is a popular method in clinics or health care centers where family care is featured. In this system the family is assigned one number and the family members within that group are assigned subnumbers to identify individual members of the family. All records then are labeled with a major number and subnumber headings that identify individual family members.

Prefix with the year is a system in which a number is assigned that includes the year treatment is received. This is not a very popular system but one that is still in use in areas where active storage is limited and inactive storage space is heavily utilized. A number is assigned for each patient, and each time the patient is admitted into the system, the year is included as the prefix number. For instance, for a patient who receives care in 1979, the record has a number that begins with 79. If a patient is admitted in subsequent years, the number will change to reflect the year of current admission.

Social Security numbering has gained popularity in many health care facilities. In this system the records are identified by the individual patient's Social Security number. Some reasons for using Social Security numbers are:

• Almost everyone has one and this system eliminates the need for keeping a number registry in the health care facility
• Fiscal reimbursement programs use this number for identification, so that many facilities are already familiar with its use
• The Social Security number has a permanence value and has been generally accepted for many other applications.

There are some disadvantages in using the Social Security number. Some individuals do not have one, particularly newborns and children, which necessitates assigning a pseudonumber that has to be changed at a later date. Social Security numbers are very lengthy, thereby increasing the possibilities for error, and, although it is illegal, many people have more than one Social Security number. It is estimated there may be as many as 4 million individuals in the United States who have more than one Social

Security number. There is also a concern among health care providers that use of a Social Security number jeopardizes confidentiality and provides easier access to outside users of data because of the possible linkage of patient and provider's records to credit information, tax information, and so on.

In comparing the numbering systems described above for selection for any one facility, once again it is necessary to take a systems approach to reach an effective decision. The type of facility, number of patients or clients involved, filing space available, availability of automated information systems, required turnaround time for retrieval of information, and many other factors must be considered in determining which type of numbering system will be utilized.

The origin of the numbering system is a file called the *number index* or *register*. The number register is a chronologic listing of numbers. This listing of numbers identifies all numbers that are issued and contains a cross-reference to the name of each patient to whom a number is assigned. The *number index* can be kept manually or it may be automated. The important factor about the *number index* is that there must be a cross-reference to all patient numbers issued to medical records. That is, whether it is an automated index or simply a file that contains the admissions and discharges for one day, there must be a separate source apart from the numbered medical records to identify which numbers have been issued and the names of the patients to whom they are assigned. The number index has importance because it contains the list of numbers that have not yet been issued and therefore is a continuing source of numerical assignment. It can be kept in the admitting department or in the medical record department, and it may be located in any number of locations in other types of facilities. The number index must always be consistent and continually checked for accuracy for it to retain its usefulness as a cross-reference when errors are discovered in the numbers on forms or records. Once a number has been assigned to a medical record, all departments that use records will have one other reference to the record in addition to the patient's name. In case of error on medication orders, lab work, or permanent filing of the record, this cross-reference and use of a number makes up an extremely effective system that provides a check to assure accuracy in processing the medical record.

The parts of a numbering system of most concern to the medical record administrator are:

1. The type of numbering system
2. The number register or index
3. Assignment of numbers

4. Methods used to imprint numbers on forms
5. Audit of number assignment
6. Audit of accuracy in imprinting

A brief description of the sequence of numbering may assist in understanding the six points listed above. The number register or index must be consistent, up to date, and capable of assigning as many numbers as needed. The numbering system must be compatible with organizational objectives, filing methods, and equipment. It must be coordinated with record storage and reflect the activity of patients and record retrieval. The assignment of numbers must be organized, supervised, and consistently monitored to assure accuracy and timeliness of numbers issued. Methods used to imprint forms must be timely, accurate, and produce legible copies. A standardized method of placing the numbers on the forms is the most effective method, regardless of whether the imprint is achieved through handwriting or electroplate, plastic card, or other automated method. There must be a continuous audit of the way numbers are issued and the way numbers are transferred to the documents. When changing a numbering system there are some guidelines that can be useful. The guidelines are particularly useful in changing from some other system to unit numbering.

First, it is important to determine well in advance just when the unit numbering is needed. It is best to attempt to tie the target date to the beginning of a calendar or fiscal year. Plan well in advance to be ready to start on the selected date. As soon as the date is selected, all the new supplies that will be needed—material, file folders, equipment for imprinting, etc—are determined. Once determined, they are ordered. Remember that folders, file supplies, imprinters, and other paper and printed products can require lengthy lead time. Training for those who will use the new system must be planned and initiated.

The actual *number assignment changeover* should start on a selected date. A new number register is used and all entries verify the starting date of the new numbering system. The original number register is retained as the major source of cross-reference regarding the original system's assigned numbers. Unit numbers are assigned to all new patients. Unit numbers are also assigned to readmitted patients. Their previous number is left on the file folder and the file folder left in place. Inserted in the file folder is a slip that records the newly assigned unit number. This is done to provide a double check on the issuance of the new number, should there be an error somewhere in the current or future process. The master patient index card is revised to show only the new unit number. The record itself is pulled from the file and all pages are renumbered with the new number. The documents that must reflect the newly assigned number are: master patient index, record and all its forms, the new number register, and the permanent file folder. Discharge analysis, disease and operation indexes, and any other registers, indexes, or files that record the original record can remain unchanged. When obtaining the individual record from these sources, the new number will be identified from the permanent file folder.

Filing Systems

The next step in the consideration of a system to retain and retrieve data is filing the data. There are several important aspects in considering an adequate filing system. Four currently used procedures of filing include *centralized*, *decentralized*, *satellite*, and *controlled-decentralized*. These are shown in Figure 7-2.

In a centralized system of filing, all information is filed in one central location. There is one file room for all data. In this system personnel methods, policies, equipment, material, and all of the components involved in an effective filing system are located and operational in one place. This allows for direct supervision, easy access for those who need the information, and an organized area for management to fulfill its role of leading, coordinating, and controlling.

In a decentralized filing system files are usually located close to the source of their active use. In a clinic, for instance, files for each individual clinic are stored in a file room located close to or in the clinic. There is no central file room where records of all clinics are filed.

In a satellite record system the majority of the records are filed in one major location but some records travel to clinics or other areas as needed and may stay in those areas for a certain period of time to be returned to the central file room only for permanent filing. In other words, while the patient or client remains under active treatment the record of the patient will remain located at the satellite clinic.

In the controlled-decentralized system all forms, requisitions, filing procedures, methods, and processes are standardized so that records in the various areas are maintained identically. Such standardization makes it easier for everyone in the organization to utilize all records regardless of their decentralized locale. Ease in using the records is accomplished by this method in addition to cost savings in purchasing forms, folders, etc.

When discussing filing in relationship to medical records or health data, it must be remembered that all types of forms, documents, cards, and other media sources related to records are also filed. Figures 7-3 and 7-4 provide a description of steps used in removing a record from the permanent file and one method of filing records that need to be completed by physicians. Included in files of medical and health records will be such records, cards, folders, and reports as the master patient index; physician, disease, and operation indexes; the medical record, both as complete and incomplete

Figure 7-2 Four Types of Filing Procedures

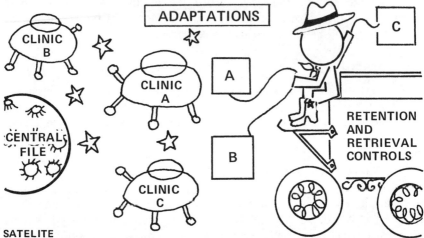

SATELITE
RECORDS REMAIN IN SATELITE
LOCATION FOR DURATION OF
ACTIVE TREATMENT THEN ARE
RETURNED TO CENTRAL
FILE — AMBULATORY CARE USE.

CONTROLLED - DECENTRALIZED
HOUSED SEPARATELY BUT CON-
TROLLED THROUGH UNIFORM
POLICIES, PROCEDURES, METHODS
& FORMS — LONG TERM CARE'
VOCATIONAL REHABILITATION,
AMBULATORY CARE.

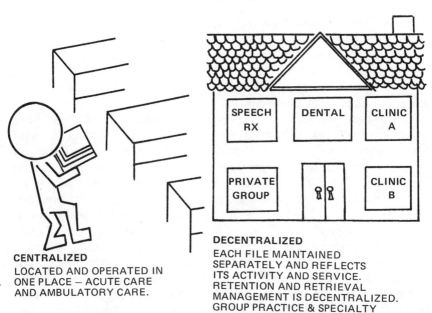

CENTRALIZED
LOCATED AND OPERATED IN
ONE PLACE — ACUTE CARE
AND AMBULATORY CARE.

DECENTRALIZED
EACH FILE MAINTAINED
SEPARATELY AND REFLECTS
ITS ACTIVITY AND SERVICE.
RETENTION AND RETRIEVAL
MANAGEMENT IS DECENTRALIZED.
GROUP PRACTICE & SPECIALTY
SETTINGS.

Figure 7-3 Steps in Record Retrieval from Permanent File

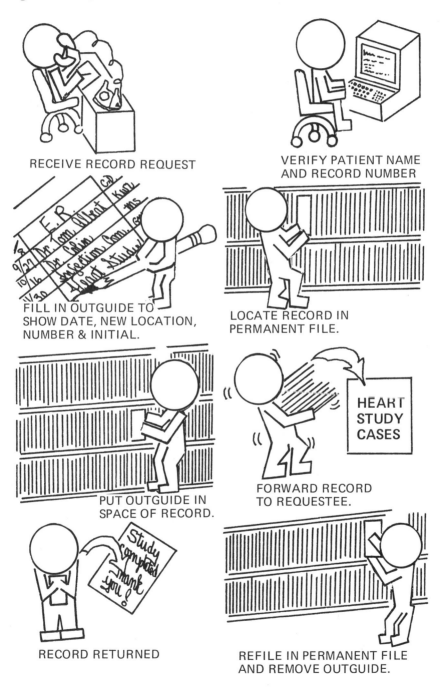

RECEIVE RECORD REQUEST

VERIFY PATIENT NAME
AND RECORD NUMBER

FILL IN OUTGUIDE TO
SHOW DATE, NEW LOCATION,
NUMBER & INITIAL.

LOCATE RECORD IN
PERMANENT FILE.

PUT OUTGUIDE IN
SPACE OF RECORD.

FORWARD RECORD
TO REQUESTEE.

HEART
STUDY
CASES

RECORD RETURNED

REFILE IN PERMANENT FILE
AND REMOVE OUTGUIDE.

Figure 7-4 Filing Incomplete Records

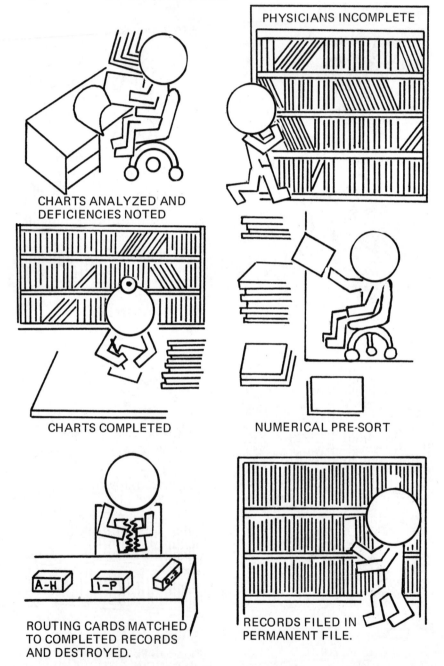

CHARTS ANALYZED AND
DEFICIENCIES NOTED

PHYSICIANS INCOMPLETE

CHARTS COMPLETED

NUMERICAL PRE-SORT

ROUTING CARDS MATCHED
TO COMPLETED RECORDS
AND DESTROYED.

RECORDS FILED IN
PERMANENT FILE.

documents; and management reports, such as inventory control sheets, requisition sheets, budgetary reports, policy manuals, forms, and paper. While not all of these items are filed systematically, all of them are accessible and easily retrievable. The files we discuss in this chapter include, in particular, the master patient index; the indexes of diseases, operations, physicians, reasons for visit, procedures, etc.; and the medical record document. It also includes special registries, such as the number registry and the pathology and radiology registries.

Once a numbering system for the record has been established and a method selected, the next consideration is the type of filing to be used. We will describe two methods of filing: terminal digit and numerical.

Terminal Digit Filing: Probably the most common type of filing is terminal digit. It is a method of filing by the last digits of a number instead of by the first digits. This varies from traditional filing in that we are used to reading numbers from left to right. In the terminal digit system one must read from right to left. For example, in our conventional numeric system, number 9361934 would come after number 9361933. In terminal digit the number would be broken down into groups of 936 19 34. The 936 would be filed behind the primary guide, 34, and the secondary guide, 19. This means that all files ending with the primary number, 34, would be together and arranged within that group by the secondary digits. The following illustrates the difference between traditional numeric filing and terminal digit filing:

Consecutive (traditional)	Terminal Digit
36,1103	237 18 01
36,1996	236 53 02
136,1998	36 11 03
136,2062	136 38 45
136,3845	242 38 56
236,5302	136 20 62
237,1801	36 19 96
242,3856	136 19 98

One of the chief advantages of the terminal digit filing system, which may be seen when the list above is studied, is that the files can be expanded more evenly under this system than with the straight numeric system. The filing can be spread out over a large filing area, so that file sections may be broken up and file personnel assigned to specific terminal digit groups. This can be done because in a terminal digit system the most recent number issued is not filed at the end of the file section. That is to say, in a file section that uses consecutive numbers filed by a straight numeric method, the files will expand in one direction only. With the terminal digit filing system expansion is spread out so that it is less likely that active (or newer) records will be bunched in one area.

The terminal digit filing system has been found to be speedy and less open to error. It takes less time to read the numbers when they are broken into small components. The numbers are less likely to be transposed and sorting is easier. Because there are no gaps in the sequence of numbers, misfiles are reduced and filing and finding are easier. The uniformity of the file section is another advantage of terminal digit filing. Identical organization in each section of the file makes it easy to distribute work for a large file area. It also allows for fixed responsibility for various sections of the file. Figures 7-5 and 7-6 illustrate terminal digit filing.

Straight Numerical Filing: The oldest and most traditional method of filing reports, documents, and other data is a simply and easily understood way to retain data for future retrieval. Records or reports are filed according to the assigned report number in chronological sequence. The consecutive sequence for the following numbers would be:

306925
458590
7238901
7980656
9021302

Anyone with the basic skill of reading numbers can quickly understand straight numerical filing. The major problem with this method is the human tendency to transpose numbers. Numbers, especially those of six or more digits, are not easily remembered in their correct sequence. Misfiles are the result of such memory tricks. Additionally, with straight numerical filing, the files fill out in one direction. Folders are not evenly distributed throughout the files, as they are with terminal digit filing. Because of the sequential nature of number assignment, all activity takes place in one area of the files. File clerks get in each other's way working in this one heavily used area.

Coding and Indexing

Coding and indexing are two major retention/retrieval functions. These avenues of entry to the data provide access in a unique way. It is unique because it identifies and compiles information components that contain essential original data for research and education. Data accessed through coding and indexing are categorized according to the major objective data elements of medical and treatment data entries. Data entries that describe diagnostic, therapeutic, and a combination of all types of care are synthesized and categorized according to basic coding systems and indexed for future retrieval. Figure 7-7 depicts the coding-indexing function.

Figure 7-5 Terminal Digit Filing Theory and Use

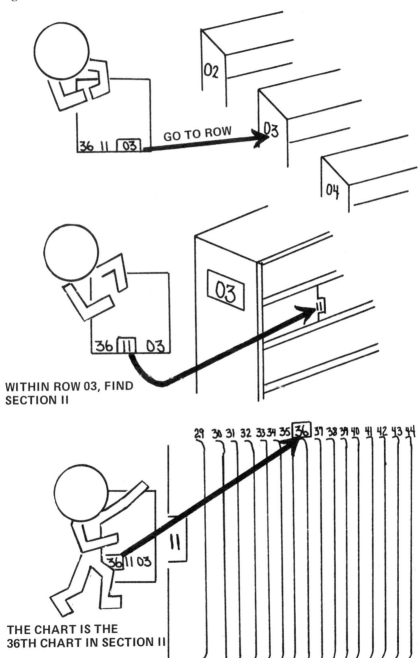

Figure 7-6 Additional Aids to Terminal Digit Filing

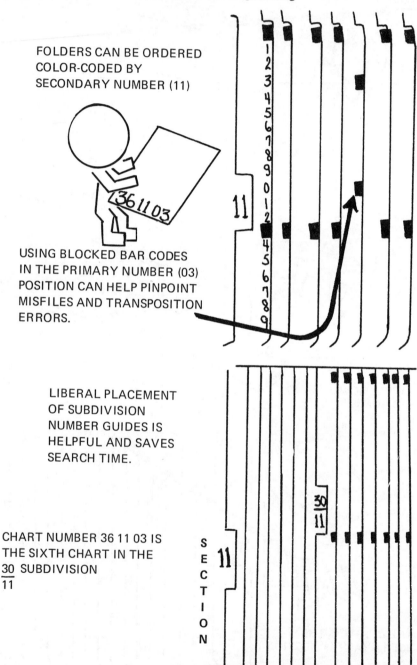

FOLDERS CAN BE ORDERED
COLOR-CODED BY
SECONDARY NUMBER (11)

USING BLOCKED BAR CODES
IN THE PRIMARY NUMBER (03)
POSITION CAN HELP PINPOINT
MISFILES AND TRANSPOSITION
ERRORS.

LIBERAL PLACEMENT
OF SUBDIVISION
NUMBER GUIDES IS
HELPFUL AND SAVES
SEARCH TIME.

CHART NUMBER 36 11 03 IS
THE SIXTH CHART IN THE
$\frac{30}{11}$ SUBDIVISION

Figure 7-7 The Coding-Indexing Function

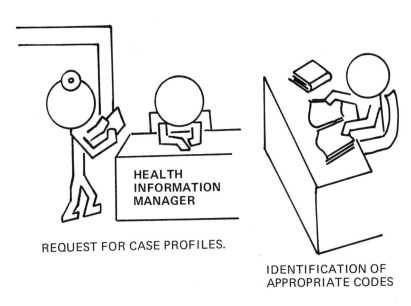

HEALTH
INFORMATION
MANAGER

REQUEST FOR CASE PROFILES.

IDENTIFICATION OF
APPROPRIATE CODES

Information Requests Satisfied Through Use of Indices.

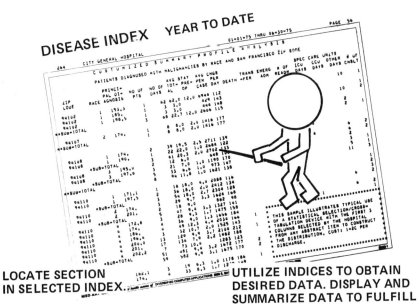

LOCATE SECTION
IN SELECTED INDEX.

UTILIZE INDICES TO OBTAIN
DESIRED DATA. DISPLAY AND
SUMMARIZE DATA TO FULFILL
REQUEST.

Coding is a numerical assignment that provides an organized approach to data retrieval. It uses a numerical equivalent or an alphanumerical equivalent to identify such data components as diagnosis, operation, procedure, reason for visit, pathologic specimens, injuries, obstetric conditions and procedures, symptoms, mental conditions, congenital anomalies, physical signs, and ill-defined conditions.

Indexing provides a listing of numbers that identify individual records coded according to the categories described above. Indexing compiles a composite source of groups of records classified under one code number. For example, all patients listed on the index card numbered 401 have been treated, diagnosed, and coded for Essential Benign Hypertension. This example utilizes the ICDA-8 Coding System. More will be explained about particular coding systems later in this chapter. Indexing was originally performed in a manual mode, but most modern health care facilities use automated techniques and equipment to store and retrieve coded material. Indexes were, in fact, one of the first functional operations in the processing of medical information to be automated.

Coding Methods: Many coding methods have been developed to capture data for all types of health information. There are coding methods for acute care, primary care, pathology specimens, procedures, and many others. These methods have evolved to provide access to particular information components and specialty aspects of health care. To be useful, coding methods must be mutually understood by all who do the coding and all who access the data through the coding method. Factors that play an important role in coding are medical terminology, nomenclatures, consideration of retrieval requests at the time of assignment of code numbers, consistency and accuracy in assignment of code numbers by all who code in *one* institution, and consistency in assignment of code number—through conformity with the coding principles and rules—by those who code in *all* institutions.

Our discussion of coding will focus on the various methods available and the purposes of those methods. Coding skill is acquired through practice coding in instructional manuals and actual complete records. Most medical record administrators and many medical record technicians do not perform the function of coding, but they are familiar with the theory of coding and coding methods currently available and have the ability to determine which method of coding is most appropriate for particular facilities. To do the latter, record professionals must have an understanding and familiarity with available coding systems and, so that they can teach or supervise others who perform coding, a working knowledge of coding itself.

Figure 7-8 demonstrates the historic evolution of the most widely used coding methods: coding for acute care hospitals.

Figure 7-8 Evolution of Coding Methods in Acute Care Hospitals

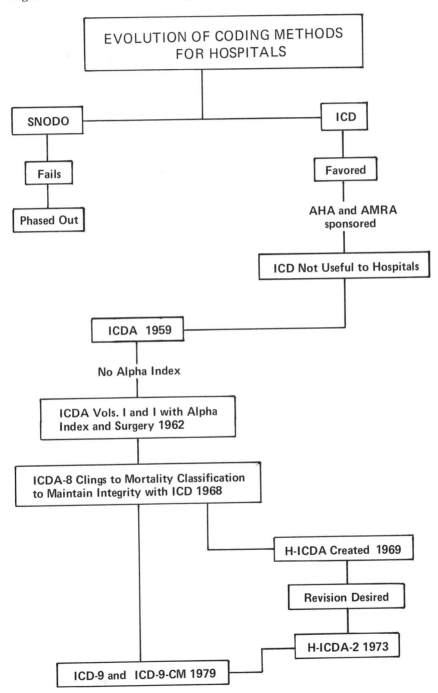

The first widely recognized and used method of coding was the *Standard Nomenclature of Disease and Operations* (SNODO). It was a very thorough method that attempted to classify every known disease that was clinically recognizable. It was later replaced by the *International Classification of Diseases*. SNODO was shelved because it tended to retain obsolete names of diseases, elaborate coding of certain diseases, problems of assigning codes for nonclinicians, and several other reasons. The *International Classification of Diseases* became the preferred system and is endorsed by the World Health Organization. SNODO primarily focused on coding and classification of the causes of death. ICDA targets the classification of diagnoses encountered in hospitals and includes categories for operations and procedures carried out in hospitals. Currently in its tenth revision, it is revised every decade. It is the required system for those U.S. health care facilities that participate in federal programs, such as Medicare and PSRO. The tenth edition was mandated to commence in January 1979. Published originally by the Commission on Professional and Hospital Activities of Ann Arbor, Michigan, ICD-9CM, the modified ICD-9 used by the United States, will ultimately become a publication of the federal government through its printing office. ICD is a basic three-digit code with four- and five-digit categories in some areas. It is a greatly expanded version of ICD-8, and some of its expansions include separate publications. These additional volumes are:

- Procedures in Medicine: surgical, nonsurgical, and diagnostic procedures
- Classification of Impairments and Handicaps
- International Classification of Diseases for Oncology
- Application of the International Classification of Diseases to Dentistry and Stomatology
- Classification of Disorders of the Eye[2]

Another method that evolved after the introduction of ICDA is *Current Medical Terminology* (CMT) and *Current Procedural Terminology* (CPT). This method is a product of the AMA and is aimed at classification of ambulatory care data. It recognized the inherent problem of the lack of standard medical terminology in both SNODO and ICDA, and attempted to conquer the terminology jinx as well as to establish useful classifications. CMT is, basically, a dictionary of preferred terms in medicine.[3] CPT is a coding method for diagnostic and therapeutic procedures in surgery, medicine, and the specialties. Its primary use is probably related to billing purposes. CPT is a five-digit code and is currently in its fourth revision. It is published by the American Medical Association.[4]

The *International Classification of Health Problems in Primary Care* (ICHPPC) is a method for use by physicians, in general and family practice, throughout the world. ICHPPC, which is based on the eighth revision of the *International Classification of Diseases* (ICD-8), is designed for (1) classification of morbidity information in the primary care setting for statistical purposes and (2) indexing, storage, and retrieval of outpatient medical record by diagnoses and problems.

Early attempts at using ICD to classify morbidity information in the primary care settings met with difficulties because basic health problems could not be adequately coded. This led to the development of more compact classifications based on ICD (i.e., the Royal College of General Practitioners Classification of Diseases in 1959, the Royal Australian College of General Practitioners Study in 1965, the Canadian Classification of Disease in 1969, and the RCGP U.S. modification in 1971.)

As the development of classifications by primary care physicians continued in various countries, an integral component was the initiation of a register of patients indexed by health problems for purposes of record retrieval in research, ease of follow up, assessment of outcome, and identification of vulnerable groups requiring special supervision and management.

In October 1972 the World Organization of National Colleges, Academies, and Academic Associations of General Practitioners/Family Physicians (WONCA) assigned a work party to develop a short tabular list based on ICD-8 and acceptable for use on an international scale by primary care physicians. This list was tested in nine countries and was based on a total of more than 100,000 patient encounters. Comments and recommendations for the more than 300 test sites were the basis for ICHPPC. In November 1974, WONCA unanimously accepted ICHPPC. Because ICHPPC is a tool that allows comparison of diagnostic descriptions, the AHA has cooperated with WONCA in the publication of ICHPPC.

The WONCA classification committee worked with the strengths and weaknesses associated with the application of ICD-8 to ambulatory care data. Because the available rubrics in ICD are too specific for many diagnostic categories seldom encountered in ambulatory care, many of the ICD categories were grouped. Additional rubrics were assigned for symptoms, important signs, and inconclusive findings based on frequency of occurrence and appropriateness of provisional diagnoses. The shift in the use of ICD from inhouse to outpatient morbidity also required additional rubrics for indexing clinical problems in the problem-oriented record. Additional changes were required to adequately emphasize whole family and individual problems, maternal and child health care, family planning, preventive medicine, and administrative tasks.

The ICHPPC contains 371 diagnostic titles divided into 18 sections that correspond with those of the ICD and other hospital classifications. It is compatible with the ICD and ICDA classifications, and the coded numbers of the individual titles were designed to correspond with those of these classifications. The diagnostic titles were selected for one of three reasons:

1. *Importance.* It was for this reason that the diagnoses Multiple Sclerosis and Tuberculosis were included.
2. *Frequency of Occurrence.* The data from the field trial were used to determine which diagnoses should be included because of a frequency distribution.
3. *Ability for the Diagnosis to Be Made in the Primary Care Setting.* Those diagnoses requiring more sophisticated facilities were excluded.

The classification as published by the AHA contains both tabular and alphabetic sections. A standardized dictionary of titles suitable for computer use is also available from the AHA. The classification is designed for coding by the health care provider, but central coding by medical record practitioners is also possible.

The ICHPPC reflects realities of primary care in its construction. In some cases, large numbers of three-digit titles of the ICD have been outlined into a single rubric for the ICHPPC. In other cases, two titles have been split from a single four-digit rubric. A section on social problems (not present in ICD) has been added to Section XVIII, and Section XVI, which includes signs and symptoms, has been expanded.[5]

Another major coding method is *Diagnostic and Statistical Manual of Mental Disorders.* Its origination can be seen in Figure 7-9, which follows. DSM-II, now in its second edition, is published by the American Psychiatric Association (APA). Some of its features are:

- A single section providing a comprehensive classification of mental disorders.
- Mental disorders associated with organic and physical factors related to other disease categories.
- Categories for mental disorders not specified as psychotic associated with organic and physical disorders, physical disorders of presumably psychogenic origin, and transient situational disturbances.
- More complete classification of mental retardation based on the recommendations of the American Association on Mental Deficiency.

It is noted that a great deal of difficulty was encountered in gaining international acceptance of and agreement on what to call a particular mental disorder, and no attempts were made to achieve any agreement on the causes, etc., of the disorder itself.[6]

Figure 7-9 Evolution of DSM from ICD

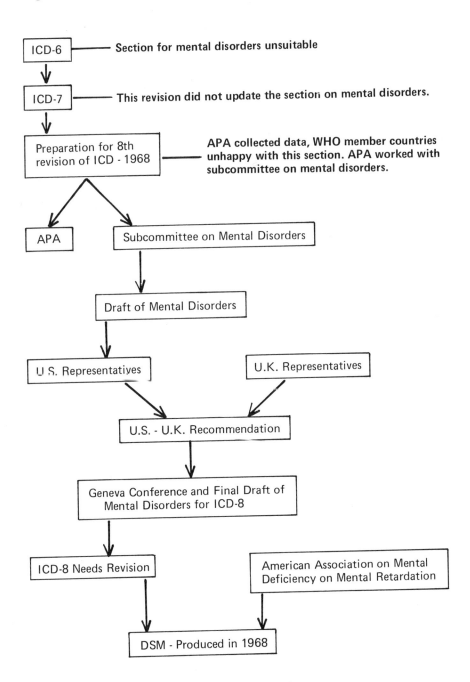

The *Systematized Nomenclature of Pathology* (SNOP) was developed over a six-year period by the Committee on Nomenclature and Classification of Disease of the College of American Pathologists. Its primary aim was to help pathologists organize and utilize their material and to assist in storage and retrieval of medical data. The first edition was available in 1965. It is now understood that those using the SNOP coding system will change to the *Systematized Nomenclature of Medicine* (SNOMED), also published by the College of American Pathologists. Training workshops in SNOMED have been offered since 1977. The College of American Pathologists first developed SNOP as a nomenclature. It consisted of four fields, including topography (anatomic site), morphology (the abnormality at that site), etiology (causative agent or agents), and function. These nomenclature fields were first published in 1965 after a field trial experience and were subsequently widely used by pathologists around the world with some 12,000 copies of the manuals sold. The initial program satisfied the needs of pathology, but it was quickly realized that subspecialty areas of pathology would require some additional terms. Once adaptations and extensions of the basic SNOP system were developed, tested, and approved, the new system became known as SNOMED. SNOMED has two additional fields, function and disease.[7]

The *Reason for Visit Classification* (RFVC) has been in use since 1973. Originated through a study known as the National Ambulatory Care Survey, the RFVC uses the following modules:

1. Symptom module (usually representing first visits)
2. Disease module (return visits with diagnosis previously supplied)
3. Diagnostic, screening, and preventive procedures (checkups, preventive inoculations, prenatal care)
4. Therapeutic procedures, process problems, and counseling (return visit initiated by physician)
5. Injuries and adverse effects module (emergency visits)
6. Abnormal test results module (return visits for test results)
7. Administrative reasons for visit (insurance physicals, return-to-work certificates)

This classification was developed to meet a need that was not being met by traditional acute care or morbidity methods and also to fill a void caused by categorization of ambulatory diagnoses, symptoms, etc. It is designed to capture the reason for the visit, not the diagnosis, procedure, ill-defined condition, or other nonspecific or specific data available through other methods of classification. The National Ambulatory Care Survey was undertaken by the National Center for Health Statistics, and the RFVC is designed to code symptoms or complaints expressed in the patient's own words. Because the survey is an ongoing project of the National Center for Health Statistics, it measures, on a continuing basis, approximately 2,000 office-based physicians' practices all over the country.[8]

Several coding methods have been briefly outlined in this section. There are many other coding methods available, and this will probably continue to be the case. No one method has ever been developed that classifies data to suit the needs of all users. To do so is very likely an impossibility until computer technology can provide such a mechanism at a cost-effective price. This is not likely, however, since some types of care are totally unrelated to others, and there is probably no need to have a system so comprehensive that it can classify every possible component of health information in one method.

Registries: Other important avenues to data collection are registries. Registries provide a synopsized group of data that categorizes a larger group of data. Some areas that use registries are pharmacies, laboratories, radiology departments, and other specialty departments. Computers have been instrumental in the design and use of registries. Whenever there is a need to retrieve data, in a chronological sequence, one entry point that is useful is a registry or index that uniquely identifies the major components needed. Familiarity with the needs of the data users, an understanding of the composition of the information components to be tapped, and a basic understanding of systems analysis provide the tools an individual needs to design a useful, current registry.

Guidelines for Data Retrieval Procedures

The most important purpose in the retrieval of data is to continually focus attention on the patient / client. The primary purpose of data retention is better patient care. Secondary purposes of data retention and retrieval must complement the primary purpose. The medical record administrator must always bear in mind that retrieval of the data is basically an activity that concerns patients and their confidential information. There must be one individual in an organization who bears the responsibility for making certain that every effort is expended to make the patient's health or medical information available when it is needed for the continued care of the patient or client. Such a person might be considered a patient advocate. This concept is part and parcel of the concept of record control. *Record control* is that part of record retention and retrieval that provides:

1. Procedural elements that assure a permanent location for data to be maintained

2. Defined limits on retrieval of the data by particular users
3. Methods to continually communicate the current location of a record

Control of data is an essential and established subsystem of the record retention/retrieval system. Included in a record control system are such components as policies, procedures, methods, and departmental working documents, such as requisition or locator slips or other intradepartmental forms and reports that facilitate the location of individual or groups of records. Record control, then, is an essential subsystem in the management of health information.

The medical record administrator provides initial direction to the development of record control. Continued direction of the record control function is provided through policies, procedures, and personnel whose efforts are coordinated toward continual control of data. In the controlling function, consideration is given to the flow of data in and out of the permanent file area. Consideration is also given to the flow of data before it reaches the permanent file area. In fact, there is always consideration of the flow of data, regardless of its status.

The medical record administrator understands data flow and its control. Therefore, this individual must bear the responsibility of developing a record control system that is compatible with the needs of data users. However, it is the medical record administrator who must also bear final responsibility for development of a record control system that works for users, providers, patients, or clients. Once again it can be seen that the medical record administrator serves in the role of patient's advocate because nonpatient users of data frequently are only concerned with their particular needs and schedule. They often overlook what the medical record administrator cannot afford to overlook: that the record in its flow through the organization must always be retrievable for patient care. For example, users of the record sometimes forget that their primary interest in the record is for research or myriad other reasons. They tend to forget that patients may, at a time that coincides with use of patient records for research or other purposes, need emergency medical care. The information that belongs to a patient must be made available for care of the patient at any time. A functioning record control system provides a method of making patient information rapidly available to all who need it. This may sound like a utopian idea, but in many health care facilities, institutions, agencies, or organizations that use health information in their continuing daily operations, instant availability of partial data or complete documents is a reality.

We have already seen that the medical record administrator bears the primary responsibility for record retention and retrieval in its subsystem of records control. Let's now take a look at the medical record administrator in retention/retrieval and outline some of the elements that are essential when carrying out this important function.

Role of the Record Manager

Functions. Develop, retain, and retrieve patient/client records in accordance with established policies that include retention, protection, and disposition of reports, forms, correspondence, and other records.

Organizational relationships. Reports to assistant administrator or administrator—administrative services; supervises assistant records manager, retention/retrieval supervisor, records center supervisor, central records clerks, microfilm technicians, forms clerks, keypunch, and CRT operators.

Interdepartmental relationships. Systems and procedures department, legal counsel, business and accounting office, all department heads, medical staff, patients, and clients.

Extradepartmental relationships. Third party payers, health planning agencies, patients/clients, legal counsels, biostatisticians, data collection representatives, physicians, hospitals, and other direct and indirect health care providers.

Responsibility for the institution. (1) Establish procedures for retention and destruction of all types of records on a departmental and facilitywide basis; (2) design and revise forms and procedures pertaining to the use of health information; and (3) coordinate problems concerning the flow of information, retention/retrieval of records, files, delivery of medical reports, and medical records.

Departmental. (1) Plan, develop, implement, and modernize record availability and departmental services; (2) maintain and control all records, including files, index cards, registers, policy manuals, microfilm or microfiche, magnetic tape, or other media used in the preparation and retention of records; (3) delegate authority through supervisors or directly to personnel for specific projects; and (4) prepare departmental and institutional manual regarding retention and retrieval of health information.

The Retention/Retrieval Manual

As we have just seen, the preparation of a retention/retrieval manual is a definite function of medical record administrators in their role as retention/retrieval managers. This manual is prepared to provide a means of sharing information about the many elements in the record retention/retrieval process. A major advantage of using a written manual is to save money when handling records. Money is saved through the use of written directions to new employees. Oral instructions alone are more likely to result in poorly performed work. A written operational manual available so that employees can read exactly what is to be completed, how it is to be completed, and what productivity level is expected is a financial and operational asset. A second advantage is the reduction of time wasted by employees redoing tasks because of errors in their first attempts at work. A third and very important advantage of the retention/retrieval manual is standardization of procedures. Standardization of records management procedures benefits the control function in the following ways:

- Duplicate functions are eliminated
- Smoother work flow is achieved throughout the entire system
- Greater understanding and cooperation are achieved by the users of the data
- Written directions and instructions provide a means for testing, revising, and improving the directions and instructions.

Some of the important elements that must be addressed in the written manual are:

1. Designate the individual who has authority for the centralized control of the record management function.
2. Identify the relationship between the records retention/retrieval function and user departments or individuals.
3. Establish uniform procedures in the origination, processing, retention, and destruction of records for the whole facility.
4. Publish instructions and guidelines for all personnel who develop, use, or retrieve the facility's records.
5. Develop an attitude among all facility employees that there is a basic principle of good records management that necessitates control of data flow.
6. Encourage employees to provide constructive suggestions concerning the retention/retrieval program.
7. Communicate changes in policies and procedures.
8. Coordinate similar records management functions and activities throughout the organization.
9. Serve as a training center or source of information for all new or transferred employees.

Contents of the manual should include:

- Retention and retrieval schedules for particular types of data
- Policies regarding the time that data may be allowed out of the central file area

- Policies regarding information available for particular users of the data
- Sample forms, such as release-of-information forms, consent forms, and summaries that are used for preparing information for external users of data
- Policies regarding the use of photocopies and the charges for those copies
- Policies regarding photocopies vs. summarizations of records
- Policies regarding release of information to patients/clients
- Policies regarding audit of the record retention function

The manual should also include as many current samples of forms, flow charts, and *retention schedules* as possible, as well as other salient information that would point out the current directions of the department.

For the manual to be a successful enterprise within the department, it is wise to include employees who are vitally involved in retention and retrieval of data in development of the written manual. Policy and procedure manuals have frequently been criticized or misused for some very obvious reasons. To prevent the misuse or nonuse of a manual, it is recommended that the writers of the manual put themselves in the place of the users of the manual; that is, try to take the approach of the individuals who read the information. This, of course, necessitates talking to, working with, or being one of the employees who actually are involved in record retention and retrieval. Another plus is a well-defined outline with bold type headings that are easily seen. Compile the manual in a format that makes additions to and deletions from it easy so that it can be continually updated. A loose-leaf binder is an excellent way to store this kind of information. The use of samples and examples to clarify policies that may seem unclear is another way to clarify what is described in the manual; dividers that clearly indicate where the information is in the manual so that it can be quickly located also make a manual a more useful document.

Let's now look in detail at some of the key items to be included in the *retention/retrieval manual*.[9] These are essential operations that must function properly for optimum levels of retention and retrieval to be achieved.

Policies: Policies are basic guides to action that prescribe the boundaries within which activities are to take place. They reveal broad managerial intentions or forecast broad courses of managerial action likely to take place under certain conditions. The policies of the retention/retrieval program will provide the framework from which all actions emanate. Policies included in the retention/retrieval program include a policy regarding the release of information. Policies and procedures to govern release of information were described in detail in Chapter 5; we will not repeat them here. Other policies considered in a retention/retrieval program are those governing retention of various types of information. There must be a policy that describes how long secondary records, indexes, and medical records will be retained. These policies will be based on the objectives of the administration and medical staff under the professional direction of a medical record administrator working closely with legal counsel for the facility. A destruction schedule will probably be controlled by a policy for any facility that prepares and uses health information. There is only so much space available to any facility, and sooner or later records will expand to a point where consideration must be given to storage in the least amount of storage space. There must be a policy, then, that addresses the length of time individual documents are to be retained and a policy regarding what will become of the documents when it is not necessary to continue retention of them. Such a policy includes directions for destruction of records, microfilming, or summarization and microfilming.

The Register: An important accessory of the manual is a register or log that records all requests for information. It lists the names of all the requesters, dates reports were requested, dates reports were sent out, and the name of the patient or client identified in the report. This register is maintained for all oral or written reports that emanate from the department. The register also is subject to a retention schedule, and there must be a distinct policy that outlines how long the register should be maintained. The register can be divided into two sections: one regarding records pulled for research purposes for physicians or other users or health care providers; the other to list reports that are provided to direct and indirect patient care providers or users for patient care or purposes other than research.

Patient-Carried Records: Another major focus for policies and procedures in the manual is the use of summaries, photocopies, no-carbon-required paper, and forms and formats that provide copies at the point of data entry. The distribution list for these copies and charges is also included in the manual. There must be a policy developed that outlines the procedure governing release of a patient's records to the patient. Many hospitals in many states now provide copies of patients' records to patients. In the past this was a very rare occurrence. The 1970s have seen an increasing request for this information by consumers. Many health care facilities now accommodate patients with full or partial copies of their records. Both the Veteran's Administration and the Army have for years furnished patients with copies of their own records and, in fact, have used the patient as carriers of their own personal health records. Such a policy is established jointly by the administration under the direction of the board of trustees or the governing body in conjunction with the medical staff, medical record administrator, and legal counsel. There are policies and procedures that describe updating records of patients who return to the facility for continuing care. In the unit filing system that we discussed earlier in this chapter, records of individuals who return for care are filed in a complete chronological document. The unit record is a compilation of information about one patient in a single source document. All admission and outpatient records are filed in one folder.

Transfer of Data: Another important policy that outlines procedures to be implemented is the transfer of data for patients who are discharged to another care facility. Information must accompany them to accommodate their treatment at the next facility. This transfer of data is carried on a handwritten or dictated summary sheet. This is often done by the direct care providers, such as physicians and nurses. In some facilities this information is transferred from the original record to an abstract report by medical record personnel. Transfer data are required, by law, for all Titles V, XVIII, and XIX patients, who include maternal and child care, Medicare, and Medicaid patients. Legislation requires that all of these patients transferred from an acute care facility to another type of facility such as intermediate or skilled nursing must have accompanying information sent with them. Sample forms are provided by federal agencies that administer these programs, or health care facilities can develop their own transfer forms to facilitate the sharing of information between the various providers of patient care.

MATERIALS AND EQUIPMENT

As discussed earlier in the chapter, the management function of establishing an effective retention/retrieval system is dependent on a four-phase cycle: the design, implementation, evaluation, and retrieval phases. In developing a system of retention/retrieval, health information management also identifies and selects appropriate materials and storage equipment. To do so requires application of the same cycle used to establish the planning phase of retention/retrieval of data entries. Table 7-1 concisely outlines what takes place.

Beginning with the data entries in a paper record system, recall that the information on paper selection, quality, stock, use, and evaluation was discussed in Chapters 2 and 4. Once the data are compiled into a paper record, the record is ready to be stored. Let's examine some of the ways in which records are stored. Included are folders, binders, and other methods.

File Folders

Six factors influence the choice of file folders: composition, cut, size, reinforcement, finish, and tabs. The folder should be strong enough to contain the record, yet it needs to be designed so that users can easily remove the record to gain access to the information.

Figure 7-10 Transfer of Patient Data for Continuity of Care

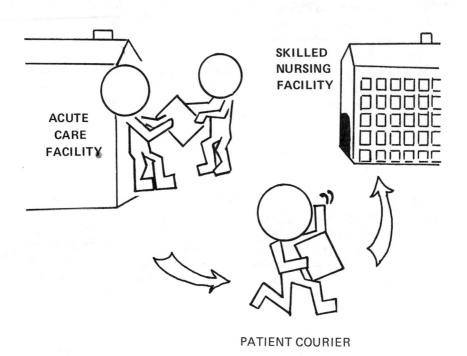

Table 7-1 Comparison of Retention / Retrieval Methods and Their Impact on Equipment Selection

Data Entries in a Paper Record System	Data Entries in a Computerized Record System	Mechanical Data Processing Methods	Subsystems Operations Within Medical Record Department
Data entries	Data entries	Data are condensed through keypunch	These activities will also require selection of materials and equipment for retention / retrieval
Entered on forms	Entered through CRT terminals	Master patient index is placed on computer output microfilm	
Forms grouped together in a logical format to make up a record	Stored on computer direct access storage device		
Record is housed in a folder	Transferred to magnetic tape for permanent storage; or	Physician's index keypunched	Operations of the department
Folders are housed in files	Processed into microfiche via computer output microfilm techniques	Disease index keypunched	Indexing
Drawer / open shelf / electrical		Special index indexes keypunched	Medical reporting activities
Can be condensed through microfilm		Key sorted on an as-needed basis	Maintenance of reports
Destroyed through organizational plans according to legal statutes	Retain in paper record folders as part of original document; or	Printed out on tabulating machine for hard copy retrieval	Special purpose files
	Filed in microfilm filing and storage units		Storage of printouts
			Microfilm operations
			Materials and supplies handling

Considering composition first, folders are made of Kraft, manila, pressboard, and patented composition. The lighter colored manila offers more visibility. It can be used for particular files, as we will discuss when we look at subsystems within a record department. The most common folder used in medical record departments is Kraft. Kraft is a darker color and doesn't soil easily. It is also stronger and better able to sustain the heavy use of a health care setting. The standard weight is determined by a point system. The standard folder adopted by many hospital medical record departments is .011 of Kraft composition.

The second factor to consider is the cut of the folder. Cut refers to the shape of the corners of the folders. They may be square or rounded. Rounded corners will stand up better to handling and will not crush or crumple with repeated filing and pulling. This factor is very important in active outpatient clinics and ambulatory care environments.

Size refers to folder body height—one half inch below the guide or guide height. Body height makes finding easier because the captions stand out better. In shelf filing where the captions are at the side, such as in open-shelf filing, a taller folder may be used. Folders for letter-size files are 11-3/4 inches wide. For legal size files they are 15 inches wide. The variety of methods available to attach the record to the folder include top-attached metal prong fasteners, side-attached fasteners, self-adhesive methods, and file backs that are inserted inside the folder itself.

Consider a file folder used in an active outpatient clinic affiliated with a hospital. One side of the folder, the right, is retained for all inpatient admission records. These records are filed with the oldest on the bottom and the most recent admission on top. There may or may not be divided indicators between admissions. If used, they can be fastened at the top of the inside of the folder with metal prong fasteners. On the other side of the folder all outpatient clinic visits can be filed, again using metal prong fasteners at the top of the folder. Variations in the positions of metal prong fasteners can affect the various users handling the paper. The most stream-lined and effective method of working with folders and papers attached within folders is one in which the document is opened, used, and closed with the least amount of stress on the papers and the folder. For instance, to open the folder, to read or write down one side of the page, and then to lift the paper up to continue writing, tumble style, is often the most efficient use of this kind of system.

The next item is the reinforcement. Folders can be reinforced along the top edge, along the tab, or along the bottom if the folder is expected to hold a great deal of material. This reinforcement feature should be carefully measured against the expected wear of the folder in relation to the cost.

The finish on folders is provided by sizing the paper from which they are made. This gives it body. The harder the finish the greater the resistance to wear and breakdown of fiber.

Tabs are the identifying extension of folders. They protrude above the back of a file folder, or they can also be placed on the side. The placement of the tab depends upon how the folders will be filed. In drawer files the tab is placed at the top, either in the middle or in sequence from left to right. In an open shelf filing system the tab is placed on the side of the folder so that it can be identified easily.

Folders can be purchased prenumbered and color coded. Decisions about prenumbering and color coding are made by the medical record department manager and should be an element addressed in the overall planning for the retention/retrieval system. For instance, records folders can be ordered that are prenumbered and color coded by year to make it easier for file rooms to purge old records at given intervals and move them to less active storage areas. For ease of use the tabs on folders should be in a standard position. This is more efficient and allows for less misfiles.

Along with the consideration of file folders must be consideration of dividers at stated intervals along shelving or file drawers. The dividers are often made up of a heavyweight fabric form of pressboard and can be used to designate alphabetic breaks in the folders or highlight numerical division within the filing system. As previously described in this chapter, for example, the terminal digital filing method, when filed on open-shelf files, will need particular guides at stated intervals. The divider guides along the shelving will direct the staff to the appropriate file number.

When folders are used, one must use chargeout devices. These can be simple cardboard ledgers that the user signs out according to date, user name, and destination of chart. Chargeout data can also be recorded right in the folder. When folders are used for chargeout information, loose papers and/or other items filed pending the return of the original record are stored in one place. This eliminates the need for duplicate handling and reduces the chance of loss of loose reports.

The variety of materials available for use as outguides is extensive. Health information managers need to examine the products available and evaluate them according to the needs of their own systems. Plastics and transparent materials are available; color-coded outguides relating to given days or time periods are available. An example worth noting is color-coded outguides to represent given clinics in an outpatient system. For instance, green chargeout cards could indicate the record has been pulled and sent to the medical clinic; orange chargeout cards could indicate the record has been pulled and sent to the urology clinic. This would immediately indicate a record's location.

Selection of folders for filing medical and health records is dependent upon the setting in which they will be used. The examples described have focused primarily on materials suitable for heavy use of the folder, such as large outpatient clinics and acute care teaching hospitals. The folder probably receives less handling by users and may be even filed alphabetically-rather than by a numbering system in small nursing homes, small area or regional neighborhood health centers, mental health clinics, and physician's offices. In these settings it may be cost-effective to use alphabetic filing. It may be as effective and more economical to use a lighter-weight folder. It may be satisfactory to use color coding by entire folder to denote alphabetic breakdown and help facilitate accurate filing.

A substitute for file folders in complex record systems is 3- or 5-ring binders. Long-term care psychiatric records and records in institutions for the developmentally disabled are often appropriate settings for these. They are strong, durable, and easy to use, both for access and for data entry. Again, the manager of the information system in each of these settings needs to make these decisions.

Medical record managers are encouraged to use a variety of resources available to their particular setting. An active outpatient clinic may have a computerized patient appointment system to effectively schedule patient load per clinic and calculate statistics on the activity level. The medical record manager in this instance should consider the possibility of automatic labeling printed out and sequenced by number so that the staff can retrieve the records rapidly. This is an example of using a partially computerized system to interface with manual components of the system. The methods and applications possible are as unlimited as the imagination of the health information manager.

Housing the Folders

Once the decision has been made on the kind of folders that will be used, the next decision is how to house these folders. Folders and binders can be stored in a number of ways. We will look at six major kinds of filing equipment that can be used to store medical record charts and folders. Drawers, files, cabinets, open shelving, storage boxes, and mechanized systems will be reviewed.

In considering the kinds of filing equipment that houses folders the reader is referenced back to the theory involved in retention: confidentiality, timeliness, and cost. How easy is it to file the material? Is confidentiality the first consideration? How much does it cost to purchase the unit and to store the information in this kind of a unit? Is there protection against natural hazards, such as fire and flood damage? How many records will the equipment hold? How much space is required as records expand, and will the file equipment selected accommodate that growth within this confined space? How safe from unauthorized use are the records in this system? These are the initial questions asked in selecting filing equipment to store records.

Drawer files are 24, 26, and 28 inches deep. The standard drawer file is 26 inches deep and will hold approximately 35,000 individual sheets in addition to the folders and guides. Four-drawer files are common because they provide maximum space within easy reach. Three-drawer files are often used for a dual purpose, a counter over which to serve the public and an area containing natural work space. When drawer files are used in an active file room, aisle width must allow for drawer opening. In cases where the standard 26-inch drawer file that opens frontward has been replaced by a cabinet designed for the drawer file to open lengthwise within the frame, the aisle space will be proportionately smaller.

Shelf files are intended for large floor areas where expansion is no longer possible or where the costs have become extensive. Shelf files are 36 inches long and can be up to seven shelves high. They occupy half as much floor-space as drawer files that have the same capacity. The space between rows of shelf files need only be 30 inches not the 54–60 inches necessary between cabinets with drawers. Open shelves cost about one-fourth as much as drawer files. Material filed on open-shelf filing can be located easily. There are variations in open-shelf filing that individual record managers would be interested in evaluating. First, there has been an addition of doors to shelf files. The doors may extend from the top of the individual shelf, pull out and downward, and thus protect the opening to the file. This allows the records stored there to remain completely encased in the file. One space-finder file houses two four-drawer files in front of the shelf to serve as a workspace. Tab Products also makes a bucket made of pressboard that is suspended on hinges in an open shelf filing frame. The bucket allows filing of up to 20 folders per bucket. Files may be easily shifted and expanded using this system. Another kind of shelving is a motorized file, such as those manufactured by Diebold and Remington Rand Corporation. This is a large encased file that houses 1,552 letter-size file inches in one unit. (A unit usually occupies 31.2 square feet.) The advantage is that the records are accessible to one person sitting at a work table attached to the motorized file. A disadvantage is in an active file room where more than one person needs to work with files at the same time.

Computerized Record System

When considering filing storage material and equipment in this application, the medical record manager must recall that data entries are entered through a CRT terminal. This may involve the selection of the CRT terminal for the department or it may simply involve working with the output in the computerized system, which may be a printer or hard-copy terminal located in the department. The information on the patient record may be stored on computer to be on-line or immediately accessible to the users. If captured this way, the information is accessible through CRT terminals to physicians and other health care providers. When the patient is no longer involved in active care the record may be transferred to a magnetic tape for permanent storage. That tape can then be stored indefinitely by recopying at stated intervals to preserve the contents of the tape, or the information on the tape can be held for a time, then processed onto microfiche using a computer output microfilm technique. That microfiche or microfilm material may then be housed in microfilm drawer files or it may be placed in individual jackets and filed with parts of the paper record system. Another consideration is that medical record data entries and computerized systems can be entered through the CRTs, stored on the computer while in use, and printed out on a printout form that itself would become the paper record form within the system. In many hospitals this is a fairly common application. Medical record departments are finding an increasing number of computer printout forms that are filed as a routine part of the medical record. We will look more closely at microfilming as an output a little later in the chapter.

Subsystems Operations within Record Departments

This section deals with the operations of the department and the purchasing of appropriate equipment. Equipment is used for handling indexing, medical reporting, treatment of particular reports and storage of printouts, etc., that are part of the routine management of a medical record or health information department.

Indexing Equipment

You will recall that a good index is designed to serve the department as efficiently and economically as possible. It should store individual pieces of information that can be retrieved efficiently. There are four main indexes kept in hospital medical record departments. These are the master patient, disease, operation, and physician's indexes. As previously discussed in this chapter, they are fundamental to all departments. Special indexing or indexes may also be used.

Indexing equipment falls into approximately five categories.

First, nonvisible loose-leaf or ledger. This is simply paper in a binder index. It can be used by someone seated at a desk. It is portable. The pages need not be removed, which reduces misfiles and dog-earing of the cards. It is less time-consuming to use than files and file drawers. It does require time to thumb through the index to locate sheets unless tabs or dividers are built into the system. The nonvisible looseleaf ledger is very appropriate in nursing homes, for indexing diseases and operations as the volume and activity level is low.

Second, a visible loose-leaf system has the same advantages that exist in the nonvisible loose-leaf system. In addition, it has guides not needed when the code numbers are visible. The code numbers themselves act as a guide when this system is used for disease and operation indexing.

Third, vertical card files are another common method of indexing. They require less space than visible files. Like card files, guides are needed. Cards have to be removed for recording in vertical card files; therefore, the chance for error or misfile is increased. Using vertical card files from a seated position is not always possible.

Fourth, physical card cabinets by Kardex can be pulled out and information posted on the cards from a seated position. In addition, the material is more accessible. It does require more space than the previously discussed methods and is more expensive to purchase.

The fifth method is use of mechanical rotary files that are scaled-down versions of the mechanized files described previously. One person may sit at a large rotating file in which all cards are contained. It has been used with master patient indexes, and disease, operations, and other special indexes. Using the system simply requires pushing a button to retrieve an individual section from which a desired card can be pulled. Less space is required than with visible card cabinets. Still, they *are* cards; they can be removed and they can be misfiled in being replaced. As indicated when discussing large mechanical files with file folders, rotary files are also limited to the use of one person at a time. In addition, if there is a mechanical failure the information is not readily available.

Ordinary file cabinets can be used to house most management reports that are maintained in the medical record department. Budgets, employee evaluations, purchase orders, records of activity, and production information within the department are all filed in file drawers. It is useful for managers to have lockable drawers for more sensitive information.

Printouts

When discussing the subsystems within a department, today's record manager must be aware of the impact of printouts. The size of the printout can be determined in the design of a system, but that may or may not involve the manager of a medical record department. What must be achieved is a method of filing the printout information so that it can be easily retrieved as necessary.

In discussing subsystems in the medical record department, the role of computer output microfilm again should be included. Master patient indexes in many hospitals have been placed on the computer output microfilm system. We will discuss this and describe its operation in more detail when discussing the role of microfilming generally.

Mechanical Data Processing Equipment

Subsystems in a department may utilize mechanical data processing methods. Data can be compressed by keypunching it. The master patient index can be keypunched and from there be placed on microfilm that can be transferred to an on-line computer to be built into an interactive master patient index system. It can be keypunched to be run off and tabulated so that more than one copy of the master patient index is available. This would be useful in health care settings where access to that information is required by more than the medical record department and where a printout of the data would be useful and facilitate the provision of care to the patient. Mechanical data processing methods are also used to keypunch disease and operation indexes in some settings. Once keypunched, these cards can be kept on file and sorted by means of a sorting machine to meet individual requests for information. The sorter can sort the cards according to requests that come in. For instance, a doctor may wish to study all of the peripheral vascular surgery performed in the past two years in the hospital. By selecting the appropriate code in the procedure book and establishing and pulling all operation and procedure keypunch cards for the past two years, they can be run through the sorter and sorted digit by digit until the specific code that reflects vascular surgery performed has been sorted out. Then these cards can be loaded into a tabulator machine that mechanically reprints the information on the card in a listed format. This affords the physician researcher a listing of all patients, titles, and procedures plus information on age, sex, length of stay, and other conditions as punched on the card. For many medical record department managers, a careful look at mechanical data processing methods might be useful. These methods can be used in the interim between working with a manually supported system and moving gradually toward an automated information system.

Practitioners need to be prepared to handle the range of systems discussed in this chapter on equipment. They need to be able to mix and match where appropriate. They need to be able to select and plan for future equipment that will meet the needs of the information flow in their particular department. As identified previously in this chapter and as discussed throughout the text, information managers must concern themselves with equipment selection based on analysis of their individual systems. They must be prepared to audit their selections on a regularly cycled basis as well.

Microfilm

In discussing the last section related to equipment for retention/retrieval of patient and health information, the reader is directed to the area of microfilming. This is a fitting summary for this chapter since all data stored by previously described methods can be retained for greater lengths of time in a microfilm state. So let's consider just why microfilming seems to be an optimum choice for many record administrators.

Microfilming can be defined as a process of photographing and reducing the film copy of a given report to a miniature of the original. The advantages of microfilming include:

- It can effect up to a 98 percent reduction in file space. There is the speed and convenience of data retrieval.

- The information can be retained right in the department and accessed through microfilm or microfiche viewers.
- The labor overhead is reduced. It takes less man-hours to sort, file, and locate a particular record and then to refile it.
- It is a secure system. You cannot alter records that are on microfilm. To duplicate the role is quite inexpensive, so it is possible to retain a backup file in a safe place outside the department. The hard-copy can be prepared from the film and can go out when needed in legal cases, for patient information transfer, or special research, while the original film remains in the department.
- A large savings in filing equipment is effected. For medical record and health information systems that are growing explosively, this can be a key issue.
- There is an easy reversion to paper. When necessary a film can be produced easily and at low cost.
- Microfilming is legally recognized. All microfilmed records are admissible as primary evidence in court.
- Microfilming is versatile. It can fit easily within existing information systems. There are a number of applications in which the microfilming process can be used. Basically the usual reduction for records is 24 to 1. It can go down to 50 to 1 and up to 5 to 1. A reel or roll equals 100 feet of film and is equal to approximately 2,000 images. The jackets for microfilm are 3″ × 5″ in size or 4″ × 6″ in size and can contain 60 images.

Remember that when you are designing a definite plan to retire your records, microfilm would be a valid, viable, and economical solution.

Let's go back for a moment and consider the various formats of the microfilming process. There is a microfilming roll, in which the record is retained sequentially. The advantage is the greatest volume stored in the smallest space. It has the lowest cost of all methods of microfilming, and saves 98 percent of storage space. It can be stored in the department so that it is readily accessible; it eliminates misfiling; it saves time that would be spent traveling to outlying storage locations when storage takes place outside the facility. The disadvantages of microfilm rolls are that they are inconvenient for study. It is almost impossible to study rolls of film. It is difficult to get the entire record on one spool. It is inconvenient when a single record on the roll is subpoenaed, and the expense of duplication must be considered. Some studies show that 50 years of commercial storage can be purchased for the same price, but this needs to be verified in the light of today's growing space costs. The unit record is not possible in using roll microfilm. You can't update an existing record on a roll of microfilm.

The next format is jacket and fiche. The advantages of this method or format are many. It is possible to study them with a reader. Research is possible; small viewers can be on the floors at the nursing stations. Jackets containing the film can be taken to court, since the fiche is limited to one record and will involve only the record subpoenaed. Since all microfilming is legally acceptable, this is a good way to handle records that may be subpoenaed. The method is adaptable to unit filing. With fiche, additional treatment and/or additional hospitalization records can be microfilmed and added to previous records in one jacket or folder. Color coding is possible with jackets and microfiche. The disadvantages are that it is more expensive than roll; there is labor involved in mounting the film; there is more possibility of loss.

A third format for microfilming is punchcard with film attached, called an aperture care. The advantages are that it is possible to have an entire record on one card, if the record is small, and other data can be instituted on the punchcard as well. The disadvantages are that the equipment is very expensive and the viewing mechanism has not been perfected.

One shouldn't discuss microfilming without a word about commercial storage. Commercial storage companies store medical records on a long-range basis. The advantages of this are the ability to provide the original records when requested, which makes the record in its original state more adaptable to research. There isn't the danger of small microfilming jackets becoming lost, and in some areas of the country commercial storage is cheaper.

Microfilming, whatever the format selected, must be assessed by the records manager. Will it be an in-house process carried on by the medical record department or will it be contract service outside the organization? In-house filming will require that camera, processor, reader, roll and jacket, reader printer, and the filing equipment—that is, the drawers and cabinets—will have to be purchased. The reader is directed to the resources available from microfilming centers and commercial companies in eliciting current, up-to-date cost figures on this equipment.

One of the more unique and most advantageous applications of microfilming is the computer output microfilm (COM) system. This is the process of translating computer-generated information into a miniature image on film. The paper reports are replaced by microfilm. Why would you want to do this?

In the COM process the computer creates magnetic tapes that contain data for report generation. For example, patient information may be keypunched on admission to the hospital. The information keypunched on punchcards can then be transferred onto a magnetic tape. These tapes are read on a tape drive and captured by a COM recorder. The film from the

COM recorder is developed. Duplicates are prepared from the original film as necessary; microfilm formats can be roll form or microfiche 4″ × 6″ film cards, containing up to 208 pages of computer output. Computer output microfilm has been used to computerize the master patient index. In a large teaching hospital computer output microfilm can be used to give each department its own copy of the master patient index. The medical record department then maintains records on all of the most recent patients registered in the index, including the current month. For patients who are new to the hospital, departments contact medical records to obtain a new number and to formally register the patient on the system. For those patients who are returning, departments could simply call for their copies of the computer output microfiche. In some hospitals the microfiche is used as a backup to on-line master patient index systems. This can include total backup for all patients registered in the facility or it can include a planned backup. For instance, all records of patients in current therapy may remain stored in the computer in an on-line mode. Six months following the conclusion of therapy, the data may be transferred onto computer output microfilm since it is no longer active. The department would then maintain the microfiche as backup.

Another example of the use of COM is the production of microfiche backups of computerized patient records. Just as the paper record can be placed on microfilm and stored, so can the computerized patient record be placed on microfilm and stored. Cost can be contained in this fashion. The overall retention/retrieval planning function for a given institution must consider the appropriate use of paper, mechanical data processing, computerized on-line systems, and microfilming as resources when constructing an individual plan for their organization. The prevailing goal continues to be the most efficient retrieval of information for the patient, for the providers, and for third parties (statisticians, researchers, medical systems planners, etc.) to benefit the overall health care delivery system.

NOTES

1. Irene Place and Estelle L. Popham, *Filing and Records Management* (Englewood Cliffs, N.J.: Prentice-Hall, 1966), pp. 54-55.
2. *ICD-9-CM* 1 (Ann Arbor, Mich.: Commission on Hospital and Professional Activities, 1978), pp. iii-xvii.
3. *Current Medical Information and Terminology, 4th Ed.* (Chicago, Ill.: American Medical Association, 1971), pp. iii-x.
4. *Current Procedural Terminology, 2nd Ed.* (Chicago, Ill.: American Medical Association, 1970), pp. iii-xii.

5. *International Classification of Health Problems in Primary Care* (Chicago, Ill.: American Hospital Association, 1975), pp. 1-6.

6. *Diagnostic and Statistical Manual of Mental Disorders* (Washington, D.C.: American Psychiatric Association, 1968), pp. vii-xv.

7. *Systematized Nomenclature of Medicine* (Skokie, Ill.: College of American Pathologists, 1977).

8. Don Schneider, and Linda Appleton, "Reason for Visit Classification System for Patient Records in the Ambulatory Care Setting," *Quality Review Bulletin, JCAH*, January 1977, pp. 20-26.

9. W. Maedke, Mary F. Robek, and Gerald F. Brown, *Information and Records Management* (Beverly Hills, Calif.: Glencoe Press, 1974).

Chapter 8

Creating an Effective Health Information System

CHAPTER OBJECTIVES

1. Identify the essential elements of a health information system
2. Relate the four principles of management to the role and function of the medical record administrator
3. Identify at least 9 reasons why a health information system is necessary
4. Cite 3 characteristics used to determine the appropriate development of a health information system
5. Differentiate between performance objectives and job descriptions
6. Identify the 4 phases of a budget
7. Differentiate between the maintenance budget and capital expenditures

ELEMENTS OF A HEALTH INFORMATION SYSTEM IDENTIFIED

In this chapter we depart from the discussion of what health information is. Other chapters have devoted their attention to the myriad elements of health data and information processing. Here we need to step outside that realm, so to speak, and look at what transforms the development and administration of that health information into a useful system. Later, there will be specific examples to demonstrate the theory and substance of a health information administration. There are many scholars and books that have contributed to the development of management theory and practice. This chapter does not attempt to be a complete treatise on management. It does outline some theories and some practical examples of management, as practiced by several hospitals and medical record practitioners. Fortunately, current literature is finding an increasing amount of published data by practicing medical record professionals who have had direct experience in the administration of a health information system. These publications and texts should be used in conjunction with this chapter so that you may have a wide exposure to all experiental management information.

A *system* has been defined as related elements that are coordinated to form a unified result; or, specifically, people, activities, equipment, materials, plans, and controls, working together to achieve a unified objective or whole. A system has also been defined as an array of components that interact to achieve some objective through a network of procedures that are integrated and designed to carry out a major activity. The components of the system may themselves be systems depending on the complexity of the parent system.

How is a Health Information System (HIS) developed? What are the components? People are the most important component of any particular system. The most important part of the "people component" is patients and clients, the sole reason for having a HIS. We classify these individuals as users of the system. For our discussion here, patients, clients, or any other consumer of health services will be classified as users of that service when they seek care from professional providers of care. The other part of the people component in a HIS is the professional and service personnel who participate in satisfying the needs of the users. These can be classified as providers of care. These individuals were described in Chapter 1 according to their various titles. For our purposes here we will categorize as providers those individuals who in any way participate in the delivery of health care, whether directly or indirectly.

There are seven important elements in the creation of a HIS: people, data, communication, leadership, organization, controls, and evaluation. Let's look at each of these and their roles in the creation of a system.

People Are the Source

The people most directly involved in developing the HIS are the medical record professionals. The registered record administrator and the accredited record technician, along with the many highly trained individuals who work in health information and medical record departments throughout the country, are the individuals responsible for managing patient data on a daily, continuing basis. The registered medical record administrator is educated through a baccalaureate degree and skilled in the areas of management, health, and biological sciences, with a specialty emphasis on management of health information in its various forms. This individual has a responsibility to develop data elements into a useful system so that patients can receive care when needed and have access to data about their care at future dates. Some of the other duties of the registered record administrator are:

- To set objectives for a health information system
- To establish policies regarding the retention and release of information contained in the records
- To establish policies and procedures to coordinate the flow of health information in the health care facility
- To maintain permanent files, that include filing and retrieval of records
- To compile statistical data, including the census, monthly and annual reports for hospitals and other users, and to prepare abstracts of records and birth and death certificates.

The medical record administrator is responsible for managing health information and to do so must be able to perform the basic functions of management: planning, organizing, leading, and controlling. The administrator must be able to develop departmental objectives, prepare a budget to support the objectives, and organize the activities, people, material, equipment, and all other elements necessary to achieve the results outlined in the objectives. Organizational skill and a facility for motivating others to work are necessary qualifications for a medical record administrator.

Data Are the Foundation

In developing an overall HIS the second important ingredient is data. We are concerned with two major types of data.

Patient Data

The first are data regarding the patient. We have discussed patient data in the form of both indirect and direct patient data. In developing HIS we are concerned with both kinds of patient data in any health care setting. We are concerned with patient data in fragmented as well as consolidated form. We are interested in patient data, whether they have been recorded or not recorded, and from the point of view of making them available, first, for patient care and second, for all other uses. Without patient data there would be no HIS.

There is a distinction between patient data and management data. In our description of a HIS that distinction is between (1) information gathered during a patient encounter with a professional health care provider and (2) data used by those who support the development, retention, and retrieval of patient data through their professional direction. The latter are management data. Also included in patient data by our definition are data gathered during a patient/provider encounter in an indirect manner. This was referred to earlier in the book as data that are not provided directly from the patient's own lips. Such indirect data would include lab reports, x-ray reports, and all other reports that are recorded without direct input or corroboration of the patient.

Management Data

The second type of data we address in discussing the need of a health information system is management data. Management data is that information that is used by providers and users as well as by patients. In particular, there are two types of management data. One is departmental management data which reflect the organizational component of the system. For instance, the reports or data needed by the entire management staff to provide a framework within which individuals and activities can coordinate desired objectives. We are speaking here of such data as policy and procedure manuals, memos, bylaws, budgets, correspondence, and individual or specialized worksheets developed for individual departmental needs. An example of this would be an inventory sheet designed to reflect exactly what an individual department has on hand for use of the employees who need the material.

The other type of management data we are concerned with that has to be addressed when we are thinking of HIS are statistical reports that will provide both descriptive and inference analyses of the activities and services provided by the institution (see Chapter 3). These statistical reports are used for planning by the administrative staff and for review of quality of care by the medical staff. The medical record administrator must be able to display statistical data in such a way that they can be easily read by those whose chief concern is patient care and whose secondary concern is review of cumulative statistical data for a variety of purposes. That is to say, statistical reports need to be presented in such a way that busy physicians who need and are interested in the utilization and effectiveness of both health care facilities and patient care can quickly read the information and move on to more important judgmental aspects. Other important points of management data are such items as the master patient index; the disease, physician and operation indexes; and production reports that reveal what various functional levels of the medical record department are performing.

Table 8-1 Major Components of a Health Information System

Kind of Plan	Distinguishing Attribute	Chief Characteristics	Sample HIS Applications	Required for Use	Common Erroneous Situation
Objective	Provides target for direction and guidance of activities	Comprehensive	To check and analyze the component parts of the medical record to see that it is complete, accurate, and useful	Interpretation for each operative level	Not precisely known or stated
Policy	Sets up the overall boundaries for activities	Broad, general, comprehensive	Copies of Patients' Records for outside users	Interpretation, judgment	Improper identification for every managerial decision
Procedure	Defines chronological series of tasks	Tailor-made to achieve specific work	Analysis of Charts (Partial Description) Deficiency Slips A. *Prepare* a written deficiency slip to indicate all deficiencies on the chart. B. Each physician has a deficiency slip. *Write* the physician's name on the top of it. If the chart needs more than one doctor to complete it, use separate deficiency slips for each one. C. *Place* slips in order with the attending physician first and other physicians after the attending, concluding with the house staff. D. Each doctor has a color-coded deficiency slip. Everywhere the physician's signature is needed (except the face sheet), *clip* a colored slip on each page where the signature is needed.	Compliance with slight interpretation required	Once established tends to remain

Table 8-1 Continued

Kind of Plan	Distinguishing Attribute	Chief Characteristics	Sample HIS Applications	Required for Use	Common Erroneous Situation
Method	Prescribes course of action to accomplish a task	Specific and detailed in how a task is to be done	ICD-9 coding, Unit Records, Terminal Digit Filing are all examples of methods used in health information settings	Compliance	Ignored or insufficient planning directed to it
Standard	Gives level of expected achievement	Tailor-made for specific work	The medical record shall contain sufficient information to identify the patient to support the diagnosis, to justify the treatment, and to document the results accurately (JCAH, Standard II, Medical Record Services).	Compliance	Not brought up to date in line with current operations
Budget	For a given period proposes financial operational expectancies into a concise format	Tailor-made for specific work. Predicts income; controls output	Sample budget is too long to include here. Budget description follows in this chapter.	Compliance with slight interpretation required	Difficult to modify as projected circumstances change
Program	Integrates diverse but related activities into a unity	Comprehensive, covers relatively large scope of facilities and activities	Implementation of the POMR for all parts of the record	Interpretation, judgment, and managerial competency	Used to identify any type of plan

An example of this is a summary of the transcription service that itemizes what kind of transcription is being done; how many reports are being typed on a daily, weekly, or monthly basis; reports that highlight increases or decreases in productivity of individual employees; and so on. Summary data used for indirect patient care would include abstracts or other types of summaries that are provided to insurance companies or other agents that pay for patient care as well as reports that go to planning or accrediting agencies.

Communication Is the Channel

Information/communication is the third element we will discuss. This important part of a HIS emphasizes all that can be known about an individual patient's encounter with a health care provider. It has to address communication between patients, providers, and users. To fully understand this particular component of a health information system, let's look at a basic communication model. Picture a sender and a receiver. In so doing, consider both parties to be active participants. There must be an active sender and an active receiver, or listener. This is especially true when we talk about the providers working as a team to treat a patient.

To get a better understanding of some of the many communication links involved in the information/communication element, let's list a variety of possibilities that involve *only* the patient/client encounter with the provider. Note the possibilities in the following listing:

- Patient/client-direct care provider
- Patient/client-indirect provider
- Patient/client-user
- Provider-provider
- User-user
- Provider-user

The above listing is important when we consider all of the complications that arise in the ordinary experience of communication between two individuals. When we increase the number of individuals involved in any particular experience of communication the possibility for error and consequent breakdown is compounded. Our purpose here, then, is to point out the possibilities for error and the consequent breakdown in any system when so many individuals are interacting in such a complex information component.

One of the most important parts of this element of the HIS is the recording and transmission of data. At this point we are describing patient/client data in their most unique form, that is, during the course of patient care or at the time of an encounter between a patient/client and a direct provider of care. This information is usually initially gathered orally; that is, in a conversation between the patient and the provider. Very soon after the oral exchange of information that same information will be transcribed or recorded, and a permanent document develops.

Teleprocessing is a modern method to record and retrieve information that was initially transmitted orally. In a manual recording system, information that was originally handwritten or oral is transcribed onto a written document. In many health care facilities providers of care use dictating equipment to convey the information gathered from the patient. Teleprocessing is the use of a computer to perform what has for many centuries been performed by hand. Data that originally was gathered orally can now be electronically stored and retrieved for future use. In many facilities where patients receive care, teleprocessing is being used for a wide variety of information storage and retrieval. CRT terminals are common instruments by which data are transmitted to a computer and are also used for retrieval of information from the computer visually displayed so that anyone can read them. In addition computers can store information that can be retrieved in a printout. The printout provides a written document of the information stored on a tape or a disk.

Another extremely important area that we must consider is information that is secondary to the patient/client-provider. We define as secondary all information that must be communicated to provide a support system for the major focus: direct patient care. Information that falls into this category includes such common everyday occurrences as telephone calls, scheduling of appointments, and discussions between providers and users. For instance, communication between physician's office personnel and insurance companies that provide payment coverage for patients, communication between health care facility management personnel describing services provided and/or requesting information about certain aspects of care for a patient's stay in a facility—all of the myriad types and forms of information from oral to written to teleprocessed. Included in this distinct part of the element of information/communication are management data. These include such important items as inventories, budgets, memos, and many of the reports that were mentioned when we discussed the second element, data. The communication aspect of this third element is as important as the information itself, and in this there must be an objective established for the communication element and the means established to carry out communication. Some of the means used to carry out communication include such items as telephones, teleprocessing equipment, transcription equipment, and personal encounters.

Leadership Is the Catalyst

The fourth element in our health information system is the leadership element. There are three areas here. The first is objectives. For there to be any kind of unified activity that progresses toward a common goal, there must initially be a description and a determination of what is needed to reach the particular objective. The objective must be measurable if it is to be useful. It must be formulated in such a manner that all participants in the system understand what is to be achieved. From this they can determine for their own sphere of activity how they are progressing toward that particular objective. For instance, an objective for the HIS might be to achieve tele-processing of all aspects of patient data processing by the end of a five-year period of time. Everyone involved in the system would need to know exactly what was expected of them and a schedule to follow in the interim between the date of establishing the plan and the five-year target date. They could, then, at various points along the way know how they were progressing toward achieving the final objective. The objective we've used is measurable and one that would provide managers with the necessary information to give effective leadership to the team.

The second area of leadership is the ability to educate. Employees, patients, medical staff, and all others involved in the organization must understand and work together to achieve the ongoing objectives of the system. There must be an ongoing education program that serves contin-ually to prepare new members of the team as well as to update information for regular members of the team. When new technologies and new methods are introduced that will affect those who work with the system, there must be an educational program to relate these innovations to their particular jobs so that they are familiar with what needs to be done.

Human relations is the third aspect of leadership, and it is extremely important. At the very center of the HIS are human beings. Motivation of individuals who work with patient care is just as important as motivation in any environment. In particular, medical record professionals must be familiar with methods of motivation when directing the efforts of those who do not have patient contact and who are, therefore, less likely to see the results of their work efforts. For instance, file clerks, transcribers, and receptionists do not often have any patient interface and only rarely have an opportunity to see the results of their clerical tasks.

Organization Is the Framework

Organization is the management principle that brings all parts together to achieve the long-term objectives. Included in organization are such important areas as planning, policymaking, developing and teaching job procedures, selecting materials and equipment, and developing methods that will work the most effectively for a particular work unit or facility to achieve the goals of the organization.

Organizational Skills Are Building Blocks

Some of the organizational skills needed by the medical record administrator are:

- The ability to schedule activities and people
- The ability to evaluate personnel
- The ability to interview and hire qualified employees
- The ability to establish educational programs for nonskilled employees who will need technical expertise in order to work with the health information
- The ability to educate others in the uses and controls needed when working with health information

Medical record administrators must have a high degree of familiarity with the confidentiality rules and regulations of the states where they practice, as well as with retention rules and regulations so that policies may be developed that allow health information to be discarded or stored effectively, both to meet the needs of the particular patient population that is being served and to comply with retention statutes. Other considerations that enter into the decision to retain information include the mobility of the patients who use the facility and the rate at which they are readmitted to that particular facility.

The medical record administrator must be able to work in a group as well as to provide leadership skills on a one-to-one basis. Committees of the medical staff and administrative committees of the facilities are groups to which the medical record administrator will be appointed. In a Medical Audit Committee, for instance, the agenda planning, scheduling and group facilitating activities are carried out by the record professional. These tasks combine leadership and organization to achieve the objective.

Coordinating Management Is an Ongoing Process

Setting objectives is, of course, the priority in establishing a unit of work that can be measured. Effective completion of this produces a roadmap for planning. Planning activities that are a part of the medical record administrator's daily routine include preparing such plans as budgets and policies. A medical record administrator must be familiar with accrediting and licensing regulations, reimbursement schedules, legal requirements of the state where the profession is practiced, state-of-the-art in health information development, and technical functions, such as coding, transcription, release of information, abstracting, indexing, audit procedures, teleprocessing, and development of personnel. Planning the activities of the department takes into account particular needs of the patients in the facility and concerns about the medical staff and its goals. As a manager, the medical record administrator operates within an approved budget. The budget is the product of the medical record administrator's familiarity with all of the items mentioned above. It is prepared jointly with the administrative staff to achieve institutional cooperation on objectives and finances that meet their combined objectives.

Understanding Information Flow Facilitates Action

To organize the people, equipment, and the activities of a HIS, the medical record administrator must be familiar with the logical flow of health information. That is, a particular job in the department must be organized so that information is processed in an orderly, speedy fashion. The medical record administrator must be aware of a particular institution's information needs and coordinate the activities and performance of developmental functions so that medical records can be available to those who need them when they need them. The ordinary course of completion of a medical record involves establishing policies that will influence the admitting department as well as all other departments who serve the patient while the patient is under care. These policies should include such things as the type of data to be collected, the format for data, guidelines for achieving accuracy of data transmittal, and controls that make sure data are complete. Such policies can influence development of the record while the patient is receiving care, so that the record can be more easily monitored when patient data are completed and the medical record is under the complete control of the medical record administrator. It is common now for the medical record department to maintain control over the early development of data entries because of the availability of record technicians who monitor information during the patient's active care. When the medical record department receives the medical record to be analyzed and completed, additional policies are needed to guide those who work on an everyday level in preparing a permanent document that will accurately reflect the care given to the patient.

Controls Are Directed to Costs

Controls is the sixth element in a HIS. The major control in the health information system is money. Nothing will go very far without money. There must be an established financial plan developed in the organizational

Figure 8-1 MRA Designs the Systems to Support Health Information Plan

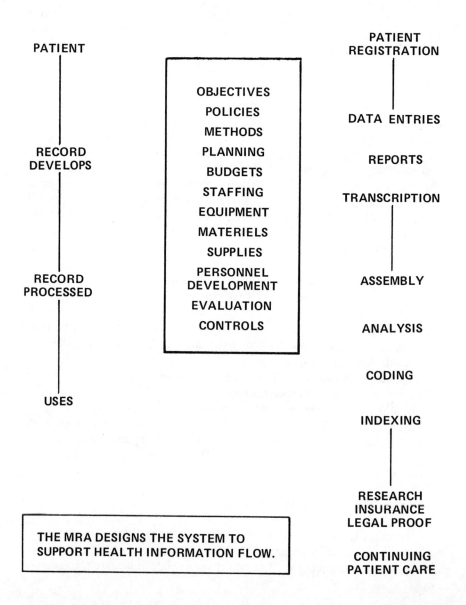

HEALTH DATA SYSTEM

PATIENT

RECORD
DEVELOPS

RECORD
PROCESSED

USES

OBJECTIVES
POLICIES
METHODS
PLANNING
BUDGETS
STAFFING
EQUIPMENT
MATERIELS
SUPPLIES
PERSONNEL
DEVELOPMENT
EVALUATION
CONTROLS

PATIENT
REGISTRATION

DATA ENTRIES

REPORTS

TRANSCRIPTION

ASSEMBLY

ANALYSIS

CODING

INDEXING

RESEARCH
INSURANCE
LEGAL PROOF

CONTINUING
PATIENT CARE

THE MRA DESIGNS THE SYSTEM TO
SUPPORT HEALTH INFORMATION FLOW.

element, and this financial plan—or budget, if you will—will have defined costs for every part of the system. There must be a factor built into the system that will monitor how much is being spent against how much was planned for expenditure. Flexible budgets will take this into account.

Controlling through Audits

The controlling function of the medical record administrator has equal importance with other functions and includes the ability to establish ongoing audits of such activities as the accuracy of data entries during development of the record while the patient is being treated. The various files and indexes that are part of the daily activities of the medical record department must also be audited. Evaluation or audits of the way the department meets planned objectives and stays within its planned financial parameters are important controls with which the medical record administrator must be familiar. Other controls that are also extremely important concern:

- Release of information for preserving the confidentiality of patient data
- Providing a retention schedule that makes patient data available when needed
- Participation in the review of medical care through establishing procedures that make the data available in a format useful for this particular function
- Accuracy of filing, transcription, selecting and transcribing codes, indexing
- Consideration of unusual circumstances and unplanned for expenditures

In the final analysis there will be only a limited amount of money available for any one activity, and this expenditure must be continually monitored. Another control in HIS is the scope of service provided. Once again, a clear definition of what types of services will be involved in this system will be developed in the organizational plan and stated in the objectives. Such questions will be answered as who will receive the benefits of the HIS, how will the system function, when will it function, and what will it cover. For instance, the scope of the service might include only patient information. The HIS could only include patient data as its focus. Perhaps management information is excluded initially and will be added in later, so that the scope of the service initially would be the health information element with plans to include management information later. The third part of the controlling element that is important is documentation. There must be documentation of all controls. That is, to effectively achieve monitoring of the system on a day-to-day basis, there must be written information for those who are doing the monitoring so they will know what it is they are monitoring and how well they are doing their jobs. They will also want to record their progress and keep these records as the planning basis for future control functions.

Evaluation Is the Measurement

The final element in a HIS is evaluation. Evaluation of the system must be established as part of the organizational objective when the initial planning is done. It is an extremely important element and includes continual review of the system, modifying the system based on changing needs and observation of the effectiveness of the present system, feedback on that effectiveness, and continual modification, review, and feedback.

THE NEED FOR HIS IDENTIFIED

Another question that we must ask in addressing development of a HIS is why the system we have just described is needed. Why do we need the HIS? First of all, we need it for patient/client care. We have described patient/client care in so much detail in other areas of the book that it may seem redundant to reiterate it here. But it is necessary to any description of why we need a health information system.

The most important reason for a HIS is to provide adequate and timely care to patients or clients. Without a system organized to collect and retrieve information that is vital to the care of patients, that care will be second rate.

The second reason for existence of a HIS is its role in supporting research. First-rate care that can achieve the goal of providing quality information to direct care providers at the time it is needed can only be achieved through an established system whose major objective is to make the information available for ongoing research. Success in research to provide new methods, new techniques, new ideas, breakthroughs in diagnosis, predictions regarding disease and populations, predictions regarding the use of drugs, can best be achieved through an organized program that pulls information together and makes it available.

Administrative functions are a third reason for having a HIS. By supporting administrative function with the system, there is a possibility that patients will receive better ancillary services, such as dietary and laboratory services, more suitable facilities, and more consideration in such sensitive areas as payment for services.

The fourth reason that a HIS is needed is for the legal protection of the patient/client and the provider. Documentation of what goes on in the care of a patient can be a boon to all parties involved in the delivery of that care. This documentation, if it is accurate, complete, and timely, can be an essential element of legal protection for every party involved.

Accrediting and licensing are the fifth reason why a system is needed. Without a system that documents in a timely manner all eventualities in health care delivery, accrediting and licensing will be slow to come and cannot be easily achieved.

Financial management is the sixth reason for having a health information. system. To properly account for services rendered, there must be a thorough and accurate system that describes those services. Financial management, then, must rely on a developed system to achieve its important function of paying for care.

Information processing is the seventh reason why we need a health information system. It is needed when a patient/client communicates with providers of care. It is equally important when data users explain to providers what kind of data they need, when they need them, how they intend to use them, and so on. For communication to be effective there must be active listening on both sides, as well as a mutual understanding by all parties of the health care delivery system. Included in the need for information processing is the documentation that provides direct patient care, proof of care, and a source for evaluation of care. Teleprocessing continues to develop software and hardware at amazingly increased speed. This development provides a continuing challenge for those in the information management professions.

The eighth reason is to justify the use of resources. Without people to develop criteria, methods to capture data to evaluate criteria, information developed to provide useful documentation, and organized leadership to develop a d control a program of evaluation, there would be no way to measure v e of resources. Expectations of quality care by consumers and delivery of cost-controlled quality care by providers will continue to provide impetus to users and providers to measure use of resources to make sure that sensible use takes place.

Ninth, for all consumers and providers of health care to function in an orderly manner there must be an organized effort on the part of providers so that consumers can use time effectively. The rigors for everyone of hectic schedules with overloading of patients for primary care, failure of providers to keep on schedule, abuse of outpatient and emergency room facilities by patients not willing to manage their time, delays in treatment because of malfunctioning equipment—all are examples of the need for effective time management.

Those who need a health information system are already familiar to us. Briefly: patients, clients, consumers, or direct care users by any title, are the primary reason for development and retention/retrieval of data. Individually, it is needed for each client's care at any level. Collectively, it is needed to provide a basis for research and education that comes around full circle and makes care of individual patients current, as based on studies of large amounts of data concerning similar diseases, procedures, symptoms, etc. To accommodate documentation for individual care, there are providers and users who must interact to provide a framework and details of a functional information system. By their interaction they build dependencies for certain elements, such as proof of care, financial statements, measurement of quality of care, and many others discussed here and elsewhere in this book.

A health information system is appropriate when any of the following three elements are present:

Coordination of patient services
Planning of health resources
Demonstration of accountability

As mentioned in Chapter 1, it is not easy to identify a health care delivery system in the United States nor is it easy to identify a HIS that is fully operational and meets the definitions of the terms in its title. However, as we have described throughout this book, major components of HIS do exist and are functioning in many sites. Not all are hospital based nor even direct-patient-care related. Any one of the three elements described above is considered a justifiable reason for development of an HIS.

Related to the reasons for establishment of HIS are the types of organizations or institutional configurations that are capable of developing and motivated to develop the HIS. There are two types:

Organizations that provide health care
Organizations that use health care information

When one considers the two types of organizations that can develop and administrate the HIS, it might seem questionable in the light of organization size, scope, and financial ability. However, it is imperative in the development and processing of information that an organized approach to the various steps in data development, control, and use take place or there can be no successful development and processing. Disorganized data in a 1,000-bed teaching hospital is no more useless than disorganized data in a family practitioner's office. Organized data in a major facility's operation is no more useful than organized data in the files of a rural public health nurse. There is no element—size of organization, scope of care provided, level of care provided, or any other—that negates the need for organized data. Any organization that uses, develops, or otherwise handles health information is eligible to participate in the development of a HIS. In point of fact, these organizations have a responsibility to develop a HIS, staff it with qualified personnel, and budget and control it accordingly.

Quantifying the Management Component

There is a thread of objectivity that runs through the components outlined in the first part of this chapter. One of the most important aspects of management is the objective description and communication of desired outcomes, plans, rationales, etc., that must be mutually understood by all those who work in the unit or organization. The materials from Cascade Hospital, reproduced as Appendixes 8A-8D at the end of this chapter describe an approach to health information in a medium-sized teaching hospital. This approach is closely allied to management by objective and demonstrates the need and use of a workable solution using objective guidelines.

Described in the Cascade information is the complete list of performance objectives for the medical record department and an indication of who is responsible to delegate the tasks necessary to meet the objectives (see Appendix 8A). Objective 5, Retaining and Retrieving Patient Data, and Objective 7, Statistical Data Utilization, target the end results and provide a reference for the tasks that are detailed in the sample procedure for analysis of discharge records. Once again, this is one hospital's approach to a HIS. There are many others.

To make the objectives useful on an everyday basis, there is a schedule that is used by the director and assistant to have a further, scheduled breakdown of tasks to carry out at various levels (Appendix 8B). Individuals are indicated as Dir., for the director of the department, a registered medical record administrator, and A. Dir., for the assistant director, also a registered medical record administrator. This schedule is kept in chronological order and they can enter their comments, dates, etc., on it at any time of the year. It is designed to be a dynamic form and has a variety of uses and methods for data entry. For example, it can be started at the beginning of the calendar or the budget year. It can be updated monthly, weekly, or quarterly, and even activities can be added as needed. It can be used in discussions with the administrator, comptroller, employees, budget committee, or other management staff. From it other reports can be generated to provide a graphic display for employees to utilize in monitoring achievements, measuring outcomes, or teaching others about departmental activities.

Two other examples are also included from Cascade Hospital. Directly related to the objectives and standards, they include a sample procedure (Appendix 8C) and guidelines (Appendix 8D) for use with the procedure.

Procedures such as the examples are usually part of a departmental procedure manual and provide a detailed account of what tasks, equipment, materials, and schedules are necessary to complete the procedure. A job description is another important aspect of an individual's reference information in accomplishing mutual objectives of management and individual. The job description is not as detailed as the procedure and identifies such information as required education or training, experience, lines of authority and designation of supervisor, and a general description of the job, as well as major job objectives.

To accomplish a list of objectives and standards such as Cascade has, one approach is to bring into focus all those who request information, act as certifiers or accreditors, and require proof of care and documentation of quality assurance. The list reproduced as Appendix 8E is a set of questions that a hospital can utilize in determining eligibility for accreditation as well as in formulating goals, objectives, policies, standards, procedures, methods, budgets, and programs. It is not all-inclusive, but will direct attention to most of the important functions necessary to an adequate and professional medical record department.

BUDGETS

Budgets are one of the most commonly described objective plans. Let's look at what a budget means in the HIS.

In discussing budget we might do well to consider the four phases of its life cycle. These would be:

1. The forecasting phase, which would involve gathering information on items that would influence the demand for or decrease of services.
2. The documentation and justification phase wherein the forecasted adjustments are made and figures finalized.
3. The administrative approval phase. In this phase the compromise between what has been requested and what is approved or allowed is established and realized, and the budget, once again, massaged and finalized.
4. The accountability phase wherein we must live within the parameters and constraints of our approved budget and be accountable for budgetary variances.

A critical element in each of these phases of the budgetary life cycle is the grasp of the upside/downside concept. The upside concept reflects factors that would demonstrate growth or increased demands on services and the cost of providing them. The downside concept would indicate adverse trends or a decline in the demand for services. The forecasting phase is perhaps the most crucial phase, in that a firm grasp of future events, conditions, and the upside/downside impacts determine the measure of budgetary adjustments to be made over previous budgets.

There are basically two types of forecasting methods to consider. These are: mechanical and analytical forecasting.

1. Mechanical forecasting, also known as historic forecasting, usually involves a straight percentage increase multiplied across the board. It can be used for yearly projections on demands and services. However, it is best to go back three years as the base from which to project.
2. Analytical forecasting employs the upside/downside concepts and seeks to project realistic figures based on the impact of demands for services. Critical factors to be considered in forecasting are future events or conditions that will affect situation, people, time, and causative controls. The health care industry is particularly vulnerable to impacts of these critical factors. The medical record administrator can readily map out an impact grid itemizing the following headings and documenting critical factors affecting them. The headings are:

> Situation
> People
> Trends
> Place
> Causative Controls

Examples of critical factors that affect situations in health care might be a change in patient days or in patient mix or in patient services. For example, the opening of an oncology unit could affect such changes. Other examples are new technology available, computer changes, and so on.

Examples of critical factors impacting people might be personnel turnover rate, availability of various levels of medical record personnel; for example, highly skilled and experienced medical transcriptionists, experienced ART's, medical audit coordinators, discharge planners, the addition of new physician specialty groups to the medical staff, additional departmental coverage, salary constraints, and merit increases.

Examples of critical factors influencing time or showing trends toward change might be increased proof of care and service demands from insurance companies. They might be trends of medical staff toward increased documentation, trends of increased utilization of transcription services, trends toward more outpatient services, increased requests for copies of patient records from attorneys, trends toward unionization, trends toward more inservice education, and so on.

Examples of critical factors influencing place are usually of geographic nature. For example, a new office building, a move to another location, an outside group moving in, sharing space or facilities with another department. One might be asked by administrative directive to share a photocopying machine with the next two departments down the hall.

Examples of critical factors that affect controls or constraints might be new legislation; the JCAH; medical audit demands; PSRO requirements; new services; changes in psychiatric legislation; changes in requirements for long-term care documentation, audits, or patient care plans; new requirements for outpatient or ambulatory care audits or statistics; and so on.

A listing of management activities performed during the forecasting phase of budget preparation would probably include the following:

- Identify the budgetary and forecasting period. This might be twelve months, eighteen months, five years, or whatever period is selected.
- Identify and gather information on future events and conditions affecting people, place, trends, controls, and situations.
- Sort out information into upside/downside influences and trace these to departmental activities and services.
- Translate or convert these impacts into measurable units: hours, people, equipment needed, dollars and cents.
- Communicate to and obtain understanding and acceptance of the forecast by all affected components of your facility. If, for example, one knows nursing service is planning to go into a heavy-scale nursing-audit activity, one can project the .5 full-time equivalent employee increase needed to do ten audits per year and obtain a signature on the justification statements. This defines the limit on the number of audits requested by nursing service and might provide half a full-time equivalent position to do the work, rather than trying to get by on existing staff.
- Write out costs debited against the budget by other departments and check into increases in cost and activity for the future; for example, messenger service, mailroom, postage, photocopying service, maintenance, accounting, taxes, and handling costs. Those kinds of things might be services that medical record administrators are unaware of that they could be accountable for.

Another consideration in budget preparation is the financial distinction between maintenance costs and new programs. By this is meant expenses to maintain the department and services exactly as they are. What increases can be identified without any change in services, personnel, supplies, etc.? What increases can be projected, considering the impacts of new changes, forecasts, and new programs?

It might be well to note here that the United States government is presently implementing the concept of zero-base budgeting, which, in effect, means a program that starts at zero and assumes that there is no present or maintenance budget upon which to build a new budget. Each ongoing activity is studied intensively, perhaps once every five years. This program is in contrast to the usual budget review, which takes the current level of spending as a starting point. It is a more intense review that starts from scratch and attempts to build up the resources that are actually needed by the activity. These studies are especially important when costs are of a discretionary type. Basic questions are raised, such as:

Should the function be performed at all?
What should the quality level be?
Are we doing too much?
Should it be performed in this way?
How much would it cost?
How much should it cost?

We'd like to point out here that while forecasting is important, there is a distinctive difference between a forecast and a budget. A budget basically has a number of general characteristics: It is stated in monetary terms. It usually covers a period of time, for example, one year. It contains an element of management commitment in that managers agree to accept the responsibility for attaining the budget objectives. The budget proposal is reviewed and approved by a higher authority than the budgetee. The budget can be changed only under specific circumstances. Periodically, actual financial performance is compared to budget, and variances are analyzed and explained.

A forecast, on the other hand, may or may not be stated in monetary terms. It can be for any period of time. The forecaster does not accept the responsibility for meeting the forecast results. The forecast results are not usually approved by a higher authority. The forecast is updated as soon as new information is received.

In the state of Washington, hospitals are obligated to work with the Washington State Rate Commission. In preparing departmental budgets, middle managers and administrators must utilize financial formulas established by the commission. The following formula is that used for medical record departments: The total number of hospital admissions per year minus newborns, plus one-eighth of the total number of outpatient visits plus ER visits.

This statistical unit is utilized to determine the dollar amount per unit of productivity and direct expenses per unit statistic. The statistical unit is divided into the totals for salaries, expenses (less capital), and productive labor. The resultant statistics are used to compare the hospital medical record department with others in a group of hospitals with similar size and services. These figures are utilized to control authorized expenses and productive hours.

For example:

Medical record unit according to formula	= 21,768
Total salaries expenditure for the year (includes expected increments)	= $224,034
Total expenses less capital	$ 36,089
Total productive hours	56,411

Therefore:

The $ figure per unit of productivity	= $11.95
OR one admission (following the formula)	= $11.95
The $ figure per hours of productivity	= $10.29
The $ figure per unit of expense	= $ 1.66

The rate commission has attempted to establish equitable formulas. It entertains directions from professionals regarding this and has periodically revised its methods to more adequately represent realistic methodology.

The Maintenance Budget

Administrative directives normally dictate what budgetary accounts, forms, and formats will be used. Once the budget period has been established (for instance, a twelve-month period), it is important to know how the facility's accounting department will report back monies spent and variances. Not only must this be understood but also how and when expenses will be debited against the department's accounts. It is to the medical record administrator's advantage to plot expenses at intervals when it is known they will occur, rather than to plot out 12 equal monthly allocations. For example, isn't it more reasonable to list a microfilming service contract every third month if you are billed quarterly, rather than to divide the annual expense by 12 months and end up with an off-balance budget for the whole year? It is also wise to know what services are charged to the medical record department by other departments, i.e., messenger service, mailroom, dietary, maintenance, painting, etc. One must be alert for any charges carried over from the previous year's budget. This can happen with certain accounting and billing practices. Bills may not be paid as promptly as one might expect and carryovers are not unusual.

At the end of this chapter sample budget forms from General Hospital of Everett are included as Appendix 8F. Examples of currently used budget requests, instructions, and expense reports are provided.

Appendix 8G is a Cost Analysis from Snow Hospital. It demonstrates how hard data can be compiled for use in describing a departmental objective. The objective in this case is modernization of equipment for the Word Processing Unit through predicted production increase. Such an objective is compatible with the objectives previously provided in the Cascade Hospital examples. Relate the Snow Hospital cost analysis to the Cascade Hospital Standards 4, Controlling, and 8, Transcription of Medical Reports.

As can be seen by the samples, there are many ways to present budgetary data, just as there are with health data. The following is a list of maintenance budget account headings that are fairly common:

General Supplies
- Folders (often largest cash outlay)
- General office supplies
- Other (Forms)

Contracts
- Microfilm Service Bureau
- PAS/SNAP
- COM/MPI

Photocopying

Travel & Education

Maintenance & Repair

Dues, Books, Subscriptions (coding books, PDRs, county medical directories)

Telephone (regular and extra lines and costs for Centrex, word processing center, couplers)

Postage (anticipated price and volume increases)

Dietary (medical staff coffee, meetings)

Intradepartmental Expenses (aspirin, bandaids, first aid from pharmacy)

Interdepartmental Income (other departments that pay for photocopying; reimbursement for cancer abstracts from regional cancer center; subpoena fees, copying fees)

Personnel/Salary

- Actual positions × salaries and anticipated staffing needs
- Shift differentials
- Merit increases/expected increments

•Cost of living allowance/inflation factors
•Replacement Costs: While sometimes overlooked, replacement costs often make the difference between a balanced budget and a salary budget that is way out of line. Replacement costs should reflect how much it will actually cost to replace an employee or cover a position in any of the following situations: vacation, holiday, sick leave, overtime, turnover, training a replacement, on-call positions. In each situation, consider who would be most likely to cover or replace. Calculate costs based on the actual projected salary of the particular individual most likely to do the work. If, for example, a medical transcriptionist becomes ill and is away from work for an extended period, is it likely that the word processing supervisor will cover? If so, how much of the salary will be covered anyway and how much will need to be in overtime? Can less expensive personnel or on-call personnel be used?

It is a common practice of a comptroller to try to automatically reduce a salary budget by virtue of turnover or attrition. Is this realistic? In most positions within the jurisdiction of the medical record administrator, it is perhaps a more common occurrence to overlap and train a new employee, in effect paying a double wage.

Capital Expenditures

Capital expenditures are often broken out into two categories: (1) New and Additional, and (2) Replacement Costs. Another way of categorizing capital expenditures is by rounding off dollar amounts.

In purchasing equipment, it is important to go beyond the obvious figures on the price tag. Consideration should be given to trade-in allowances, freight and delivery charges, taxes, packing, installation charges, hook-ups, training or instruction charge, assembly charges, etc.

The practice of trying to identify and isolate cost centers is becoming more and more prevalent, particulary in light of such agencies as state rate commission. Whenever possible, it is often useful to understand and control at points where costs are accrued. Can you break out and isolate your costs? Is it possible to push for a separate department accounting budget for an area like a word processing center? Separating personnel costs, salaries, forms, equipment expense, contracts and leases, photocopying expense, mailing costs, reference books, and supplies for this area from those of the whole department can affect greater budgetary control. Can further cost refinements be pinpointed by costing out services to Radiology, Oncology, ER, Pathology, etc.?

REFERENCES

Drucker, Peter F. *Management: Tasks, Responsibilities, Practices*. New York: Harper & Row, 1974.

Gibson, James L.; Ivancevich, John M.; and Donnelly, James H., Jr. *Readings in Organizations: Behavior, Structure, Processes*. Dallas, Texas: Business Publications, Inc., 1976.

Haney, William V. *Communication and Organizational Behavior*. Homewood, Ill.: Richard D. Irwin, Inc.

Littlefield, C.L., and Rachel, Frank. *Office and Administrative Management*. Englewood Cliffs, N.J.: Prentice-Hall, 1970.

MacGregor, Douglas. *The Human Side of Enterprise*. New York: McGraw-Hill Book Co., 1960.

Massie, Joseph L. *Essentials of Management*. Englewood Cliffs, N.J.: Prentice-Hall, Inc., 1971.

McCool, Barbara, and Brown, Montague. *The Management Response: Conceptual, Technical and Human Skills of Health Administration*. Philadelphia, Pa.: W.B. Saunders Co., 1977.

McFarland, Dalton E. *Management Principles and Practices*. New York: Macmillan Co., 1974.

Newman, William H.; Summer, Charles E.; and Warren, E. Kirby. *The Process of Management: Concepts, Behavior and Practice*. Englewood Cliffs, N.J.: Prentice-Hall, Inc. 1970.

Appendix 8A

Cascade Hospital
Washington, USA

Medical Record Department

GOAL

The goal of the Medical Record Department is to further the growth and development of the hospital according to its stated goals through the coordination and maintenance of a clinical data bank. Data for all hospital patients are to be retained and retrieved for the use of those who participate in the patient's care and other authorized parties. This will be accomplished by the following objectives.

1. *Planning*: Develop and utilize ongoing planning mechanisms designed to accomplish the department's goals.

   Standards:

   a. Using facility-wide forecasts provided by Administration, finer forecasting is performed on an annual basis to determine manpower, material, and fiscal resources required for the calendar year (Director).

   b. Annual and quarterly objectives are developed incorporating programming, scheduling, and budgeting (Director).

   c. Progress is measured against plans quarterly (Director and Assistant Director).

   d. Policies and procedures are reviewed annually to determine continued relevancy. (2) Recommendations for policy changes are made, and procedures are revised as needed (Director d.1. and d.2.; Assistant d.2).

2. *Organizing*: Determine work to be performed so that it can be accomplished effectively and efficiently.

Standards:

   a. The department's organizational chart is to be reviewed annually (Director).

   b. Specific objectives are developed annually for and with department staff, and reviewed periodically (Director).

   c. Position descriptions are prepared for all department staff, and revised as needed (Assistant).

3. *Leading*: Develop the technical and professional expertise of departmental staff by recognizing capabilities, directing new and continuing challenges, and compensating appropriately.

Standards:

   a. Annual evaluations and quarterly evaluations to demonstrate improving communication and acceptance of new objectives (Director and Assistant).

   b. Merit increases are proportionate to employees' continued improvement in performance consistent with the hospital's merit review criteria and departmental expectations (Director and Assistant).

   c. Continued promotions are granted to deserving and qualified employees, and qualified employees are directed into professional standing through continuing education as such promotions are feasible.
(Director = Approval, wage, and administrative functions)
(Assistant = Recommendations and continuing education)

   d. Methods of selection, placement, and training are continually improved to the maximum benefit of both department and employee (Assistant).

4. *Controlling*: Measure performance and results of all components of the Medical Record Department against understood and accepted plans, evaluating exceptions to plans and securing prompt and effective corrective action so that plans are achieved and continued improvement is ensured.

Standards:

a. Understood and accepted objectives, programs, schedules, and budgets are utilized at all levels of the Medical Record Department in conjunction with the related performance standards necessary to access progress and evaluate results against plans. (Director)

b. A consistent, logical reporting system that will provide to the Director of Medical Records prompt, accurate information to measure actual performance compared with standards is developed and used at all times. (Assistant Director)

c. Acceptable limits of variance within which accountable employees can correct their own mistakes are established and timely corrective action taken. (Director and Assistant)

d. All exceptions outside understood and accepted limits of tolerance are reported and explained immediately to the Director of Medical Records with recommendations for corrective action. Verbal exceptions reports, explanations, and recommendations are verified in writing within six working days of initial submission. (Assistant Director)

5. *Retaining/Retrieving Patient Data*: Provide facilities and systems for the preservation of clinical records in a manner in which they are readily accessible.

Standards:

a. Record processing is to proceed efficiently as to allow completion in a reasonable period of time (Assistant).

b. Routing control procedures are refined to allow rapid location of information (Director and Assistant).

c. Filing systems are updated to ensure maximum benefit in accessibility (Director).

d. Equipment and systems to assess automated information are updated according to need (Director).

e. Criteria for the completion of medical records are to be reviewed for adequacy, effectiveness, and compliance with JCAH standards and consistency with the current medical staff bylaws on an annual basis (Director and Assistant).

6. *Release of Clinical Information*: Safeguard the confidential nature of clinical information while cooperating with other health facilities, private practitioners, social agencies, and third parties in the sharing of such information in the patients' best interests and with proper authorization.

Standards:

a. Requests for clinical information are answered following the guidelines of confidentiality and with proper authorization. Priority is given to requests concerning the ongoing health care of the patients. (Director)

b. With the aid of legal counsel, release of information practices and policies are periodically appraised and updated. (Assistant Director)

c. The Medical Record Department staff is periodically reappraised of codes of confidentiality and changes in medico-legal aspects of release of clinical information. All MRD staff are bound by the ethical code of the American Medical Record Association in areas concerning confidentiality and unethical practices. (Director and Assistant)

d. Requests for information will be accomplished within a reasonable period of time. (Assistant Director)

7. *Statistical Data Utilization*: Provide assistance to the administrative, medical, and clinical staffs in the meaningful utilization of data abstracted from clinical records.

Standards:

a. To ensure relevancy, thorough understanding of the need for particular data is to be established when compiling the requested information (Assistant).

b. Compilation of such data is to be maintained as an important function, but not at the sacrifice of the foregoing objectives (Assistant).

    c. Monthly statistical reports required by Administration will be processed on a timely basis; the content of which will be reviewed annually for relevancy (Director and Assistant).

    d. The hospital's annual statistical report will be generated by this department and the content will be reviewed for relevancy by the Medical Record Department and Administration (Director and Assistant).

8. *Transcription of Medical Reports*: Provide transcription services to the medical staff for various reports contributing to the medical record.

    Standards:

    a. Dictation/transcription equipment and systems are to be maintained at a level of proficiency so as to provide maximum service (Director).

    b. The quantity and caliber of transcription staff are to be maintained at a level so as to provide maximum service (Director and Assistant).

    c. Analysis of the quantity, quality, character, and trends in production, numbers, and types of reports will be reviewed quarterly and annually (Director, Assistant and Central Dictation Supervisor).

9. *Improvement of Interdepartmental Relationships*: Continually identify and evaluate the ways in which the Medical Record Department can be of service to other areas of the hospital.

    Standards:

    a. Policies exercised by the Medical Record Department affecting other departments are reviewed annually, revised if necessary, and periodically recommunicated (Director).

    b. Requests for new services will be evaluated in light of foregoing objectives. Those requests related to ongoing patient care will be given priority (Director).

    c. The members of the departmental staff will be evaluated quarterly and annually for effective communication utilized in dealing with other departments and the public (Director and Assistant).

10. *Tumor Registry*: Maintain a tumor registry that will contain information on all carcinoma cases diagnosed and treated, with particular attention given to their followup and survival histories to assist the medical staff in their study and successful treatment of cancer.

Standards:

a. All carcinoma cases of in and out patients diagnosed and treated, with the exception of those followed by the Adult Leukemia Center, are identified and entered into the Tumor Registry. (Assistant Director)

b. All primary carcinomas are abstracted and entered into the Cancer Surveillance System regional automated registry. Our affiliation with the CSS is reviewed annually by Administration to determine the need for continuing our participation in a regional registry. (Assistant Director)

c. A patient index of all abstracted carcinoma cases is maintained to ensure maximum accuracy in patient identification, data control, disease by site, and retrievability. (Director and Assistant)

d. Followup is performed on all carcinoma cases and completed within one month of their anniversary date of initial diagnosis, and secondary and metastic cases are completed upon discharge. (Director and Assistant)

e. Tumor Conferences of the medical staff are held monthly for the continuing education and effective cancer treatment skills of the medical staff. The medical staff, with the assistance of the Tumor Registry, provides carcinoma information on the activity of carcinoma cases by site, longevity, survival rates, and modalities of treatment. (Director and Assistant)

Health Information System Schedule for Cascade Hospital

Exhibit 8B Health Information System Schedule for Cascade Hospital

Date: April 1979

Medical Record Department Objectives and Activities	Acct	Schedule			Budget	Comments (OK V.E.)
		Start	Finish	Time Req'd		
1. *PLANNING*: Development of Master Schedule of activities for the Medical Record Department in 1979.	Dir.	April	April	2 weeks	—	Completed
Evaluation and revision of microfilming policies and procedure.	Dir.	July	July	2 weeks	—	

Date: April 1979

Medical Record Department Objectives and Activities	Acct	Schedule			Budget	Comments (OK V.E.)
		Start	Finish	Time Req'd		
Refinement in standard cited in objectives.	Dir.	Jan	Dec	—	—	Continued project
Objectives are reviewed and revised as necessary.	Dir.	Jan	Dec	—	—	Continued project
The investigation of the advisability of establishing a maintenance contract for the reader/printer will take place.	A. Dir.	Aug	Aug	1 month	—	
2. *ORGANIZING*: The job descriptions of Director and Assistant are evaluated and redefined.	Dir.	Jan	Jan	3 weeks	—	Completed
The department's organizational chart is reviewed.	Dir.	Feb	Feb	1 week	—	Completed
Specific objectives are developed and reviewed periodically.	Dir.	Jan	Dec	—	—	Continued project

Date: April 1979

Medical Record Department Objectives and Activities	Acct	Schedule			Budget	Comments (OK V.E.)
		Start	Finish	Time Req'd		
Job descriptions and procedures are reviewed and necessary changes made.	Dir.	Aug	Oct	3 months	—	
Development of inventory listing, depreciation, and replacement schedules will take place.	A. Dir.	April	June	2 months	—	
3. *LEADING:* The Quality Assurance Program for all employees is implemented with monthly conferences for each employee.	Dir.	Jan	Jan	4 weeks	—	Completed
Refinements are made in the Q.A.P. as necessary and safety awareness is realized.	Dir.	Jan	Dec	—	—	Continued project
Monthly departmental meetings are conducted with an agenda and documented minutes.	Dir.	Jan	Dec	—	—	Continuous
Annual and quarterly evaluations take place.	Dir.	Jan	Dec	—	—	Continuous

Date: April 1979

Medical Record Department Objectives and Activities	Acct	Schedule				Comments (OK V.E.)
		Start	Finish	Time Req'd	Budget	
In-service education is offered to all personnel in this department to enhance professional expertise.	A. Dir.	Jan	Dec	—	—	Continuous
Enhancement of caliber of supervisory staff in Central Dictation and department proper.	Dir.	Jan	Dec	—	—	Continuous
Learning opportunities are made available to ARTs to prepare for medical audit and enhance professional expertise.	Dir.	Jan	Dec	—	—	Continuous
New procedures are developed and documented for training new personnel.	A. Dir.	Aug	Aug	2 weeks	—	
Reanalysis and reclassification of admit and discharge clerk position takes place.	A. Dir.	Mar	April	1 month	—	
Reanalysis of duties of weekend evening clerk position takes place.	A. Dir.	May	June	1 month		

Date: April 1979

Medical Record Department Objectives and Activities	Acct	Schedule			Budget	Comments (OK V.E.)
		Start	Finish	Time Req'd		
4. CONTROLLING:						
Work measurement and standards are developed for Medical Record positions.	Dir.	July	Dec	6 months	—	
Management by Objective tools are developed, understood, and utilized to obtain adequate controlling performance.	Dir.	Jan	Dec	—	—	Continued project
Objectives, programs, schedules, and budgets are used as performance standard to measure progress.	Dir.	Jan	Dec	—	—	Continued project
Routine reporting to the administrative head is to be maintained as a means of performance measurement.	Dir.	Jan	Dec	—	—	Continuous
Close attention is given to the Operating Budget reports.	Dir.	Jan	Dec	—	—	Continuous
Installation of sun and bug screens as requested in budget.	A. Dir.	April	June	2 months	$470	

Date: April 1979

Medical Record Department Objectives and Activities	Acct	Schedule			Budget	Comments (OK V.E.)
		Start	Finish	Time Req'd		
5. *RETAINING/RETRIEVING CLINICAL DATA:*						
Boxing of old records to make room for 1979 records takes place.	A. Dir.	Jan	Oct	8 months off & on	—	
Microfilming of records through 1973 takes place.	A. Dir.	Jan	May	5 months		
Microfiching of records through 1975 takes place.	A. Dir.	May	Nov	6 months		
Expansion of the terminal digit filing system takes place.	A. Dir.	May	June	1 month		
Compatible microfiche and medical record numbering systems are implemented.	Dir.	May	Dec	—	—	Continuous
Refinement in loose sheets charting procedures are made with special emphasis on Clinical Lab activity.	A. Dir.	Mar	June	3 months		

Date: April 1979

Medical Record Department Objectives and Activities	Acct	Schedule				Comments (OK V.E.)
		Start	Finish	Time Req'd	Budget	
Medical Record automated systems are evaluated and redesigned.	Dir.	Jan	Oct?			Continuous
Approval for revision of Medical Record Data Processing systems is obtained.	Dir.	Jan	?			
Medical Record revised data processing systems implemented and operational.	Dir.	?	?			
6. *RELEASE OF INFORMATION PERFORMANCE:* The department staff is periodically reappraised of codes of confidentiality and changes in medico-legal aspects of release procedures and policies.	Dir.	Jan	Dec			Continuous
Legal opinion re: legal requirement for attending physician to chart in record all psych release of information incidents is sought.	Dir.	April	April	1 month	—	

Date: April 1979

Medical Record Department Objectives and Activities	Acct	Schedule				Comments (OK V.E.)
		Start	Finish	Time Req'd	Budget	
Psychiatric legislation is investigated with legal counsel and appropriate procedural changes made.	Dir.	April	May	1-1/2 months	—	
On-call hire is added to staff to assist in Business Office requests. May need to be made permanent authorized 1/4-time position.	Dir.	April	April	2 weeks	—	
Medical staff campaigns to provide final diagnoses to assist in cash flow.	Dir.	Jan	Dec	—	—	Continuous
Refinement of correspondence procedures to hasten processing time takes place.	A. Dir.	April	June	3 months	—	
Data Processing Medical Record program design takes place to provide an automatic listing of available diagnoses to the Business Office.	Dir.	April	April	1 month	—	Completed

Date: April 1979

Medical Record Department Objectives and Activities	Acct	Schedule			Budget	Comments (OK V.E.)
		Start	Finish	Time Req'd		
7. STATISTICAL DATA UTILIZATION PERFORMANCE:						
Implementation of new statistical forms for reporting hospital monthly statistics takes place.	A. Dir.	Jan	Jan	1 week	—	Completed
Refinements are made in reconciling statistics with Data Processing by improved communication, constant audit, and corrections procedures improvements.	Dir.	Jan	Dec	—	—	Continuous
The 1978 annual statistical report is completed.	A. Dir.	Jan	April	4 months	—	Completed
The annual statistical report is presented to the Administrative Council for opinions re: relevancy and possible additions and deletions.	Dir.	April	May	1 month	—	

Date: April 1979

Medical Record Department Objectives and Activities	Acct	Schedule			Budget	Comments (OK V.E.)
		Start	Finish	Time Req'd		
Medical audit needs and our capacity to assist are evaluated in conjunction with the Health Care Review Center (HCRC).	Dir.	Jan	June?	6 months	—	
Clarification of the role of the Research Committee and their authority and time demands is obtained.	Dir.	April	May	1 month	—	
Data Processing revisions in the Medical Record programs are implemented to eliminate manual retrieval and search efforts.	Dir.	Jan	?	—	—	
8. *PATIENT IDENTIFICATION AND DATA CONTROL PERFORMANCE:* Position of admit and discharge clerk evaluated for relevancy and possible reclassification.	A. Dir.	Mar	April	1 month	—	

Date: April 1979

Medical Record Department Objectives and Activities	Acct	Schedule			Budget	Comments (OK V.E.)
		Start	Finish	Time Req'd		
Delays in updating the Master Patient Index are experienced due to receiving late reports from Clinical Lab and from the floors are decreased and outpatient reports are processed in a timely basis.	A. Dir.	April	June	2 months	—	
Conversion of 275,000 patient identification cards in the Master Patient Index. Cards reduced to approximately fifteen 3" × 5" microfiche through a computer-on-microfilm application. See budget request.	Dir.	April	Dec	8 months	$16,000	Continuous
Acquisition of Xerox supplies cabinet as requested in budget.	Dir.	April	April	1 month	$75	
Acquisition of Microfiche Kit as requested in budget.	Dir.	May	May	1 month	$203	
Acquisition of Microfiche Storage Cabinet as requested in budget.	Dir.	May	May	1 month	$433	

Date: April 1979

Medical Record Department Objectives and Activities	Acct	Schedule				Comments (OK V.E.)
		Start	Finish	Time Req'd	Budget	
8A. *RECORD PROCESSING AND COMPLETION PERFORMANCE:* Criteria for the completion of medical records are reviewed for adequacy, effectiveness, and compliance with JCAH standards and consistency with medical staff bylaws.	Dir.	Jan	Jan	1 month	—	Completed
The closure of the 1978 computer files will take place and manual runs for the disease, operations, and physicians indices will be made.	Dir.	Jan	April	4 months	—	
Placement of ARTs on the floors to perform deficiency analysis, utilization review certification requirements, and chart completion procedures.	Dir.	July	Aug	1 month	—	HCRC?
Data processing design and approval for Incomplete Medical Record Audit subsystem is obtained.	Dir.	Jan	?	?		

Date: April 1979

Medical Record Department Objectives and Activities	Acct	Schedule			Budget	Comments (OK V.E.)
		Start	Finish	Time Req'd		
Implementation of the above.	Dir.	Jan	?			
Elimination of routing procedures through the use of the subsystem.	Dir.	?	?			
Controls established on types of record deficiencies through subsystems.	Dir.	?	?			
Refinement of abstract procedures and elimination of abstract filing procedures through subsystem and abstract redesign.	Dir.	?	?			
Decrease in average shelf-life of incomplete record by 50%.	Dir.	?	?			
Decrease in numbers of incomplete medical records by 50%.	Dir.	?	?			
Bringing record completion performance into compliance with JCAH standards will take place.	Dir.	?	?			

Date: April 1979

Medical Record Department Objectives and Activities	Acct	Schedule			Budget	Comments (<u>OK</u> V.E.)
		Start	Finish	Time Req'd		
Suspension criteria and practice to be reconciled with bylaws and actual practice.	Dir.	?	?			
8B. *TRANSCRIPTION OF MEDICAL REPORTS PERFORMANCE:*						
To increase productivity of Central Dictation staff by revising clerical functions, thereby decreasing the overtime and on-call utilization in 1979.	Dir.	Jan	April	4 months	—	completed
Acquisition of the Emergency Room endless loop recorder.	Dir.	Jan	April	4 months	$2,030	
Acquisition of secretarial posture chairs.	Dir.	Feb	Feb	1 week	$390	
Reduction in Xerox utilization through MT/ST forms.	Dir.	Feb	Feb	1 month	—	
Approval of Secretary I "sliding" positions.	Dir.	Mar	Mar	1 month	—	

Date: April 1979

Medical Record Department Objectives and Activities	Acct	Schedule				Comments (OK V.E.)
		Start	Finish	Time Req'd	Budget	
Obtain approval for the playout clerk position in Central Dictation to realize savings in personnel.	Dir.	April	May	1 month	$460/mo	
Installation of E.R. endless loop recorder.	Dir.	April	May	1 week	—	
Obtain approval of 1.O F.T.E. to perform E.R. transcription.	Dir.	April	April	1 month	$570/mo	
Commencement of E.R. dictation services will take place.	Dir.	—	May	—	—	Continued project
Stabilization of Central Dictation staffing and elimination of unauthorized labor.	Dir.	Jan	May	5 months	—	
Verification of large miscellaneous category of reports transcribed to be classified (Increase of 67% realized in 1978).	Dir.	Jan	Dec	—	—	Continued project

Date: April 1979

Medical Record Department Objectives and Activities	Acct	Schedule				Comments (OK V.E.)
		Start	Finish	Time Req'd	Budget	
Enhancement of management skills of supervisory staff.	Dir.	Jan	Dec	—	—	Continued project
9. *IMPROVEMENT OF INTER-DEPARTMENTAL RELATIONSHIPS:* Initiation of change to permanent medical record number assignment will take place.	Dir.	Jan	Dec	—	—	Continuous
Quality Assurance Program will take place to assist in evaluation of interdepartmental relationships and problem solving.	Dir.	Jan	Dec	—	—	Continuous
Work with the chairmen of the Medicine and Surgery Departments re: chart completion and final diagnoses availability.	Dir.	Jan	Dec	—	—	Continuous
Survey or questionnaire will be sent to the Medical Staff re: Medical Record Department performance.	Dir.	Oct	Oct	1 month	—	—

Date: April 1979

10. TUMOR REGISTRY PERFORMANCE:

Medical Record Department Objectives and Activities	Acct	Schedule			Budget	Comments (OK V.E.)
		Start	Finish	Time Req'd		
The decrease of the percentage of delinquency in the followup of cancer patients will take place.	Dir.	Jan	Dec			Continuous project
The Tumor Registry will be current in terms of new cases abstracted and entered in the computer for the Cancer Surveillance System.	Dir.	Jan	Oct	2 months		Continuous project
The Tumor Registry will be approved following an inspection by the American College of Surgeons upon the completion of the above.	Dir.	Oct	Oct	1 week		
The effective replacement of the present Tumor Registrar will take place and the new individual adequately trained.	Dir.	Mar	Mar	3 weeks	—	Completed

Date: April 1979

Medical Record Department Objectives and Activities	Acct	Schedule				Comments (OK V.E.)
		Start	Finish	Time Req'd	Budget	
SPECIAL ASSIGNMENTS:						
Conferences with HCRC re: URC, chart completion, and medical audit requirements.	Dir.	Jan	June?	—	—	
Approval of Consent Manual.	Dir. & A. Dir.	Jan	?			
Publish an article in professional journal.	Dir.	Dec	Dec	1 month		
Utilization Review Committee—Review surgical components of in-patient plan.	A. Dir.	Jan	Dec			Continuous

Cascade Hospital
Procedure for Analyzing

Objectives

- To check and analyze the component parts of the medical record to see that it is complete, accurate and adequate.
- To check and complete statistical information on Medical Record Abstract sheets.

Materials Needed

1. All charts for patients discharged the previous day should be assembled and an abstract completed on each chart.

2. Blue pen, red pen, pencil, and brown felt pen.

3. Stamp pad, CONSULTATION stamp, HISTORY AND PHYSICAL stamp, ink pad, and colored tags.

4. Service Classification Guide.

5. Coding books, Abstracts.

6. Deficiency slips.
   a. White (Med. and Surg.)
   b. Blue (OB. and NB.)

7. Blue expiration tags and red complication tags.

8. Lists for keeping track of Medicare charts without Medicare recertification stickers, patient care charts, deaths within 24 hours of surgery, infections and complications.

Special Instructions

1. Medicare Recertifications: This is the first thing you will do when you prepare to analyze a day of charts. Make sure you have all the charts for that day. Go through the discharge list for that day and find all the Medicare patients for that day. Now, go through those progress notes counting

the days from admission. Make sure there is a Medicare recertification on the 12th day, the 18th day, the 30th day and every 30 days after that. These must be completely filled out by the physician. Most of these stickers will be on the charts by the time you get them. If you do have to put stickers on, date them with the correct date, that being the 12th, 18th, 30th, etc., day of the stay. Then on your list you will mark down how many Medicare patients were in 12 days or more. Opposite that you will mark down the number of charts you had to put stickers on. On the front of this list you will find a breakdown of floors. You mark how many charts needed stickers and check them in on the listing of floors.

2. Patient Care Committee Review Stamps: After doing the Medicare review, go back through the stack and look for charts having the Patient Care Committee Review Stamps on them. These will be found in the lower right hand corner of the face sheets. Tally them up on a list according to the floors and keep a running daily tally.

3. Surgery Deaths Within 24 Hours of Surgery: Go through all the death charts and make a list of all those charts of patients who died within 24 hours after surgery. These charts will later be reviewed.

4. Complications and Infections: This is a somewhat open category. In determining complications and infections there are several things to rely on in the chart. These are:

   a. Front Sheet: The doctor may write the complications somewhere on the front sheet. Read it carefully to see if something is stated to be a complication. If so, write it on your list of complications and infections.
   b. Progress Notes: These will be the best sources for discovering complications. Read through each note carefully and anything that does not appear to be normal, or at least normal for that particular illness, should be written down on the list.
   c. Lab Sheets: These are particularly helpful in picking out infections (urinary tract, wound infections, pneumonia, etc.).
   d. See Guidelines for Determining Presence and Classification of Infections in Charts for detailed assistance.

Some commonly encountered infections and complications:

1. *Urinary tract infections*: Usually discovered in the Urinalysis by an increase in WBCs after catheterization. Also the Microbiology section if the urine grows bacteria in the culture and a sensitivity is done.

2. *Pneumonia*: Usually discovered in the progress notes and also possibly in an x-ray stating something about consolidations being present. Should also be found in a positive sputum culture.

3. *Wound Infection*: Usually found by a positive wound culture and also probable mention in the progress notes.

4. *Paralytic Ileus*: Should always be stated as such in the progress notes.

5. *Wound Separation*: Should be mentioned in the progress notes.

6. *Hemorrhage*: Should be mentioned in either the progress notes or the operative report. Complications should be tagged with red plastic tags. They should be written on the complication–infection list and indicated with a brown circle in the date column if they were entered on the Abstract (only enter those you are sure of), and if not entered on the Abstract, that should be indicated in pencil by writing "not abstracted" on the list in the date column. Those not abstracted should be pulled for the Infection Control Nurse to review, who will help you to decide.

5. Listing Cancer Cases: As you go through and analyze the chart you should be picking up all cancer cases, old and new. These should be entered in the green steno book and should include the discharge date, name, number and an * for new cancer and a ✓ for an old cancer or a recurrence. Second primaries should be entered with a red star as these are few.

6. Nursing Deficiency Notices: There should be a nursing note for every shift (3) of every day the patient is in the hospital. As you are scanning the nursing notes, if you see a place where the nurses have not charted you should make out a nursing deficiency note. These you should make in triple copy. Copy 1 you will send to Nursing Service, copy 2 you keep for one week and if the floor still has not completed this deficiency you will send them a second notice and in one more week if they have still not completed the deficiency you are to send up the third notice with a note indicating that their cooperation as soon as possible would be appreciated.

Analysis Procedure

1. Deficiency Slips:

a. Use the deficiency slip to indicate all deficiencies on the chart.

b. Each physician has a deficiency slip. Write the physician's name at the top of it. If the chart needs more than one doctor to complete it, use separate deficiency slips for each one.

c. Place slips in order with the attending physician first and other physicians following, concluding with the house staff.

d. Doctors have a colored tag for their deficiency slips and everywhere their signature is needed (except face sheet) there will be the same colored tag on the left edge of the page where their signature is needed. If you should run out of colored tags (7 colors) you can overlap two different colored tags to make more colors.

2. Quantitative Analysis:

(Work on one chart at a time)

  a. Face sheet

     1. Admitting diagnosis: If there is an acceptable admitting diagnosis typed on the upper half of the face sheet by the admitting department you may write in, in ink, by the admitting diagnosis space, "As Above". If there is not an acceptable diagnosis there, you must ask the attending physician for one.
     2. Final diagnosis: All charts need a final diagnosis.
     3. Operation: If any procedure was done on the patient the physician should record it on the face sheet.
     4. Complication: All complications should be recorded on the front sheet.
     5. Death charts: Cause of death should be recorded on all death charts.
     6. Physician signature: All face sheets must be signed by the physician. If a house officer signs it, it must be co-signed by the attending physician.
     7. Enter names of all consultants in the space provided.
     8. Enter service and special statistics in indicated space.

        a. CA for cancer patients
        b. PL for plastic surgery
        c. NT for normal tissue

     9. Death charts: fill out + or − 48 hrs. death and if or if not an autopsy was performed.

History and Physical Exam

  1. If written by an Intern or Resident, it must be co-signed by the attending physician.

  2. We would like to have a heart and lung check for patients in under 48 hours. For patients in over 48 hours we would like to have a complete history and physical. For patients who enter for the same condition within 30 days we would like to have an interval note. Check the Progress note for a possible note adequate to serve as a History and Physical. If one of these is in the chart, use the H & P stamp in the margin next to the note.

  3. If there is no history and physical anywhere in the chart, put a blank one in, writing the patient's name and number at the bottom and ask the attending physician for an H & P, put a blank Short Stay H & P in the chart and ask for a Short Stay H & P.

  4. All H & Ps must be signed by the physician.

Consultation Sheet

1. Consultations are required on all first C-sections.
2. They are also required on the following cases:

a. Curettages or other procedures by which a known or suspected pregnancy may be interrupted.
b. Operations performed for the sole purpose of sterilization on both male and female patients.
c. Cases on all services in which according to judgment of the physician:

1. The patient is not a good medical or surgical risk.
2. The diagnosis is obscure.
3. There is doubt as to the best therapeutic measures to be utilized.

3. Check for required consultations.
4. If the consultation is not recorded, route to the consultant for completion.
5. A satisfactory consultation includes an examination of the patient and the record. A written opinion signed by the consultant must be included in the medical record.
6. If you find a note adequate to be called a Consultation in the progress notes, stamp in the margin with the Consultation stamp and this will be acceptable.
7. All Consultations must be signed by the Consultant.
8. Write in the names of all consultants in the space provided on the face sheet.

Laboratory and Bacteriology

1. Use these to check for complications and infections.

a. Use Urinalysis to check for increased WBCs, indicating an infection.
b. Use Hematology sheet for checking on increased WBCs indicating possible complications such as pneumonia.
c. Use the Microbiology sheet to detect such things as wound infections, septicemia, urinary tract infections.

Special and Diagnostic Reports

1. These include X-rays, EEGs, EKGs, etc.
2. These reports should all be signed.

3. If you find either X-rays or EKGs that are not signed, attach a note asking that they be stamped with the signature and return to the X-ray Department and the EKG Department.

Anesthesia Record

1. No record is required for a local anesthesia.

Operative Report

There must be a report for each surgical procedure performed.
1. Report must be signed by the physician.
2. Minor surgery performed in the Emergency Room is recorded on the Emergency Room Record.

Post Anesthesia Record

1. No record is required for a local anesthesia.

Progress Notes

1. If over 48 hours and there are no progress notes route to the doctor for completion.
2. All charts, over 48 hours, must have a discharge summary signed by the physician. If under 48 hours, a discharge note is necessary, signed by the physician. (Exception—House Staff and Clinic charts to be signed by residents only).
3. Check for documentation of complications.
4. Death charts—expiration note by pronouncing doctor or House Staff.
5. All progress notes must be signed. Use colored tags.

Physicians Orders

1. All verbal, telephone and written orders must be signed by the physician. User colored tags.
2. On routing orders a mimeographed signature is acceptable if recorded in the Administration Office.
3. All charts must have a discharge order signed by the physician or House Staff.
4. All orders should be written in ink and not pencil. If pencil is used, return it to the physician to be rewritten.

Graphic Charts

1. Check for any suspicious temperature spikes that may indicate a complication. (A slight increase in temperature is normal 48 hrs. post op.).

Nurses Notes

1. Check for nurses admit note—date, time, signature.
2. Check for discharge note and signature.
3. Check for falls and other accidents—The Director of Nursing Service (DNS) should have an incident report for any such occurrences. Write a note indicating the name, number, date of discharge, date of accident, and what the accident was and send it to DNS in care of the Safety Office.
4. Death charts—check for name of pronouncing doctor, time, date and disposition of remains and belongings, and also if there was an autopsy performed.
5. If nurses notes are incomplete, route the deficiency slip to nurse and indicate date, floor, shift, and what is missing. Then fill out a nursing deficiency notice (3) and send to Nursing Service.

Service Classification

1. Determine the service assignment based on the final diagnosis and procedures performed, using the Service Classification Guide and/or the Disease Classification in *Textbook and Guide to Standard Nomenclature of Diseases and Operations*.
2. Write the assigned service in the indicated space on the face sheet.
3. Beside the assigned service add the special statistics if any.

   a. Cancer CA
   b. Plastic PL
   c. Normal Tissue NT
   d. Normal Appendix NA

Clinic or House Staff Charts

1. All clinic and housestaff charts are completed by the resident assigned to the case.
2. Face sheet is to be co-signed by the attending physician assigned to the case.
3. History and Physical to be co-signed by the attending physician on the case.
4. Clinic summaries are required on all charts except New Borns.

OB and NB

1. OB Delivery charts require:

a. Admitting diagnosis
b. Final diagnosis
c. Pre-natal history
d. Delivery record
e. Discharge Summary only if it was an abnormal delivery or complications were encountered
f. If first C-section, consultation required.

2. New Born charts require:

a. Admitting diagnosis
b. Final diagnosis
c. New Born physical
d. Discharge Summary only if abnormal child.

Appendix 8D

Guidelines for Determining Presence and Classification of Infections in Charts

If the physician indicates in the chart that an infection is, or has been present, then the information is recorded unequivocally, as infection, whether or not additional supporting data are present in the chart.

In the absence of such specific information, the examiner must then make a judgment as to whether the information represents an infection. The presence of an infection at the time of admission is usually easily established. However, greater difficulty is usually experienced in determining the presence and classification of infections that develop after admission. The following guidelines are directed towards clarification of the latter situation. These criteria are intended to be used for the purpose of identifying and classifying infections. Hopefully, infections detected by these criteria will correlate well with actual clinical diagnosis. In some instances, suspected infections that do not meet these criteria will correlate well with actual clinical diagnoses. In some instances, suspected infections that do not meet these criteria will nonetheless be sufficiently established on clinical grounds to require therapy.

Nosocomial infections express themselves clinically and in hospitalized patients in whom the infection was not present or incubating at the time of admission. When the incubation period is unknown, an infection is called nosocomial if it develops at any time after admission. An infection present on admission can be classified as Nosocomial but only if it is directly related to or is the residual of a *previous* admission. Both infections with endogenous organisms carried by the patient and with organisms originating in the animate or inanimate environment are included in the definition. When thus defined, *the term "nosocomial infection" will include the vast majority of potentially preventable infections* while admittedly including some infections that may be regarded as inevitable.

Application of specific guidelines requires that the clinical and laboratory data be reliable. *There must be a high degree of certainty as to when the*

551

clinical manifestations of the infection in question had their onset. Additionally, when the diagnosis of infection depends on bacteriologic identification or organisms, colony counts or other laboratory procedures, it is essential that these procedures be reliably performed on adequately collected and promptly delivered specimens.

It must be emphasized that in a given patient with an existing culture established nosocomial infection, two situations can commonly arise which must be considered as new, individual, nosocomial infections: (1) The appearance of clinical infection *at a new and different site*, even though with the same organisms as the original infection, must be considered as a new nosocomial infection. (This would probably represent self-infection.) (2) Conversely, the appearance in culture of *new and different organisms* from a previously described site of nosocomial infection must be considered as a new individual nosocomial infection if there is a coincident clinical continuation or, particularly, deterioration in the patient's condition.

The following guidelines are for the classification of nosocomial infections in specific sites, offered as a practical application of the principles already stated.

URINARY TRACT INFECTIONS

The onset of clinical signs or symptoms of urinary tract infection (fever, dysuria, costovertebral angle tenderness, supra-pubic tenderness, etc.) in a hospitalized patient in conjunction with *one or both of the following factors* (if available) *developing after* admission is sufficient for the diagnosis of nosocomial urinary tract infections:

1. *Colony counts* of greater than 10,000 pathogens per ml* or visible organisms on an unspun sediment of fresh urine.
2. Pyuria of greater than 10 WBC's per high power field.

If a patient with a prior negative urinalysis and/or culture develops clinical symptoms of urinary tract infection while hospitalized, and neither urinalysis nor urine culture have been repeated, he should be considered to have a nosocomial urinary tract infection. Also, as described above, the appearance in culture of new organisms in an existing urinary tract infection together with clinical continuation or deterioration constitutes a new nosocomial urinary tract infection.

Asymptomatic Bacteriuria is applied to those persons having colony counts of greater than *100,000 organisms per ml without previous or current manifestations* of infection; such asymptomatic urinary tract infections

---

*A carefully collected midstream urine specimen is adequate for examination.

should be classified as nosocomial if an earlier urine culture was negative at a time when the patient was not receiving antibiotics. If a patient is admitted to the hospital with a urinary tract infection, subsequent culture of a new pathogen in numbers greater than 100,000 organisms per ml should be regarded as a new infection.

SURGICAL WOUND INFECTIONS

Any surgical wound which drains purulent material, with or without a positive culture, is considered to be the site of a nosocomial infection. The source of the organism, whether endogenous or exogenous, is not considered.

RESPIRATORY INFECTIONS

Clinical signs and symptoms of a lower respiratory infection, (cough, pleuritic chest pain, fever and particularly purulence, and fever) developing after admission are regarded as sufficient evidence to diagnose respiratory infection, whether or not sputum cultures or chest X-rays are obtained.

Other conditions which may result in similar signs or symptoms (congestive heart failure, post-operative atelectasis, pulmonary embolism, etc.) may often be differentiated by the clinical course of the patient; however, even if such entities are suspected to be present, the diagnosis of lower respiratory infection is made in the presence of one or more of the following: purulence, positive sputum culture or suggestive chest X-ray. Super-infection of a previously existing respiratory infection is considered to be a new nosocomial infection when a new pathogen is cultured from sputum and clinical or radiologic evidence indicates that a new organism is associated with deterioration in the patient's condition. Care must be used in distinguishing super-colonization from super-infection.

SKIN AND SUBCUTANEOUS INFECTIONS

Any purulent material in skin or subcutaneous tissue first developing after admission is regarded as indicating a nosocomial infection. Whether or not a culture is positive, negative, or has not been taken. This category includes nonsurgical wounds and burns, as well as various forms of dermatitis and decubitus ulcers. In patients who are admitted with skin or subcutaneous infections, a change in pathogens cultured from the infected site is regarded as a nosocomial infection if continuing purulent drainage can be attributed to the new pathogen. *Cellulitis* caused by bacterial agents is usually not accompanied by purulent drainage; in such instances primary reliance must be placed on *clinical judgment* which may be confirmed by cultures of tissue fluid aspirates.

BACTEREMIA

Any culture-documented bacteremia that develops in a hospitalized patient who was not admitted with evidence of bacteremia is regarded as a nosocomial infection, unless the organism has been judged to be a contaminant. Such nosocomial bacteremias may occur in the absence of recognized underlying infections, or originate from a site of nosocomial infection, or from manipulation of a site which was infected at the time of the patient's admission (i.e., catheters, drains, incision and drainage . . . etc.)

OTHER SITES OF INFECTION

Intravenous Catheters and Needles

Purulent drainage from the site of an intravenous catheter or needle is regarded as a nosocomial infection, even if no cultures are obtained. Inflammation of such sites, without purulent material or strong clinical evidence of cellulitis is not regarded as an infection unless a positive culture is obtained from the catheter tip or from aspirates of tissue fluid.

Gastroenteritis

Clinically *symptomatic gastroenteritis* having its onset after admission and associated with a *culture which is positive for a known pathogen* is regarded as nosocomial gastroenteritis. If the incubation period for the pathogen is known (i.e., salmonella, shigella, etc.,) the interval between admission and the onset of clinical symptoms must be greater than the incubation period. Alternatively, nosocomial gastroenteritis may be diagnosed if a prior stool culture, obtained after admission, was negative for the pathogen in question.

Endometritis

Purulent cervical discharge accompanied by *either* a *positive* culture for pathogens or *systemic manifestations* of infection is regarded as nosocomial endometritis if the onset occurs after admission.

Many other possible sites of nosocomial infection must sometimes be considered. Application of the general principles outlined above, however, will generally make classification of these infections possible. It must be reemphasized that CLINICAL IMPRESSIONS / DIAGNOSIS (*if* available) *almost always supersede laboratory or radiological data.*

DEFINITION OF INFECTIONS LISTED

Urinary: Infection present if above 10,000 bacterial colonies per ml. urine are isolated.

Wound: Report infection if purulence and/or cellulitis is present.

Lower Respiratory Infections: Pneumonia, bronchitis, bronchiectasis, pulmonary tuberculosis.

Upper Respiratory Infection: Common cold, sinusitis, pharyngitis, laryngitis, otitis media, croup.

Cutaneous: Abscesses, ulcers, paronychia, secondarily infected traumatic wounds, etc.

Abdominal: Infectious diarrheas, gastroenteritis, cholecystitis, diverticulitis, appendicitis, hepatitis.

Gynecological: Endometritis, salpingitis, septic abortion, etc. REPORT ALL ABSCESSES.

Appendix 8E

Determining Accreditation Eligibility

1. Registration or certification numbers for RRA/ART.
2. Documentation of a continuing education program for all medical record personnel.
3. List of abbreviations for use in the medical record; evidence of medical staff approval.
4. Written policies and procedures, including those related to confidentiality and security of medical records and their content.
5. Evaluation reports of all medical record consultant visits since the last survey.
6. Letters of authorization for use of signature stamp.
7. Samples of consent forms in use.
8. Medical audits completed or in progress since last survey.
9. Statistics reflecting the following as of the date of survey:
    a. The average number of patient admissions and discharges per month for the preceding 12 months;
    b. The total number of delinquent medical records (beyond the grace period stated in the medical staff rules and regulations); and
    c. A breakdown of the delinquent records by deficiency, i.e., transcription deficit, lack of signature, lack of clinical resume, lack of timely history or physical examination, or other record deficiencies (e.g., operative notes missing, verbal orders not signed).
10. The number of delinquent records as of 30, 60, 90, and 120 days prior to the survey.
11. The number of months (at the time of the survey) for which disease and operative indexing is backlogged.

Please respond to each of the following statements by inserting an "X" on every appropriate line (–).

1. A unit medical record is maintained for each patient:
    — a. Yes
    — b. No
    NOTE: If "no," please state the corrective action being taken or the method used to attain the equivalent _____
    _____
    _____
    _____

2. The following records maintained in this hospital are included in the unit medical record:
    — a. Inpatient
    — b. Outpatient
    — c. Emergency patient (nonadmitted)
    — d. Hospital-based home care program patient

3. Completed inpatient medical records routinely contain:
    — a. Patient identification data
    — b. Medical history of the patient (including relevant past, social, and family histories)
    — c. Inventory of body systems
    — d. Emergency room treatment, if admitted through the emergency room
    — e. Report of the physical examination
    — f. Diagnostic and therapeutic orders
    — g. Evidence of appropriate informed consent
    — h. Clinical observations (including progress notes, nursing notes, and consultation reports)
    — i. Reports of procedures, tests, and results
    — j. Conclusions at termination of hospitalization, including:
    — 1. All relevant diagnoses
    — 2. All operative procedures performed
    — 3. Clinical resume
    — 4. Final progress note, as required
    — 5. Necropsy protocol, where applicable

4. The problem-oriented medical record is used:
        a. Yes,
    — 1. On a hospital-wide basis
    — 2. For inpatients
    — 3. For outpatients
    — 4. By some departments/services (please specify) _____
    _____

    __   5. By some nursing units
    __   6. By certain physicians
    __ b. No

5. Obstetrical records contain all available prenatal information:
    __ a. Yes
    __ b. No (please explain) _____

    _____

6. The medical record of each surgical patient documents a current, thorough physical examination prior to the performance of surgery:
    __ a. Yes
    __ b. No

7. Individuals authorized to accept and transcribe verbal orders are identified by title or category in the medical staff rules and regulations:
    __ a. Yes
    __ b. No

8. Individuals who may accept and transcribe verbal orders include:
    __ a. RN
    __ b. LPN/LVN
    __ c. Other (please specify) _____

    _____

9. The medical staff has defined the categories of verbal orders that are associated with a potential hazard to the patient and that must be authenticated by the responsible practitioner within 24 hours:
    __ a. Yes
    __ b. No

10. Evidence of appropriate informed consent required for a procedure or treatment includes:
    __ a. Patient identification
    __ b. Date
    __ c. Procedure or treatment to be rendered
    __ d. Name of the individual rendering the procedure or treatment
    __ e. Authorization for anesthesia, if indicated
    __ f. Indication that alternate means of therapy and the possibility of risks or complications have been explained to the patient
    __ g. Authorization for tissue disposal
    __ h. Signature of any witnesses

11. There are written policies and procedures for the following special consent situations:
    __ a. Sterilization
    __ b. Abortion
    __ c. Evaluation or treatment of an unconscious patient

— d. Evaluation or treatment of an unaccompanied unemancipated minor

— e. Photographing of patients

— f. Observation of surgical procedures

12. Medical record entries may be made by authorized:

— a. Medical staff members

— b. House staff members

— c. Nursing service personnel

— d. Therapeutic dietitians

— e. Specified professional personnel (please specify) _____

_____

13. Reports of professional consultants reflect an examination of the:

— a. Patient

— b. Patient's medical record

14. When oxygen is prescribed for newborn infants, its use is recorded in the medical record:

— a. At least as a concentration percentage

— b. At regular defined intervals

— c. In accordance with the written policy of the newborn nursery

— d. Showing that it was initiated and terminated on order of a physician

15. Medical record entries relating to postanesthesia recovery include, where appropriate, the:

— a. Vital signs

— b. Patient's level of consciousness on entering and leaving the recovery area

— c. Status of infusions

— d. Status of surgical dressings

— e. Status of tubes, catheters, drains

— f. Name of physician responsible for the patient's release

16. The responsible practitioner records and authenticates a preoperative diagnosis prior to surgery.

— a. Yes

— b. No

17. Operative reports are dictated or written immediately after surgery.

— a. Yes

— b. No

18. Reports from the clinical laboratory, nuclear medicine services, and radiology services are filed in the medical record:

— a. Within 24 hours

— b. After 24 hours (please explain) _____

_____

19. Medical record requirements have been established for organ transplantation procedures involving:
    __ a. Live donors
    __ b. Brain-wave-death donors
    __ c. Cadaver organs
20. The clinical resume recapitulates for each patient:
    __ a. The reason for hospitalization
    __ b. The significant findings
    __ c. Procedures performed and treatment rendered
    __ d. Condition on discharge
    __ e. Instructions to the patient and/or family
21. Complete necropsy protocols are made part of the medical record within 90 days.
    __ a. Yes
    __ b. No
22. Written consent of the patient or his legally qualified representative is required for release of medical information to persons not otherwise authorized to receive this information.
    __ a. Yes
    __ b. No (please explain) _____
    _____
    _____

23. Medical records may be removed from the hospital's jurisdiction and safekeeping only in accordance with a court order, subpoena, or statute, as stated in written:
    __ a. Hospital policy
    __ b. Medical staff policy
24. All medical record entries are dated and authenticated.
    __ a. Yes
    __ b. No (please explain) _____
    _____
    _____

25. Abbreviations and symbols permitted in the medical record:
    __ a. Have been approved by the medical staff
    __ b. Have only one meaning each
    __ c. Are listed in a readily available explanatory legend
26. The medical staff rules and regulations specify that following discharge of the patient, medical records shall be completed:
    __ a. Immediately
    __ b. Within 15 days
    __ c. Within 30 days
    __ d. In more than 30 days (please explain) _____
    _____

27. The following are employed with supervisory responsibility:
    — a. RRA, full-time
    — b. RRA, part-time
    — c. ART, full-time
    — d. ART, part-time
    — e. Qualified registrar (military facility)
    — f. None of the above
28. A qualified medical record consultant evaluates the medical record department at least quarterly and renders a written report.
    — a. Yes
    — b. No (please explain only when item 27f has been checked) _____
    _____
    _____

29. At least one supervisory individual is participating in a preparatory course leading to eligibility for accredited status.
    — a. Yes
    — b. No (please explain only when item 27f has been checked) _____
    _____
    _____

30. There is documentation of the participation of all medical record personnel in the following education programs related to their activities:
    — a. Orientation of new personnel
    — b. On-the-job training
    — c. In-service education
    — d. Outside opportunities for at least supervisory and management personnel
31. Medical records may be obtained by the medical staff from the medical record department:
    — a. At any time
    b. For a limited time:
    — 1. Monday through Friday, during normal working hours
    — 2. Monday through Friday, after normal working hours
    — 3. Saturdays
    — 4. Sundays and holidays
32. Microfilmed medical records are:
    — a. Readily accessible to the medical staff
    — b. Reviewable through equipment that is convenient for medical staff use
    — c. Not readily available to the medical staff at all times (please explain) _____
    _____
    — d. Not applicable, since no medical records are microfilmed

33. The disease and operative classification used is:
    ___ a. *International Classification of Diseases*, adapted
    ___ b. Other (please specify) _____

    _____

    _____

34. Internal quality control measures are used for assessing proficiency in:
    ___ a. Abstracting medical record information
    ___ b. Coding medical record information
    ___ c. Applying medical record information to patient care evaluation programs
35. The role of medical record personnel in the following is defined:
    ___ a. Patient care evaluation activities
    ___ b. Committee functions
    ___ c. Use of automated data processing systems

Appendix 8F

Budget Forms Used by General Hospital of Everett (Washington)

Personnel Budget Request Form Instructions:

Form P-2 (Rev. 79) is designed to assist in budgeting for personnel in 1979. For purposes of requesting FTE's it is essential that columns (2) and (3) be completed.

Each cost center to which personnel time will be charged in 1979 must be completed in the "Personnel Budget Request Form." Fill in the blanks for Department, Unit, Cost Center and Budget Year. If possible relate your department, or unit's activity to FTE's in the current year. This will give a base upon which the budget year FTE's can be calculated. For example:

1978 Estimated Treatments	42,800
1978 Estimated FTE's	14.10

$$\frac{14.10}{42,800} = .00032944 = \text{current year indicator}$$

Next determine the activity for this cost center in the budget year. If the hospital has made statistical projections for your department or unit use those, unless you can justify another. Using the projected budget year statistic, multiply it times the current year indicator. For example:

$$.00032944 \times 44,000 \text{ (79 estimate)} = 14.50 \text{ FTE's.}$$

This new FTE figure provides an indication of what your FTE request should approximate. In order to hold the increase in the cost of health care down, each department and unit should strive to provide more service with the current levels of staffing. If the activity in your area is constant then you should strive to provide a constant level of service with fewer personnel.

Every employee of the hospital falls into one of the following personnel categories:

01 Management and Supervision
02 Technician and Specialist
03 Registered Nurse
04 Licensed Practical Nurse
05 Not Used in General Hospital of Everett
06 Non-Physician Medical Practitioner
07 Other Salaries and Wages (All personnel not included in the above categories, i.e., nursing assistants, secretaries, clerks, housekeeping personnel, etc.)

The FTE's required for your department or unit should be allocated by personnel category on Form P-2. The example is for illustration only. Unless it is helpful for you, days, evenings and nights do not have to be separated.

It is not necessary that columns (5) and (6) be completed. These can be done by the business office.

If you are requesting a change in program which would result in more personnel, fill out a "New Program or Program Change" budget form and use an additional Form P-2 (Rev. 78). Clearly mark the additional form as "New Program Request". The form used to record the personnel request for your current program should also be marked with "See addendum for additional request".

Supplies and Expense Budget Request

Explanation: There is a computer printout for each cost center within the hospital. Supplies and expense requests for budget year 1979 are to be placed on the printout.

Instructions: The printout is designed to cover a four year period: the "SECOND PRIOR YEAR", 1976; "PRIOR YEAR", 1977; current year, 1978; and budget year, 1979. Included on the form is information relating to 1976 and 1977 actual's, 1978 budget figures, and 1978 first 6 months actual.

Requests for FTE's are to be requested on Form P-2 (Rev. 78). The FTE related dollars will be calculated in the business office.

After reviewing the information on the printout, project total supplies and expenses by category for all of 1978 into the column "CURR YR PROJ TOTAL". To get the 1978 projected totals, the figures in "CURR YR 6 MO ACTUAL" can usually be doubled. In categories where documented changes in use are occurring, one time payments have been made, or will be, and/or other definite factors affecting expenses are known, other adjustments may be necessary to get reasonable 1978 estimates.

After projecting 1978 dollars, project total supplies and expense dollars for current programs into 1979.

DO NOT project any increases from one period to the next for inflation. The Accounting Department will adjust your budget figures for expected price increases. Your projections should concentrate on expected dollar increases or decreases in the cost of supplies and expense for reasons *other than inflation*, such as:

1) Usage changes—could be either up or down
2) Contract changes, additions, deletions
3) Lease or rental changes, additions, deletions
4) Price changes unrelated to inflation—For example, advances in technology can cause prices to go up or down
5) Requests for additional supplies, services, rentals, etc.

It should also be understood that these projections should be based on the *status quo* and *should not* reflect additional needs relating to new program or program change requests. Additional supplies and expense needs relating to new programs or significant program changes are to be listed separately on the "New Program or Program Change" budget form and transferred to the "BUDGET YR NEW PROG" on the computer printout.

After projecting 1978 and 1979 dollars, run totals for each column. To check for reasonableness divide the dollars for 1978 and 1979 by the projected total workload units for the two years, respectively. A check with the "Productivity Report" for the cost center involved will provide information concerning 1977 actual, 1978 budget, and 1978 actual year-to-date ratios of supplies and expenses to workload units. Your figures for 1978 and 1979 should approximate those on the report, or be less.

If workload units have not been projected and are needed for your cost center, you may contact Mr. Belcher for assistance. If the projections previously received appear unreasonable or inaccurate do not hesitate to discuss them with Mr. Judy or the appropriate Assistant Administrator, and Mr. Belcher.

Appendix 8G

Snow Hospital
Cost Analysis of
Transcription Services
Medical Record Department
July 27, 1977

PRODUCTIVITY

CURRENT STAFFING PATTERN		PROPOSED STAFFING PATTERN	
Day Shift:	4.0 FTE	Day Shift:	3.0 FTE
Evening:	1.5 FTE	Evening:	1.5 FTE
Current:	500-600 lines per day	*Proposed*:	900-1000 lines per day
Reasons:	a) Use of inappropriate Word Processing Equipment.	Reasons:	a) Use of electronic technology and elimination of complicated coding for recording material.
	b) 5.5 hours per day spent in non-productive transcription time.		b) Simultaneous input/output.
			c) Automatic formatting.
			d) No media handling.
			e) Visual display of material.
			f) Indexes and updates Transcription Log.
			g) Unattended printout at rate of 540 words-per-minute.
			h) Uninterrupted printing of multi-page documents.

ASSUMPTIONS

1. Continued increased workload for transcription due to influx of new physicians into community, increased hospital services and need for transcription services in other hospital departments.
2. Increased emphasis on maintaining complete and accurate medical records for continued patient care, patient care appraisal and medico-legal matters.

3. Skilled medical transcriptionists will continue to be in high demand. Few medical secretaries can adapt well to the versatile hospital transcription work.
4. Anticipation of continued increase in labor costs at a rate of 9% per year.

SNOW HOSPITAL

COST ANALYSIS OF TRANSCRIPTION SERVICES

RATIONALE: PROPOSED SYSTEM

1. Maximum utilization of skilled and highly paid medical transcriptionists and elimination of current non-productive transcription time, with an increase of production to *at least* 900-1000 lines per day.
2. Cost savings with installation of Linland Word Processing Equipment and reduction of 1.0 FTE medical transcriptionist, at an immediate rate of $3,608 (annual basis). Overall projection for 5 year forecast results in a savings of approximately $64,384 during the 5 year period.
3. Minimize turn-around time due to concurrent input/output capability of equipment.
4. Improved transcription services to the Medical Staff and the hospital, providing faster turn-around time and letter-perfect reports, both original and copies.
5. Improved working environment due to elimination of current problems with noise level in department. This would eliminate the need to proceed with plans to enclose transcription area with acoustical modular units, at a proposed cost of $4,400.
6. Reduction of clerical duties for transcriptionists and improved management information since transcription log and production rates are stored within system and available in printed format as necessary.
7. Establishment of productivity standards for transcription for improved management of this area.
8. Stabilization of staffing for transcription area.
9. Opportunity for all transcriptionists to work on more efficient equipment which would be beneficial to employee morale and further their skills as transcriptionists.
10. Minimize down-time and repairs on equipment because of electronic technology and solid-state components. Current rate of service calls at 2-3 per month on Mag-Card machines alone.

11. Elimination of overtime for transcription, which is currently costing approximately $800 annually.

12. Availability of two used Selectric typewriters (valued at approximately $200) to other areas in the hospital as needed.

13. Increased productivity and development of standards provided with this equipment (as well as other benefits) would provide us with the capability of meeting increased demands on the transcription area due to the influx of new physicians into the community and the expansion of other hospital services. Additionally, the Medical Record Department could potentially provide expanded transcription services to other areas in the hospital, thus eliminating the need to provide personnel and equipment in these areas.

14. Utilization of equipment for providing routine reports (statistical reports, lists of delinquent records and physicians, to name a few examples) and other types of information that can be stored and provided in printed, updated format as necessary.

SNOW HOSPITAL
COST ANALYSIS OF TRANSCRIPTION SERVICES:
5 YEAR FORECAST

	1978	1979	1980	1981	1982	1983
CURRENT SYSTEM						
Labor (Salary & Fringe Benefits)	$72,200 5.5FTE	$78,697 5.5FTE	$85,779 5.5FTE	$107,780 6.5FTE (+1.0 FTE)	$117,480 6.5FTE	$128,054 6.5FTE
Equipment (Includes Service and Maintenance Agreements)	$ 5,050	$ 6,610 (+2 typewriters)	$ 5,300 (Increased Maintenance)	$ 6,080 (+1 typewriter)	$ 5,550 (Increased Maintenance)	$ 5,550 (Increased Maintenance)
Supplies	$ 2,600	$ 2,834	$ 3,089	$ 3,367	$ 3,670	$ 4,000
Renovation of Space		$ 4,400				
TOTAL	$79,850	$92,541	$94,168	$117,227	$126,700	$137,604
PROPOSED SYSTEM						
Labor (Salary & Fringe Benefits)	$59,448 4.5FTE	$64,798 4.5FTE	$70,630 4.5FTE	$ 76,987 4.5 FTE	$ 99,481 5.5FTE (+1.0 FTE)	$108,433 5.5FTE
Equipment (Includes Service and Maintenance Agreements)	$14,718	$14,718	$14,718	$ 14,718	$ 14,718	$ 14,718
Supplies	$ 2,076	$ 2,263	$ 2,467	$ 2,689	$ 2,931	$ 3,195

Salvage of Typewriters	− $ 200					
Shipment of Mag-Cards	+ $ 100					
ANNUAL TOTAL	$76,142	$81,779	$87,815	$ 94,394	$117,130	$126,346
ANNUAL SAVINGS	$ 3,708	$10,702	$ 6,353	$ 22,833	$ 9,570	$ 11,258
TOTAL 5 YEAR SAVINGS	$64,484					

Chapter 9

Using Computer Technology as a Primary Tool in Health Record Systems

CHAPTER OBJECTIVES

1. Recognize actual and potential role of computer technology in establishing and maintaining health information systems
2. Identify performance competencies that health information professionals need in order to plan and implement appropriate computer applications
3. Relate the process of systems analysis to the development of computer applications in health information
4. Identify the four-phased sequence of systems analysis
5. Prepare written progress reports for documentation of long-range systems planning
6. Recognize the range of complexity in computing health information
7. Differentiate between direct and indirect computer impact on patient records
8. Identify 4 long-range strategies for computer applications in health information systems

COMPUTER TECHNOLOGY—AN IMPORTANT RESOURCE

The computer is a challenging tool. The medical record profession needs to make skilled use of its capabilities in many ways. It has the potential to enhance and extend the use of patient information in significant ways. It also has direct impact on health care costs. Computer applications in health care have increased the availability and accessibility of health information. These applications exist in hospitals, ambulatory care settings, long-term care settings, and specialty clinics. Data collection networks, coordinating patient information among several individual health care agencies, are also well established. Virtually every technical function identified in this text as an appropriate activity in establishing and maintaining an effective health information department has been computerized. Many of these are computerized in low-cost applications, using batch methods such as punch-cards. Others have made use of teleprocessing developments and use on-line methods to accomplish their objectives.

Health Information Managers Need to Focus on Many Factors

The questions below are examples. They will continue to be issues in exploring new developments and reviewing and updating current technological applications.

- Can hospital computer systems be identified and defined?
- What systems in medical record departments and related areas are computerized? Can we define common elements in them?
- What standards can be identified in computer applications?
- How do existing computer applications, such as those listed below, influence the patient record?
  — Record formats
  — Printout summaries of laboratory tests
  — Computerized histories and physicals
  — Computerized discharge summaries
  — CRT screen displays for patient registration
- Does the problem-oriented record facilitate computerization of patient records?
- What is an encounter form? What are some basic elements found in different kinds of encounter forms?
- How well are commercial shared computer services programs such as Shared Computer Systems and others meeting current needs? Do these programs have applications for ambulatory care or long-term care?

Review the description of health information systems functions shown as Exhibit 9-1. How do these systems relate to the questions we have just listed? Which ones are likely to be developed in or for hospitals? What other health care settings can you identify?

Exhibit 9-1 Health Information Systems

I. Scheduling and Communications

Optimal patient care involves an enormous amount of information exchange, for the purpose of bringing together various resources (people, information and material). Such a communications system is the backbone of any medical information system; it is the element which links all the other subsystems together. The logistics of in-patient and out-patient scheduling is also a part of this function, involving the allocations of ancillary services as well as admissions and discharges.

II. Administrative Management

Good administration of medical facilities and services demands both retrospective and prospective analysis of vital management information such as patient accounting, cost accounting, medical staffing, facility usage, census, budgeting, inventory control, and preventive maintenance. It includes the capability of creating simulation models of the operating health care system, for analysis, planning and redesign. It covers all levels of administrative information, from individual patient encounters to that necessary to manage the largest government facility.

III. Patient Data Base Acquisition

This includes various techniques for the acquisition and processing of all elements of the patient's history, physical examination and progress notes. It also embraces all other methods used to develop the basic patient data base, including consultant reports and those elements contributed by support personnel, such as nurses' observations and various types of physicians extenders.

IV. Nursing Services

This subsystem includes all processes which directly support the nursing care team in administering patient care. For example, it incorporates the scheduling and prompting of direct nursing care functions, including shift change summary reports on each patient's care and condition. It also includes the regeneration of all doctor's orders on demand, and any nursing station administrative functions not covered specifically in another subsystem.

Exhibit 9-1 Continued

V. Patient Support

All components which involve patient comfort or therapeutic adjuncts to nursing care are combined in this subsystem. This includes inhalation therapy, occupational therapy, and physical therapy as well as central supply. It also includes the food service components, incorporating areas such as menu planning, nutritional accounting, and the food control elements of procurement, inventory, preparation, and cost accounting.

VI. Diagnostic Support

This subsystem brings together all the components directly supporting the diagnostic workup. Though a somewhat heterogeneous grouping, most elements include the acquisition of an analog signal, analog to digital conversion and an automatic or semiautomatic interpretation. This refers to such areas as electrocardiography, electroencephalography, pulmonary function, and newly emerging elements such as electronystagmography or electromyography. Support for Nuclear Medicine is also included with this group as is computer assisted diagnostic consultation.

VII. Laboratory

All elements of the clinical laboratory fall into this subsystem involving areas such as chemistry hematology, microbiology and urine analysis. In addition, it encompasses other elements of pathology including histopathology (cytology) and gross specimen analysis involving areas such as autopsy reporting and forensic pathology. It includes aspects of quality control, trend analysis, laboratory instrument monitoring, and positive control of each specimen of body fluid. Blood banking is also a part of this subsystem.

VIII. Pharmacy

The information aspects of therapeutic agents and their usage are all grouped under this subsystem. These include drug inventory control, prescription formulation, maintenance of a formulary, and appropriate aspects of clinical pharmacology such as usual dosage, orders checks and reminders, contraindications and hypersensitivity reactions. Appropriate aspects of clinical toxicology and acid-base (fluid) therapy are also components of this subsystem.

Exhibit 9-1 Continued

IX. Radiology

Components involving diagnostic radiology include facility and technician scheduling, patient preparation notices and reminders, techniques for reporting and interpreting individual roentgenograms and film file inventory control. Therapeutic radiology includes support for treatment calculations (including isodose curve plotting), generation and maintenance of patient treatment schedules as well as tabulation of results (Tumor Registries).

X. Patient Monitoring

These components all involve the integration and presentation of large (continuous) amounts of physiometric data by sophisticated instrumentation in environments such as the Intensive Care Units (general, cardiac, burn), Recovery Rooms, Delivery Rooms, or Emergency Rooms. It includes as well, functions which are not online, such as Dynamic Cardiography.

XI. Medical Library

The Medical Information System requires a capability to maintain and update a large number of relevant computer displays, including those for input of various elements of data, those which incorporate "capsules" of important medical reference information, and those which parallel the physician's diagnostic logic process. Such an enormous requirement demands a separate subsystem, which is closely aligned with the more commonly recognized reference information generation function of the Medical Library, and suggests a new and appropriate role for this valuable resource.

XII. Health Records

The capturing of information by each of the above subsystems generates a data base quite comparable to the current patient medical record. This subsystem refers to the advanced information management components which are associated with this information, such areas as prospective and retrospective statistical analyses and the generation of various types of output reports. This last function includes the development of statistical compilers and other techniques for the on-going correlation and auditing of health information parameters such as diagnoses, therapy and the tracking of the clinical progress of disease (Epidemiology). It also includes components involved with the nomenclature and coding of disease processes as well as techniques to monitor the quality of care being administered.

Source: *Computers in Medical Practice*, Society for Computer Medicine. Reprinted with permission.

Medical record administrators and medical record technicians must be prepared to function along a continuum of developing technology. It will require effective decision making to establish the most beneficial patient information system. This may be a paper record system or a partially or fully computerized patient information system that includes technical support. The decision-making process will not be limited to selection of the most effective method for establishing and maintaining patient information. It will also extend to cost analysis, user acceptance, dynamics and constraints of change, and performance review. Health information managers will need to draw on skills and competencies keyed to developing technology. To do this they must form a knowledge base and translate specific information from that base into action plans to meet their particular objectives.

Skills That Focus on Developing a Knowledge Base

Specialized knowledge will be required. This will include:

- The ability to develop and maintain an understanding of data coding, information storage and file design in medical computing including, logical structure in application programs and physical structure in data storage.
- The ability to identify elements of data processing. This includes information flow through a computer system, beginning with the source document, data entry, processing cycle, storage, access, printout, and information distribution.
- The ability to communicate in data and teleprocessing terms that will facilitate working with computer systems professionals in cooperative planning and in operating particular computer applications.
- The ability to analyze computer programming, to read and follow the logic flow that the programmer uses in writing a program. This includes the ability to prepare procedures in a precomputer format. For instance, the use of playscript (technique) procedure writing clearly describes the sequence and identifies the source of the action for steps in the procedure. This assists programmers to identify the programming activities.
- An awareness of current technology that includes functional operations within medical record departments as well as hospital computer systems, health data networks, and the role of teleprocessing in handling patient information in these systems.
- The ability to continually monitor developing computerized patient records. A particular focus on problem-oriented medical record computerization and its effect on patient record processes and evaluation should be included.

- The ability to work with clinical algorithms and decision support system models and their interface with patient records.

Once the knowledge is acquired, it needs to be applied. This can be done in two ways. First, long-range planning must be undertaken so that each individual application will be capable of interfacing with other applications as well as of accommodating the future needs of the organization. Second, systems analysis must be employed to assist in making decisions about initiating individual computer applications. Systems analysis is a major activity that is a form of problem solving directed to computer solutions. However, it is not intended to always result in a computer solution. Improper or poorly planned information flow in any health care setting will only be weakened by technology unless the design and plan itself is improved or corrected. Computers will never counteract bad management practices. Medical record administrators and technicians need to base planning for technology on sound organizational and systems principles. Given the knowledge in computer potential that we have considered necessary, it is likely that patient information managers would be expected to:

- Prepare strategies for planning and implementing computer applications in a given health information department. This includes identification of immediate benefits to providers, operational benefits to department staff and employees, and patient benefits, such as supplying information in a more expedient fashion so that care can be improved.
- Develop a comprehensive data security policy and recommend support procedures for maintaining the confidentiality of patient information.
- Identify output descriptions for planning applications in a comprehensive way so as to facilitate system design. This goes beyond identification of objectives. This goes to the product definition at a functional level; that is, what must be available through the computer application to carry on the health care within that facility.
- Calculate cost benefits of computer technology for their department and measure that calculation against cost projections for their existing systems whether it be manual, partially computerized, or a commercially developed application, such as discharge abstract systems.
- Design an interim patient record that is a microfiche or hard-copy record made up primarily of computer generated output in those settings where patient information is maintained on the computer until discharge or cessation of treatment.
- Employ the principles of data capture, data organization, clinical decisions (the use of data to direct medical care) and medical research.

Mumps programming techniques and developments and uses of
SNOMED and other tools will need to be drawn from basic educational areas and applied to individual applications.

SYSTEMS ANALYSIS PROVIDES A MAP

To apply specialized knowledge to the performance expectations we have
just listed, systems analysis for computer applications must be employed. It
builds on specialized knowledge of data processing for effective planning.
Using computers as tools is increasingly important in planning and processing health information for individual and collective use. Systems analysis
for computer applications consists of four major phases.

- One, the study phase includes fact finding, problem identification, and
  feasibility analysis.
- Two, the design and resource allocation phase identifies resources,
  both human and machine, that will be set aside for application on the
  particular project that is targeted in the study phase.
- Three, the development and conversion planning phase incorporates
  program writing, debugging, staff training, and preparation of user
  manuals for system, program, and user activities.
- Four, the operation and review phase incorporates actual system
  changeover and postinstallation performance review activities.

We can define systems analysis as a problem-solving method for applying
the knowledge and processes required for planning and implementing computer-based systems in health and patient information handling.

Skilled use of the tools and techniques of systems analysis guarantees effective systems designs. RRAs and ARTs will use methods and procedures
explained in Chapter 8. Management tools will remain the origin of all
systems planning, whether computer related or not. The applied management skills of systems analysis in computer applications is particularly
keyed to enhance communications with the data-processing professional.
Let's look more closely at the four phases in developing a computer application.

The Study Phase

The study phase is a fundamental examination of the operation that
needs to be improved or evaluated. A primary component is problem identification; that is, a clear formulation of the problem involved in the manual
operation. Problem formulation is accomplished through fact finding, in

which all users of the operation are polled to see how they use it and what problems and strengths they have observed in the existing process. Next, constraints are clearly laid out. One example of a constraint is a specified cost limitation. Another may be limitations of staffing. Others may include working with existing computer installations in the hospital and recognizing that any new application must interface with the existing application.

Formulation of objectives for the proposed system is next. The health information manager must determine the general and specific objectives of the operation to be computerized and translate those objectives into computer-related objectives. Describing percentage improvements for a comparison of the proposed solution with the existing operation is one example. Another would be:

> Given an authorized request for a medical record, medical record retrieval time would be reduced from 20 to 5 minutes.

Preparing output descriptions is the next step that completes objective-setting by defining performance criteria. For instance, two output descriptions built from the objective we have listed as "reduce retrieval time from . . ." could be:

- A printout produced in the main file room that automatically prints all chart requests in two-part labels. The labels include patient number, name, requesting party, authorization code number (which tells the staff the requester is authorized to have the chart), date, and time of the request. One label is placed on the outguide and one on the chart.
- An activity summary produced at the end of the day that lists the number of charts requested, distribution of request frequency, and a list of all charts not returned for that day.

Another example of an output description would be a partially completed discharge abstract format that can be called up on the CRT screen in the medical record department. It is used for review, completion of coding, and final chart abstracting verification before being sent to the Professional Standards Review Organization to meet reporting requirements.

The RRA must determine what outputs will be necessary for any proposal. Printouts, screen displays, management reports, audit trial reports, and other specific products that the proposed system must produce are spelled out at this time. Output descriptions define the functional requirements of a system that have been formulated through the objectives.

Once the elements of problem identification, objectives, and output descriptions have been worked out, the move into feasibility analysis is made. This is the process that examines, identifies, and ranks alternative solutions to the problem. This includes different types of equipment.

Table 9-1 lists steps in performing a feasibility analysis. Feasibility analysis also prepares cost analysis reports. This includes careful cost analysis of the existing system, including the use of equipment, supplies, and staff time for carrying on the operation, and comparing that to cost projections for selection of computer equipment, programming, development time, and projected staff time for the computer solution. This staff time projection may call for no immediate reduction in staff but may include a cost avoidance factor that limits the need for new staff for the operation in question.

How do we do this projection? Several resources are used. Hourly programmer costs can be determined. The cost of equipment to purchase, lease, or rent can be determined. Table 9-2 provides comparison of cost for computer equipment by rental, lease, or purchase. The cost of run time for applications included in the programs can be provided by the data processing department within the organization, or through a user manual in a time-sharing operation. Determination of service requirements for the equipment will also give a cost indicator. It's important that the health information manager conduct a feasibility analysis and project results far enough into the future to show long-range effects of this application. It is also important that the feasibility analysis indicate how the proposed system will satisfy constraints that have been previously identified. This means that if a medical audit proposal for computerization does not interface—that is, connect easily or with reasonable modification to existing computer applications within a hospital, such as computerized census reporting—then the proposal will be examined more critically.

At the conclusion of these steps there should be a formal study phase report prepared by the RRA manager and/or systems team members, or task force team members conducting this study phase analysis.

Sometimes all of the study phase activities are coordinated and conducted under the term and concept of feasibility analysis. The same steps are included, that is, problem identification, fact finding, identification of constraints, formulation of objectives, description of output, cost analysis, possibility of interface with existing systems, and projected time for making the system capable of meeting the needs of the organization. In this case, the results of the feasibility analysis are formally prepared in a written document. This document is then made available to the administration, which makes the decision whether to move on.

Table 9-1 Steps in Feasibility Analysis

1. DEVELOP EXISTING GENERAL SYSTEM FLOW CHARTS FROM PERFORMANCE DEFINITIONS IN STUDY PHASE.

2. DEVELOP SYSTEM CANDIDATES (e.g. DISCHARGE ABSTRACTS).

3. PREPARE DETAILED DESCRIPTION OF CANDIDATES – INCLUDE SPECIAL FEATURES.

4. TARGET MEANINGFUL SYSTEM CHARACTERISTICS – HOW WELL DO THE CHARACTERISTICS MEET THE NEEDS?

5. IDENTIFY COST ELEMENTS FOR EACH CANDIDATE.

6. WEIGHT PROJECTED CANDIDATES PERFORMANCE AND COST ELEMENTS USING SIMPLE RANK SCALE ei 1-10 AND DISPLAY.

7. RECOMMEND BEST CANDIDATE.

Table 9-2 Comparison of Purchase, Lease, or Rental Options

Disadvantages	Advantages
Rental	
1. Danger of obsolescence reduced	1. Most expensive in long run
2. No large capital outlay required	2. Rental costs may increase periodically
3. All responsibility rests with the manufacturer (single contact)	
Lease	
1. Significant cost savings over rental	1. User is committed for a long time period which reduces flexibility
2. No large capital outlay required	
3. Lease costs remain fixed over life of contact	
Purchase	
1. For the long range, generally the least expensive method	1. Large capital outlay required
2. Tax advantages can be accrued by the owner	2. Less flexibility to meet changing needs
	3. Danger of obsolescence

Design and Resource Allocation Phase

The second phase is directed to design and resource allocation. This consists of building a plan to carry out the specifications determined in the study and feasibility analysis phase. It includes allocation of staff time and projected tasks from data processing. Project assignments for programmer analysts, application programmers, and data processing management staff should be established and time set aside to work on the project. Required reference manuals are identified, such as the operations manuals, user manuals, and program documentation manuals. In addition, during this phase equipment functions that will be required to carry out the objectives and produce the output descriptions listed in the first phase are identified. This equipment function description should be reviewed by health information user managers to verify that plans are coordinated. Appendix 9A is an example of how equipment capabilities are determined by output descriptions. The example is drawn from the PROMIS program, which has computerized the patient record with on-line access.

Notice how the design specifications clearly define how the programs (software) and the equipment (hardware) will make the outputs available in the required manner. For instance, access and response to patient records are identified.

By looking at equipment functions and comparing the variety of kinds of equipment available, another facet of review can be provided. Vendors can provide assistance. In this process a hospital or health facility may be seeking bids for a system to be built to specifications for their particular organization. Exhibit 9-2 illustrates some components of a request for a proposal that could be used in this particular application. A health information manager who is working with outside computer resources will need to understand what must be identified in a request for proposal (RFP) that will be sent to vendors.

Remember that the system requirements are identified in the study phase. Objectives constraints, and output descriptions are combined to identify the performance specifications required to solve the original problem. The hardware and software elements listed in the model are determined by the study phase. The purpose of computer systems is to collect, process, store, and retrieve data for the users. Data and information needs of the user must be comprehensively mapped out if effective system design is to take place. Whether a design plan is prepared by outside vendors or written by the data processing division within the health organization, there will be a formal written report. This report should be submitted to the users with particular items that they will be using in their day-to-day operations carefully marked for their analysis and further review. Effective management planning will

Exhibit 9-2 Selection of a Computer System

The first step in selecting a computer is to prepare a request for proposal for prospective vendors. In addition to the specific information requirements in each setting, an RFP will include both broad and detailed data processing needs, such as the following:

Hardware

- The CPU shall include 6 timesharing terminal ports with capability for expansion to 16.
- Removable disk storage capability with an online capacity of at least 50 million 8-bit bytes.
- On-line printer with the following minimum capabilities:

  1. 600 lines/minute alphanumeric printing speed
  2. 132-print-position line
  3. 64-character printing unit

Software

- Programming languages: The vendor may make recommendations regarding programming languages. However, minimum requirements are:

  1. For business data processing: COBOL or RFP II.
  2. For on-line programming: Basic, or interactive FORTRAN or APL.

- Languages must conform to ANSI standards or, where appropriate, to detailed definitions in Section VI of this specification.
- The operating system shall have the capability for simultaneously serving as:

  1. A timesharing system supporting interactive computing from terminals
  2. A batch processing system accepting programs from any input device for a queued batch processing operation.

- The disk storage file structure shall be standardized so that files created through one language can be processed by programs in any of the other languages without format conversion.

588   MEDICAL RECORDS IN HEALTH INFORMATION

Exhibit 9-2 Continued

Other Requirements

- The vendor must provide six person-weeks of education and training on the proposed system for XYZ employees.
- The vendor must make available to XYZ test time on a computer similar to the one proposed. This is to allow for program preparation and testing prior to delivery of the computer.

Also included as part of the bid specification are projected time schedules.

---

require that this be reviewed and confirmed as meeting the specifications set forth in the first phase of systems analysis before moving into the next phase.

Development and Conversion Planning Phase

First, developing the activities of the external system is initiated. Implementation includes writing and debugging programs, purchasing equipment, testing equipment, and preparing operating manuals for system operators, programmers, and users. Second, the conversion plan is defined, including installation of hardware and personnel training. The conversion plan for the manager of the particular application should include review of all user manuals and system documentation to see that they are clear and understandable. Then performance testing is needed; that is, a dry run of the particular application to see if the results produced match the specification laid out in the study phase.

The development phase often includes PERT charts, which display the tasks that are being performed to meet the stated objective, and GANTT charts, which show how closely the plan for bringing the system into fruition is being followed. These charts will be helpful to the information manager in determining how well the proposed change for the operation is being carried out. System testing will require input data for participating in evaluation of system test results. For example, a set of discharge information needs to be provided to be entered on-line for an interactive inhouse discharge analysis system. The results of the on-line entry, the reports produced, and the turnaround time can then be measured against specifications defined in the study and problem identification phase. In this time period test results are compared with the previous system to measure accuracy.

Training the managers who will be responsible for the overall functions within the department should be underway also. Operators and programmers who will need to be working with the system for debugging, upgrading, and program revisions will also participate in training. Training and demonstrations are carried out for users who deal with day-to-day operations of the system. Medical staff and other allied health personnel who may need to understand the functions of the computer application and how those functions will affect their day-to-day activities should be kept informed. As with the first two phases, the third phase should include a formal written report of the activities that have been carried out, including the results of training. This is a critical concern to health information managers if the staff is to be adequately oriented and prepared to make the change to the new system.

The Operation Phase and Review Phase

The operation phase is defined as the time period when the changeover from the old system to the new system occurs. It comprises system changeover, in which the new computer systems operations are observed and data taken to validate the operation, and performance review activities. Performance review boards or postinstallation audit committees are formally identified teams that gather and evaluate information on current operating performance to measure against the original specific performance objectives. The performance evaluation must be carried out at intervals and must be prepared to correlate performance with original or revised specifications. This is the process required to justify costs, validate planning, and coordinate any activity with other computer application planning that would be involved in an overall long-range plan for the organization. The RRA would be involved in gathering statistics showing reduction in clerical time and related activities accomplished by the new system and increased production, where this occurs. For instance, in computerized word processing systems, the output or production levels may increase threefold after the introduction of a computerized system.

The last concept we wish to discuss in the operation phase is the concept of the management of change itself. This means open communication between the manager of the health information department and the staff as well as other departments within the organization. First, people need assurance that the necessary operations are being carried out. Second, managers must clarify that technology will be more likely to result in changes in procedures rather than in elimination of positions. Third, problems that occur in the system will have to be evaluated and resolved by cooperative effort from employees, the departmental manager, and systems people themselves, so that the routine operations of the department can be effectively carried out. The management of change requires skill in human relations. Skills in positive reinforcement and in eliciting cooperative involvement of the departmental staff will create the attitude and enthusiasm needed in moving to a computerized system and can effectively facilitate its overall improvements to the delivery of health care within the organization.

Systems analysis that we have described is based on the four general phases of bringing up or developing a computerized system. Health information managers must be conversant with systems analysis and be able to actively engage in all phases. Designing particular formats, reviewing proposals, evaluating the operations, and making recommendations for changes are all elements. The role of system audits and methods for improvement and upgrading are also key elements.

COMPUTER TECHNOLOGY AND A MEDICAL RECORD DEPARTMENT

Let's examine a scenario of the major functional operations that have been computerized in a hospital medical record department. It is intended to offer the student a mental picture of the options and opportunities that are available. This is not to recommend universally that these applications be planned and developed for any individual organization but to prepare learners to use the knowledge of existing applications and build on that knowledge to individually plan improved systems within their own organizations. This systems improvement may include computer components or it may not. If properly carried out, the systems analysis process will clearly identify when computer solution alternatives are appropriate and when they are not. In addition, the systems analysis process, which is simply a particular form of problem-solving technique, will help practitioners evaluate existing computer installations or existing proposals and plans for such installations. They should feel comfortable in requesting involvement and participation and asking to review documents and formal planning instruments, such as GANTT charts, that will clearly indicate the evolution of the technology in their organization.

Medical Record Practitioners and Information Science

It is impossible for medical record practitioners to become skilled information scientists without directing major portions of their effort and interest to this area. It is possible for them to become active managers of computer applications within their particular setting. Each time they communicate in data processing jargon and ask questions that help explain how one term fits with another, they are building their own network of information.

The health information manager must fully understand the process involved when establishing a computerized record system and the questions that need answering before the process starts. What information will the computerized record contain and are these data readily available on the source document? What mode of input will be the most efficient for the operation? Keypunch machines and data cards, hard-copy or CRT terminals, or optical scanning equipment are all options. How will particular files be accessed and updated with additional data? Will there be a need for a hard-copy printout at any point in the process? What is the most economical storage device for the system's historical data and how often will it be accessed? These are a few of the questions that must be examined when considering computerizing a specific function or activity.

Recall the list of specialized knowledge requirements on pages 580 and 581. In the following pages we will examine some functional operations in a medical record department that have been computerized. See if you can identify functional outputs, interim record examples, and indications of long-range systems planning. We will initiate our review by considering the functional operations in two broad categories:

Direct Impact vs. Indirect Impact on Patient Records

Direct impact activities are those activities that are a part of processing every record:

- Admission and discharge functions—MPI (Master Patient Index)
- Census
- Chart assembly
- Chart analysis—adequacy and completeness—deficiency notification and follow-up
- Discharge analysis for statistics
- Disease and operation coding and indexing
- Special study reporting
- Filing and retrieval
- Insurance reporting for reimbursement
- Files purging, microfilming and/or destruction

Record resource activities are those activities that use individual records or groups of records to carry out the function. They may be related to an individual patient or to particular groups of patients.

- Medical reports and insurance
- Utilization review
- Medical audit

- Tumor registry
- Research retrieval
- Word processing—central dictation
- Medical staff projects
- Special study reporting

Medical record departmental activities can be viewed in these two categories. The first category is composed of activities in which the record acts directly upon the activity or the activity requires information from the record.

The first of these is *admission and discharge functions.* This function consists of recording the fact of admission and the fact of discharge of a patient on a master patient index. Master patient index operations have been computerized in on-line patient registration. This process makes use of a CRT computer terminal to enter and store information for on-line retrieval through that terminal. When patients enter the admitting department, the admitting clerk asks if they have been patients previously. Patients' names are then verified by typing in the names on the CRT terminal. If the patients have been in the hospital before, their names will appear on the screen along with the hospital numbers assigned to them. If the patients have not been there previously, the clerk may call for a registration screen display. They may type in something like "pt/reg" to indicate patient registration is about to begin. The screen then displays a form indicating the information that should be filled out on admission. The clerk then types information from patients directly onto the terminal. When the information has been completed, the clerk pushes a transmit key to send the data directly to the computer. At that point it may be disseminated to other departments in the hospital. This would include dietary, housekeeping, lab, x-ray, business office, and any other departments that may need to know when new admissions are entering. Hospitals that are participating in a preadmission program, in which scheduled surgeries are planned ahead so that patients can provide preliminary information, can sometimes carry out this process prior to patients' entries into the system. In this case when patients enter the admitting department, their names are typed and the information is indicated on the screen along with appropriate date of admission. At that time the admission clerk need only verify that a patient is entering the hospital and again key the transmit button to disseminate the information. The admission will actually happen at the admitting department through a patient registration or patient admission process.

The discharge function of notification that the patient is going to be discharged may be carried out by nurses on the nursing station. They may step to a CRT terminal and key in a patient's name, date of discharge, indicate to where that patient is being discharged, and transmit. Again, the process is repeated. The information is disseminated to the departments that need to know that that patient is leaving the hospital on that day.

The second activity discussed is the *Census.* Each census entry actually is a building block in a structure that begins with the admission function itself. Each time a patient is admitted the name is added to the list that makes up the census report. If the system is an on-line hospital system, then each time a patient's name is added the file is automatically updated. Someone may be admitted at one o'clock and the information transmitted to the computer. At two minutes after one the radiologist, who wishes to check the current census, keys CEN. to retrieve the information for display on the CRT screen. This display will include the person who has just been admitted. Computerizing the census can be an extension of an on-line admitting process, as has been stated, or it can be a batch process. In a batch process, the patient is admitted and sent to the care unit. The admitting information is keypunched and held. Each night reports come from the care units that provide an accounting of the number of patients in the hospital on each unit. All counts are collected and tallied by the computer in a batch mode. Recall that the census is run daily, and lists of admissions, discharges, transfers, and deaths are included in the census report. When it is computerized it is beneficial for the entire hospital. Census printout reports can be duplicated easily and sent through intrahospital mail, or census information can be displayed on a CRT video screen for immediate availability to those who need the information.

The next function is *chart assembly.* Earlier in the text we described the El Camino Hospital system in Mountain View, California. This system has a primarily computerized patient record up until the time of discharge. At the point of discharge the information that has been stored on the computer is printed out, assembled, and sent to the medical record department. The chart assembly at El Camino is assisted by the computerization process.

Sometimes chart assembly is combined with another function, the *chart analysis* process, that verifies completeness and abstracts basic data for statistical reporting. This system has been computerized for a long time. We have used the method of individual abstracts upon discharge to collect a basic discharge data set that can be transmitted to PSRO for reporting. Hospitals have participated in the PAS program, the Med-ART Program, and other discharge abstracting services. (See Exhibit 9-3.) These systems have allowed hospitals to complete an abstract form, upon discharge. These forms are then sent to the abstracting company in groups of 100 or 200, as designated by the company. If you examine the abstract form you will see items of information that later are compiled to produce a standard set of reports for the record department. This will include the following activities.

Exhibit 9-3 Case Abstract for Commercial Discharge Abstracting System

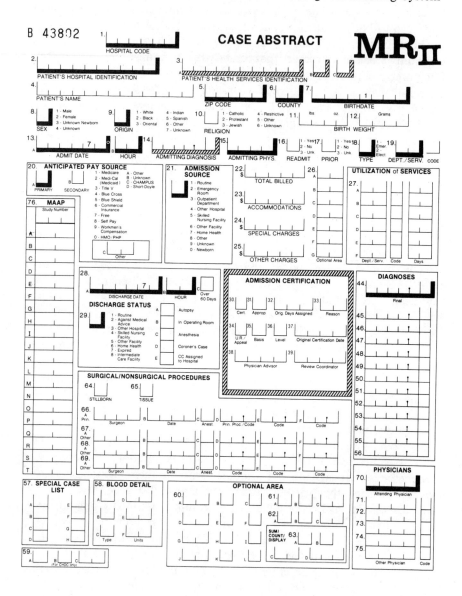

- *Discharge analysis for statistics*
- *Disease and operation coding and indexing*
- *Special discharge data studies*

The selection of discharge abstracting systems and participation in these systems is a primary concern for the medical record managers today. They must evaluate the nature of the system, the cost per discharge to their department. They must determine how their staff can be trained to carry out functions and if the reports provided by the abstracting company are prepared in a timely and useful manner. They must ascertain if the information is actually used by the medical staff and other interested persons within the agency. Note the visual on CPHA professional activity study in Figure 9-1. This figure illustrates the growth and expansion of discharge abstracting service by the Commission on Professional and Hospital Activities (CPHA). It indicates how CPHA's reporting operations have expanded to try to meet the needs of the health care delivery system.

Chart analysis for deficiency notification follow-up is another system that has been computerized in many departments. This can include completion of an abstract form for keypunch or it can include directly entering the information about chart deficiencies under a physician's name that is called up on a CRT screen. When the patient's information is keyed in under a physician's name, this automatically stores the information so that lists of incomplete records can be printed out and that list made available in a timely fashion, perhaps daily, for each physician on the staff. It also provides for production reports on the total number of chart deficiencies for each physician on the staff and can group those deficiencies according to services, such as medicine, surgery, cardiology, and so on.

Filing and retrieval is another activity that directly affects every individual record. Computers have been used in this function. They provide printout lists for retrieving charts for clinic appointments. They have also been used to prepare lists for purging files that are no longer active.

Insurance reporting for reimbursement is usually carried out for each record at time of discharge. Many hospitals now incorporate this in the coding system they use on discharge. Once the diagnosis has been coded, it is automatically sent to the insurance carrier along with discharge data.

The second group of functions involve record resource activities. These activities are those that use individual records or groups of records to carry out functions. They may be related to individual patients or to particular groups of patients. *Medical reports and insurance* is an example of using individual records to complete requests for information. *Utilization review* is an example of the use of group and individual records to carry out the process. *Medical audit* also uses groups of records in a sampling mode to

Figure 9-1 CPHA Growth Re-creating Technological Changes and
Resultant Report Sophistication

CPHA [COMMISSION ON PROFESSIONAL AND HOSPITAL ACTIVITIES]

1950

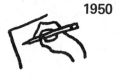

- Manual comparison of individual, non-standardized reports

- Interhospital study of routine, traditional statistical reports

1953

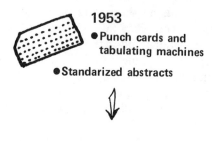

- Punch cards and tabulating machines
- Standarized abstracts

- Simple interhospital studies Monthly statistical reports
- Disease, operations and physicians indices
- 13 hospitals participating

1977

Magnetic Tape

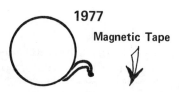

- Quality Assurance Monitor
- Length of Stay Study Study of Patient Charges
- PAS Profiles
- Concurrent Review Study
- Medical Audit Program
- Medical Care Evaluation
- Special Studies

- 2200 hospitals
- 150,000,000 cases
- 17,000,000 added annually

1990's

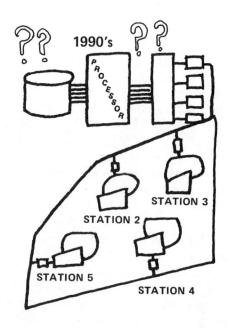

STATION 3
STATION 2
STATION 5
STATION 4

carry out the process. *Tumor registry* involves tracking follow up for patients who have tumors. It usually involves reporting outside the agency as well as tracking within. *Research retrieval* for medical staff studies involves pulling records by groups to look at given problems. *Word processing* and *central dictation* units are functions within medical record departments that process, through dictation systems, actual information on the patient record. Computer impact exists in this area in the form of CRT terminal data entry equipment where medical stenos type dictation directly into computer terminals with excellent error correction capability by insertion of items or lines where appropriate. This information, once it has been proofread, is then printed out on an impact printer. Computerized word processing systems are based on microprocessor technology. Other record resource activities include *medical staff projects,* such as data collected to participate in medical staff committees, and special study reporting.

COMPUTER IMPACT ON THE PATIENT RECORD

Information formerly handwritten and typewritten is now available on computer printouts that offer more concise and readable data to record users. Computer printouts are commonly a part of hospital, clinic, and nursing home records. History and physical examinations, summaries of laboratory findings, diagnostic test results, medication records, physician orders, nursing history and assessments, and discharge summaries have been computerized. Consider Exhibit 9-3. Imagine the time saved for technicians, for example, when lab results are automatically printed out in paper form ready to be filed in the patient record. If you look at a physician's orders computer printout in a nursing home you may notice that it corresponds with the medication administration form. These forms may be created at the same time. This kind of computer application is frequently used in skilled nursing facilities where physicians review and renew all orders on a monthly basis. Use of the computerized system allows more readable information to be maintained and frees the nursing staff from hand-transcribing the medication administration record. The nursing staff can audit the information once and make corrections in less than half the time it took to review both forms in the handwritten record.

Collecting patient histories has been done with the help of the computer for some time. By having the patient complete a questionnaire prior to seeing the physician, information is more readily available and the doctor can spend time with the patient more effectively. Computer-assisted history-taking may be accomplished by patients completing questionnaires that are later keypunched and printed. In another method, the patients can review

Exhibit 9-4 Indirect Data: Laboratory Report

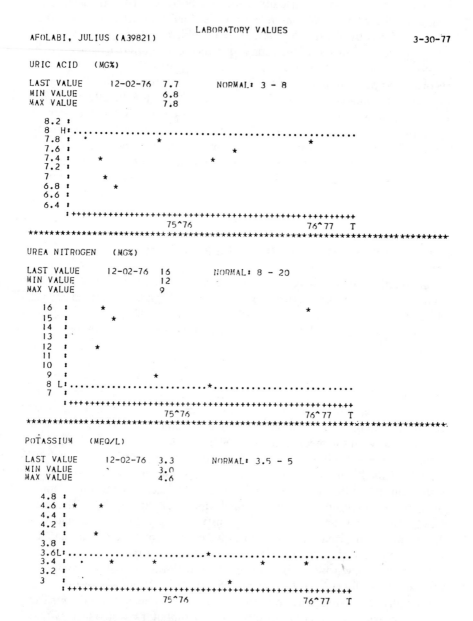

```
                              LABORATORY VALUES
AFOLABI, JULIUS (A39821)                                          3-30-77


URIC ACID   (MG%)

LAST VALUE       12-02-76   7.7       NORMAL: 3 - 8
MIN VALUE                   6.8
MAX VALUE                   7.8

   8.2 :
   8   H:..........................................................
   7.8 :   .               *                           *
   7.6 :                                    *
   7.4 :       *                        *
   7.2 :
   7   :       *
   6.8 :         *
   6.6 :
   6.4 :
       :+++++++++++++++++++++++++++++++++++++++++++++++++++++
                 75^76                        76^77    T
********************************************************************************

UREA NITROGEN   (MG%)

LAST VALUE       12-02-76   16       NORMAL: 8 - 20
MIN VALUE                   12
MAX VALUE                    9

  16  :       *                              *
  15  :         *
  14  :
  13  :  .
  12  :     *
  11  :
  10  :
   9  :           *
   8  L:...........................*.........................
   7  :
      :++++++++++++++++++++++++++++++++++++++++++++++++++++++++
                 75^76                        76^77    T
********************************************************************************

POTASSIUM   (MEQ/L)

LAST VALUE       12-02-76   3.3      NORMAL: 3.5 - 5
MIN VALUE                   3.0
MAX VALUE                   4.6

   4.8 :
   4.6 : *     *
   4.4 :
   4.2 :
   4   :     *
   3.8 :
   3.6L:...........................*.........................
   3.4 :   .     *        *                *        *
   3.2 :   .
   3   :                          *
      :++++++++++++++++++++++++++++++++++++++++++++++++++++++
                 75^76                        76^77    T
```

Reprinted with permission: Jenkin, M.A., M.D.,
A Manual of Computers in Medical Practice,
The Society of Computer Medicine, 1977.

questions with an interviewer, who enters the information on a form display on a computer terminal. In still more advanced examples patients answer questions directly by operating the terminal. Studies have proved that the information is consistently more reliable than handwritten notes taken as part of a routine medical examination by a physician and written or dictated as patient history.

In some cases all patient information is stored in the computer and a minimal paper record is maintained. The doctor or technician requests information via computer terminal and the data are displayed on a screen. There may be a printer attached so that the image may be copied or information may be used directly from the screen. The reader should review such programs as the Kaiser computerized record model, the Co Star ambulatory care system, and others for in-depth analysis and review. An example of a fully computerized patient information system is used at Ottery St. Mary's Practice in England. The system was designed by Ottery St. Mary's doctors in conjunction with a systems analyst of the Exeter Community Health Services computer project.

In this system the records are displayed on a TV-like terminal placed beside the doctor's desk. The terminal has a typewriter keyboard for input and a screen for display. The terminal is connected by exclusive lines to the computer center of the Royal Devon Exeter Hospital in London. The secretary begins the record when the patient registers. The patient has a health center number by which the record can be recalled for future reference. This number links the screen display summaries, display of medication, and display of extension that form the records. In this system doctors work directly from the terminal. They can review the patients' previous medication. They can also make additional entries to records at that time. Information is then stored on computer and is available when they wish to call for it in the future. It is also possible in this system for doctors to delete obsolete or trivial information from existing records and transfer it to backup storage directly through the terminal. When they delete information through the terminal, the information is pulled off the computer and then stored on microfilm so that it can be recalled if necessary. In the El Camino Hospital in Mountain View, California, the paper record is produced upon discharge of the patient. This record includes dictated histories, physical and discharge summaries, computer printouts of all laboratory tests and physicians' orders, medication administration, selected nursing histories and assessments, plus discharge plan. It is a composite of computer printout forms and dictated chart forms that is assembled and treated as a standard medical record upon discharge. Some computer applications not only print out documentation of the process, such as the physician's orders or the results of a laboratory test, but actually generate computerized interpretation of the test itself. Electrocardiograms and radiology are both areas in which computer technology has been developed. Students will need to investigate computerized tomography.[1]

The concept of computerized axial tomography was initially developed by Cormack, in a remarkable paper published in the *Journal of Applied Physics* in 1963. He described the idea of making measurements of the x-ray transmission "along lines parallel to a large number of different directions" so as to obtain a sequence of x-ray transmission profiles. He carried out an experiment in which he used a gamma-ray source, collimating the beam to a width of 7 millimeters, and measuring, with a Geiger-Muller counter, the intensity of the transmitted beam at 5 mm intervals over a 12.5 centimeter scan-pass length. The subject of his scanning experiment was an aluminum cylinder surrounded by a wooden annular ring. He proceeded to calculate the absorption coefficients by means of the scanning process, and found that his experimental results agreed with the actual absorption coefficients of the materials within three significant figures. Cormack noted that his results were applicable to the field of radiology, but at the time a practical implementation was thought technically infeasible, probably because of the large size of the computer necessary at that time.

Hounsfield designed the first commercial instrument capable of obtaining images useful for medical purposes. First marketed in 1973, the Hounsfield device could scan only from the ears up to the top of the head, since it required that a water bag surround the portion of the head being scanned. The machine produced a low resolution picture with an 80 × 80 matrix of picture points and required 15–20 minutes of computer processing to produce a picture after the mechanical scan was completed. The display, furthermore, was an oscilloscope on which a moving green line swept out the picture in 10 seconds, necessitating time-exposure photography to produce a permanent picture record. The algorithm used was Hounsfield's own derivation, based on successive approximations, and required that all of the scan data be first stored in the computer's memory before the picture reconstruction process could begin.

We at Georgetown were privileged to be involved in the next significant development in the history of computerized tomography. Our invention of the ACTA Scanner (Automatic Computerized Transverse Axial Scanner) made possible for the first time the tomographic examination of any section of the body. The prototype ACTA Scanner was in clinical operation at the Georgetown University Hospital and on the market by February 1974. This revolutionary whole body scanner had no need for an intervening medium like a water bag, and produced a high resolution picture with a 160 × 160 matrix of picture points for the body. The ACTA used a convolution algorithm for reconstruction, a process which allows simultaneous computations during the mechanical scan, thus generating an accurate cross section image immediately upon completion of the mechanical scan. The reconstructed picture was displayed on dual television monitors, one black-and-white, the other color. Since 1975, all computerized tomograph scanners have been patterned after the ACTA Scanner.

We can pause here and focus on four distinct computer applications identified in this chapter.

- Computer network systems that connect information throughout various departments in the organization
- Computer applications of functional operations in medical record departments
- Computerized patient records that fully or partially replace the paper records
- Computerized tomography that uses technology to interpret data in diagnostic tests

How medical record administrators and medical record technicians will work with these will depend on their knowledge and application skills in data processing. Systems analysis and long-range planning are the activities required.

LONG-RANGE STRATEGIES FOR COMPUTER APPLICATION

Today's health information practitioners are working with computer technology along a continuum from simple keypunch applications to very sophisticated teleprocessing networks. One of the challenges of this profession is to identify exactly where along the continuum your particular health care setting fits. You will recall that the requirements for developing, establishing, and maintaining an effective health information system were laid out in Chapter 8. Now Let's build on those concepts and focus on the medical record practitioner's leadership, partnership, or consumer role. There are four strategies.

1. Medical record departments use computer technology through contracts with computer companies. Discharge abstracting systems that offer comprehensive statistical reporting and indexing are examples of this. Additional package systems that can be purchased include registration, admission, discharge and transfer systems, clinical appointment scheduling systems, record control systems, and others.
2. In some hospitals and clinics total information system projects are underway. The Virginia Mason Hospital in Seattle is developing a Hospital Computer System. The Seattle U.S. Public Health Service Hospital is developing PHAMIS, Public Health Automated Medical Information System, which will computerize the Ambulatory Care Record. It's useful to realize that there are many other facilities that have undertaken the goal of a total hospital information system. In this situation medical record administrators may be working with communication networks, on-line data retrieval, and/or computerized printouts that comprise the record itself. Such a system may have pharmacy, radiology, clinical laboratory, admission and billing, and utilization review procedures on computer. The patient record may or may not be computerized. The master patient index is often an on-line component of such a system.
3. The medical record practitioner may be working in a setting which has many applications but no comprehensive total computerized system that encompasses all departments or that forms a network between them. Even in this situation practitioners will do well to plan for applications within the department that could be supported by microprocessing equipment and a budgeted programming position.
4. Medical record practitioners may be working in alternative settings with heavy applications in teleprocessing networks. Here they are dealing with data entry through summary of clinic visits. They may be dealing with data retrieval through specialized reports and registry. They may be working with clinical algorithms or decision-support systems that assist physicians in arriving at diagnoses and in solving problems for individual patients.

The role of practitioners is to be able to plan for technology just as they would plan for expansion of a department to meet patient, hospital, and community needs. Along with the four situations that have just been described, there are approximately four *roles* that RRAs and ARTs must be able to handle.

First, they must be consumers. They must be able to understand products that are presented to them. This includes sophisticated computer technology. There are word processing systems that use microprocessors to computerize the central dictation subsystem within a department. Practitioners need to understand enough about systems and computers to understand what the product is that is presented, how to analyze its benefits, and how to ascertain its costs. This means developing an awareness of terminology and jargon that is part and parcel of computer technology itself.

Their second role is that of team members, functioning via task force or special planning committee that plans for specific applications of computers within the department—in fact, within a hospital setting. Here the record practitioner might be a member of a team that includes other department heads and the systems analyst for data processing to develop long-range plans and strategies for implementing computer systems within the hospital. For example, current systems may include billing and payroll. What is the first system that will be added to this? On-line patient registration is one example. The purpose of the team role is to focus on the planning function so that it will include all departments within the hospital and so will thoroughly identify the information flow within the hospital.

If patient registration initiated through a preregistration process is placed on the computer, that simple decision is not so simple. From the decision to place patient registration for outpatients and/or inpatients on the computer, a number of other subsystems can be built. Once patients are registered, they can be added to a census. The census can become part of the computer process. The admission and the discharge lists produced each day can be part of this system. Once patient registration, admission, and the census are on the computer, it is not at all difficult to add the components of PSRO screening and utilization review (UR). This can be done in a simple fashion, using keypunch equipment to produce a daily listing for the UR coordinator, to make the rounds of the hospital. It may involve a more sophisticated system that includes listings for the UR coordinator, activity schedules for the physicians so they know the utilization of their own patient loads, and activity schedules for the UR committee so they have overall information on utilization of services for Titles XVIII, XIX, V federal beneficiaries.

A third role for the health information manager is as a long-range planner for operational systems within the department. This may include computerizing a record control system and a decision to use computer output microfilm rather than on-line methods. It can certainly include planning for computerized word processing systems. The following list is an example of operations within a health information service or medical record department that can be planned and coordinated using microprocessing equipment.

- Record control
- Tracking the medical record to and from the main file area

- Physician and other health provider deficiency system
- Providing individual and summary reports on documentation standards by practitioners throughout the hospital for JCAH reporting
- Research medical audit procedures providing screening operations for the overall quality assurance program for the hospital
- Computerized applications of medical reports that are established predetermined data sets for standardized reports for the medical record department, either to send to specific agencies, such as cancer or tumor institutes, or for individual transfer of information to carry on medical care at optimum levels
- Special statistical applications that use already developed software in data base management mode

  — To provide data analysis and retrieval
  — To provide tools for management to make decisions about services within the organization (whether they are hospital ambulatory care setting or network facilities)

The fourth role that the medical record practitioner might fill is that of a liaison among existing health data centers. An example of this would be a mental health network, such as the Mississippi Multi State Information System, which plans for storing and interchanging information through teleprocessing and data networks. Another example currently in operation now is the Shared Computer Systems Corporation, operating out of King of Prussia, Pennsylvania, where a central host computer stores the data and information is transmitted over phone lines. Teleprocessing techniques are used to process the data, retrieve it, and handle support systems for operations within the agency.

Figure 9-2 summarizes the six critical issues identified by Melville Hodge in designing the El Camino system and is another way to view the overall picture of long-range systems planning.[2] These issues are certainly reflective of the ideas and applications we have examined in this chapter. The challenge is for you to draw from the many resources to meet your organizational objectives.

NOTES

1. Robert S. Ledley, "Computerized Tomography: A Progress Report," *Computers in Health Care: Are They Worth It,* Proceedings of the 8th Annual Conference of the Society for Computer Medicine (Minneapolis: Society for Computer Medicine, 1978).

2. Melville H. Hodge. *Medical Information Systems* (Germantown, Md.: Aspen Systems Corp., 1977), p. 66.

Figure 9-2 Six Critical Decision Steps to Consider for Medical Information
Systems

Reprinted with permission: Hodge, M.H.,
Medical Information Systems, Aspen
Systems Corporation, 1977.

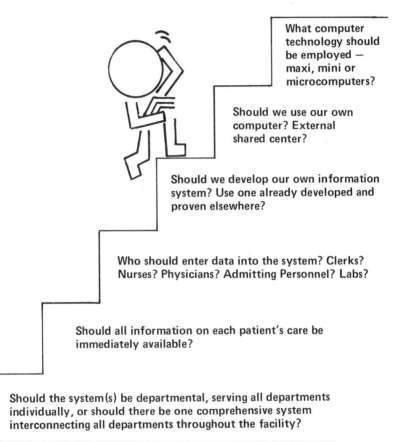

What computer
technology should
be employed —
maxi, mini or
microcomputers?

Should we use our own
computer? External
shared center?

Should we develop our own information
system? Use one already developed and
proven elsewhere?

Who should enter data into the system? Clerks?
Nurses? Physicians? Admitting Personnel? Labs?

Should all information on each patient's care be
immediately available?

Should the system(s) be departmental, serving all departments
individually, or should there be one comprehensive system
interconnecting all departments throughout the facility?

REFERENCES

Collen, Morris F., ed. *Hospital Computer Systems.* New York: Wiley & Sons, 1974.

Gabrieli, E.R. *Potential of Medical Computing.* Buffalo, N.Y.: Journal of Clinical Computing, 1975.

Grams, Ralph R. *Problem Solving, Systems Analysis, and Medicine.* Springfield, Ill.: Charles C Thomas, 1972.

Hill, Nancy S., ed. *Computers in Health Care: Are They Worth It?* Proceedings of the 8th Annual Conference of the Society for Computer Medicine. Minneapolis, Minn.: Society for Computer Medicine, 1978.

Hill, Nancy S., ed. *Effective Performance in the Dynamic Health Care Environment,* Proceedings of the 7th Annual Conference of the Society for Computer Medicine. Minneapolis, Minn.: Society for Computer Medicine, 1977.

Hodge, Melville H. *Medical Information Systems.* Germantown, Md.: Aspen Systems Corp., 1977.

Jenkin, Michael A., ed. *A Manual of Computers in Medical Practice.* Edina, Minn.: The Society for Computer Medicine, September 1977.

Koss, Neal, ed. *Common Goals: Working Together,* Proceedings of the 6th Annual Conference of the Society for Computer Medicine. Minneapolis, Minn.: Society for Computer Medicine, 1976.

Appendix 9A

PROMIS System Design

III. THE SYSTEM DESIGN FOR PROMIS

A . Technologic characteristics:

A PROMIS system designed to help solve four major problems facing medicine today (lack of coordination, failure to record logic, dependence upon human memory and lack of meaningful feedback loops on the everyday practice of medicine) must have three technologic characteristics:

1) Responsiveness: It must be very responsive and allow the information originator to be directly interfaced using a touch sensitive CRT computer terminal;

2) Reliability: It must be very reliable so that it is continuously accessible and usable as an information utility; and

3) Access to large files: It must allow access from any terminal tied to the system (if confidentiality allows) of all patient records kept within the system and of a large, structured, medical information data file used for the generation of the patients record and to provide the medical guidance in decision making.

These three characteristics are the major architectural elements of a PROMIS system.

B. Design characteristics:

The characteristics of the design approach followed by PROMIS Laboratory to implement this architecture are:

1) Build the system so it is modular and scalable (i.e. expandable or contractible).

2) Build the system so it has minimum redundancy yet under various types of failure can still operate.

3) Build the system out of reasonably inexpensive components (i.e. mini-computers) that are technologically updatable without having to modify the application software.

4) Build the system so that the difficult systems problems can be solved (i.e. the access to the distributed POMR file) while the system is still reasonably small and well understood.

5) Build the system out of "off-the-shelf" components or at least "mostly-off-the-shelf" components. (If anything must be built that is not now a standard product, get it from a manufacturer who will make it a standard product.)

6) Build the system using recognized software development approaches which increase programmer productivity, decrease debugging time and allow all software to be maintained by a team instead of the individual who originally wrote it. These approaches include language processors that allow "structured" (go-to-less) programming and the use of decision tables as an integral part of the program specification process.

7) Build the system so that all application and medical content programming is done in a higher order language that has machine independent characteristics. This will help maintain the software base if the hardware base is changed.

8) Build the system so that all software tools required to compile, edit and debug all application software are available within the same hardware and operating system base as the health care delivery systems base. This is a corollary to "top-down" program development (where commonly used pathways are exercised very early in the software development cycle) since the commonly used pathways in the total system are used to get the application software developed. This helps increase the reliability of the system very quickly.

Many of the above characteristics should enhance the exportability of the final system.

C. The major elements of the new system design—the PROMIS technology.

   1. general information

      The new technologic approaches at the highest levels involve multiple nodes tied together in a (limited) network. The network is limited in the sense that the functions to be performed are very well defined. Each free standing node (VARIAN-75 CPU with associated peripherals) will handle the frames (i.e. the medical content to be displayed) and medical record files for the segment of the health care facility(ies) served by its terminals. Internode communication will facilitate retrieval and storage of patient information from the other segments of the health care facility(ies) served by other nodes. In the event of a node failure another node will be able to pick up the failed nodes functions (i.e. by switching terminals and moving the patient record files).

   2. increased capacity

      The technologic approaches employed using the latest hardware technology allow much greater capacity than the CDC 1700 system.

      a) The central memory of the V-75 (VARIAN-75) can be increased up to 1 million words (maximum on CDC was 64,000).

      b) The secondary memory (disk storage) can be increased up to thirty-two 46 million character disks (maximum on CDC was 45 million characters).

      c) The network approach allows for modular growth up to several hundred terminals (CDC limit was 28).

   3. increased flexibility

      The design of the new PROMIS Programming Language (PPL) and supporting software environments allow much more flexibility in the programming of applications. For example:

      a) Limits on size of patient record on the CDC system, of order and problem list files are virtually eliminated.

b) "Memory buffer pool" design allows utilizing more central memory without reprogramming for increasing responsiveness or permitting more terminals to be added.

c) PPL frees programmer from most of the concerns about physical characteristics of data, allowing concentration on the medical logic.

4. distributed data base improvements

The distributed patient POMR record design allows tailoring of the system capacity to handle a wide range of loads, while maintaining reliability and continuous access. The frames and programs are duplicated on each node with this approach and the medical records are located where most heavily used across the network.

5. CATV transmission system improvements

The PROMIS terminal communications system allows installation of terminal taps in many locations and terminals can be plugged into any tap. This permits great flexibility in system usage—including portable terminals for "rounds." The communications medium is a standard two-way CATV network which can be used for entertainment TV, closed circuit TV, paging and other communications simultaneously with the computer-to-terminal signals and the computer-to-computer signals. See Appendix 10.

6. PROMIS terminal improvements

The PROMIS terminal allows a more flexible touch-screen format (no longer a rigid two column screen), greater screen capacity (1,920 characters instead of 1,000 as on the CDC) and more levels of enhancement of the displayed text (upper and lower case plus intensified video and inverse video instead of only upper case on the CDC). (See Appendix 9)

IV. THE IMPLEMENTATION APPROACH FOR THE PROMIS SYSTEM

A. The tasks:

The implementation of the new PROMIS system has been underway for over a year. The VARIAN-75 computer was installed in September of 1974. The implementation can be divided into seven major areas, although some areas must be completed before other areas can begin. Certain tools cut across these areas (e.g. system performance monitoring, data back-up and restartability) and will be implemented at the most expeditious point.

1) basic system software tools

Basic system software tools are required to develop the application software. This includes such tools as:

a) A system programming language for development of all other system software tools. This language is a preprocessor to the assembler. It facilitates writing of "structured" code and easy access to the firmware enhanced instructions in the V-75.

b) A CRT based source entry/editor.

c) Utility routines to dump to tape from disk and conversely and for disk to disk copies.

d) A PROMIS file system that extends the Varian supplied one in many ways including:

i) Files are not limited to 32,760 sectors but can be extended up to over 2 million blocks.

ii) Files do not have to be contiguous blocks of space but can extend across multiple areas and across multiple storage devices.

iii) Files can be expanded as needed without major maintenance.

iv) Files can have individual blocks assigned/released.

e) A CRT based binary entry/editor for any file in the system. This is only used in extreme cases but it is essential for some problems.

f) A warning panel which provides visual and audio signals of various software controllable system conditions which require operator action.

g) A hardware monitoring device to measure the percentage of utilization of up to 8 system resources simultaneously.

2) PPL

The development of the PROMIS Programming Language compiler, run-time routines and environments:

a) PPL compiler consists of a scanner, a parser and a code generator

b) PPL run-time routines consist of:

  i)   Terminal I/O processor.

  ii) Block (Disk) I/O processor.

  iii) Error I/O processor.

  iv) The sentence I/O routines.

3) Frame Editor

The development of frame editing, printing, searching and other management tools written in PPL. (All medical content will be kept within frames in the system; and since all entry of new medical content will be done by individuals who are not computer programmers, the tools for use must be "high level" and easy to use.)

a) A CRT based "frame-editor" allowing selection mode of modification of old frames and entry of new ones as well as keyboard entry when necessary. A family of these frame editors will have to be written for each type of medical data to allow individuals to directly interface the system without using computer programmers to enter the frames. The frame editor is table driven to facilitate modification and handling of multiple data types.

b) A "frame-printer" allowing externalization of all frames. This will allow outputting of not only single frames but also pathways of them for ease in understanding and use. This will be useful also for printing reports using data kept in the frames.

c) A frame searcher using the complete frame library or major sections as input, that will be able to find all the frames which satisfy a search request. This can be used to find all frames which, for example, contain the same medical words, that are written or modified by the same person or that refer to the same internal code of a specific problem or procedure.

d) Other tools, specific to certain classes of frames, to facilitate maintenance.

Chapter 10

Evaluating Patient Care through Documented Health Information

CHAPTER OBJECTIVES

1. Identify the role of evaluation in health care delivery
2. Describe the role of medical record professionals in health care evaluation programs
3. Recognize appropriate federal and legislative terms and relate their application to health care evaluation
4. Differentiate between utilization review and medical audit
5. Describe a method for carrying out a medical audit
6. Relate the history of medical care evaluation to current methods in carrying out medical care evaluation activities
7. Differentiate between outcome and process audits
8. Relate the AMRA PSRO position statement to current and future roles of health information managers
9. Understand the role of profile analysis as a major element in evaluation
10. Describe various ways computer technology has been used in health care evaluation

INTRODUCTION TO EVALUATION

Health care delivery is a major business in the United States. The cost of health care has accelerated from 38.9 billion in 1965 to 118.5 billion in 1975. This triple increase is worth noting. There are three major issues in health care delivery today. First, health planners, legislators, and patients themselves expect competency of health care providers in all instances. They view this as a right, just as they expect a right to competency in other professional services. Lack of competency causes both patients and providers to consider liability. Patients/clients seek assurance that competency will be a guarantee within the health care system. Second, the economic necessity of controlling exploding costs within the health care system has necessitated an accountability of services. This accountability addresses the values of services provided, the practicability of offering all kinds of services, relating services to the needs of individual patients, and planning levels of care for all patients. Third, a program of continuous assessment by allied health professionals to educate themselves and their profession to meet the needs of the future has come to fruition. Nurses, physical therapists, nuclear medicine technologists, respiratory therapists, psychologists, alcoholic treatment counselors, and other professionals in the helping professions are evaluating their own services. They are looking at the services that they currently provide and are considering how the current and future educational programs will fit into the overall health care system. Will they meet the needs of future patients? To do this successfully, to consider issues as they are raised, to justify the very passage of legislation that guarantees patients' rights as we are now defining them, the individual patient record is considered the primary source of evaluation. Individually and collectively it is the information system.

The manager of a health information system (HIS) must demonstrate competency to perform the following tasks.

- Determine the legal status of health care appraisal. This includes identifying the publishing sources of national, state, and local laws and applying the laws to the health information system. It also includes, in appropriate settings, determining and applying the role of accreditation by the Joint Commission on Hospital Accreditation (JCAH) in mandating patient care evaluation programs.
- Develop a clear understanding of patient care evaluation and apply the principles to a particular setting. Settings include hospitals, skilled nursing facilities, ambulatory care, and specialty clinics.
- Define and explain the audit cycle role and function, including the definition of terms, to other health care professionals.
- Demonstrate the ability to actively participate in audit committees within the organization. This participation ranges from a member role in criteria selection and definition to a committee facilitator role in coordinating overall audit activities.
- Construct an effective management framework to establish and maintain an audit program in the organization. This should satisfy audit requirements established by the accrediting and certifying agencies that conduct organization reviews.

- Prepare individual adaptations of existing audit models to fit particular needs. This means imaginative analogy. For instance, design an audit program for a particular application to assess the care given, review it in an orderly fashion, and present findings in a reasonable format so that the health professionals in the agency can carry on the auditing process.
- Employ appropriate statistical methods for data collection and display of audit results. This involves the ability to understand and use sampling techniques and the innovative use of graphs, charts, and other techniques that facilitate communication of results.
- Represent the organization by preparing written appeals to fiscal intermediaries to justify cases that have been denied. This involves skilled information analysis with patient records.
- Utilize communication skills in working with personnel, in in-service training, and in monitoring overall audit processes. This focuses on the primary purpose of audit itself: to enhance staff's participatory interest by providing meaningful feedback incorporated into continuing education for direct application in patient care.

Major points of the above listing are summarized in Figure 10-1.

HISTORY OF MEDICAL CARE EVALUATION

A careful review of the history of medical care evaluation will assist us to create a map of progress in health care evaluation. Look at the historical evolution of medical care evaluation shown as Exhibit 10-1. Notice the variety of sources that have been responsible for elements in the concept of health care evaluation. The variety of terms and methods devised along the way should be considered as the foundation for the goals and objectives we have today.

In the 1930s there was an extreme shortage of health facilities and health services, because of uneven distribution of resources and a lack of sufficient health manpower to satisfy health care needs.

In 1935 the Social Security Act provided for federal support of state and local public health programs. The Hill-Burton legislation (PL 79-725)[1] was enacted in 1946 to pump federal dollars into the economy for the specific purpose of creating building programs for new health care facilities and expansion programs for existing ones. This targeted the establishment of hospitals and clinics as a major step in providing health services.

Basic mechanisms available for medical care evaluation were essentially the property of the JCAH through the 1950s and early 1960s. In 1965 the Regional Medical Programs were created (PL 89-237).[2] These programs

Figure 10-1 Competencies the Health Information Manager Must Demonstrate

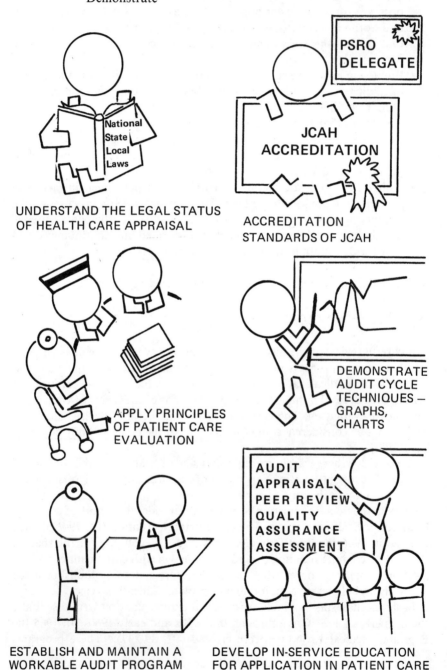

UNDERSTAND THE LEGAL STATUS OF HEALTH CARE APPRAISAL

ACCREDITATION STANDARDS OF JCAH

APPLY PRINCIPLES OF PATIENT CARE EVALUATION

DEMONSTRATE AUDIT CYCLE TECHNIQUES – GRAPHS, CHARTS

ESTABLISH AND MAINTAIN A WORKABLE AUDIT PROGRAM

DEVELOP IN-SERVICE EDUCATION FOR APPLICATION IN PATIENT CARE

Exhibit 10-1 Evolution of Medical Care Evaluation

		Effects
1910	Flexner Report evaluated quality of undergraduate medical education in the U.S. and Canada.	Closed 60 of 155 medical schools then in existence.
1912-1916	The study of surgical outcomes was undertaken by E. A. Codman and was recommended to the American College of Surgeons (ACS) as a means of measuring patient care.	Codman recommendations were not followed. The idea of evaluation was incorporated into the standards movement.
1913-1919	The ACS established the Hospital Standardization Program (HSP).	This targets the first formal quality assurance effort for evaluation by means of a peer review concept in a voluntary accreditation program.
1940s	The ACS calls for tissue committees.	This was followed by other committees for review of specific aspects of care in hospitals. Deaths, transfusions, infections, and antibiotics were identified. These were incorporated into the overall HSP.
1952	Establishment of the JCAH.	Evolution from the ACS to the Voluntary Accreditation organization—incorporated the active review of medical care through standards.

Exhibit 10-1 Continued

1953   The Commission on Professional and Hospital Activities (CPHA) and the Professional Activity Study (PAS) began as a cooperative study among 13 southwestern Michigan hospitals.

Formally stated its purpose was to be the study of hospital and professional activities for the improvement of patient care. It established a component of its program called Quality Assurance Monitor (QAM). This program introduced an abstracting program using hospital medical records of discharged patients. Data collected in this process were used in the QAM.

The QAM Program Was Used To Develop The Only Comprehensive Retrospective Monitoring Device For Use In Hospitals

1956   P. A. Lembeke performed an audit of records of patients on whom major gynecologic surgery was performed. The major purpose was to identify unnecessary surgery and feed back the results to the surgeons.

This was the origination of the term Medical Audit— used to describe the assessment of medical care using process data from medical records.

Medicare Legislation Impact 1965

1967   Utilization Review (UR) is required by Medicare/Medicaid in Conditions for Participation for Hospitals. 405.1035 required a UR plan to provide a review of:

This emphasized analysis of patterns of care:
—using data from outside service (such as PAS studies)
—in cooperation with the fiscal intermediaries
—through internal studies of medical records

—admissions
—duration of stays
—professional services furnished

This Added The Term Utilization Review To The Existing Terms

1970	DHEW Publications—State Operations Manual HIW-7, U.R. appendix E.	This more clearly defined review component. Extended duration reviews examined an individual patient's length of stay. Special studies concentrate on the facilities practices in patient care, both administrative, and medical practice being objects for study.
1970	JCAH Medical Staff Standard III.	The medical staff organization shall strive to create and maintain an optimal level of professional performance of its members, through the appointment procedures, the delineation of the medical staff privileges and the combined review and evaluation of each member's clinical activities.

We can say here that the earliest forms of medical care evaluation to be used widely were variations of the technique of case-by-case assessment using process data from medical records, developed by many and grouped under the name of Medical Audit.

Generally, hospitals and the JCAH considered the various programs of medical audit, peer review, and patient care appraisal to satisfy the intent of the Medicare/legislation.

Exhibit 10-1 Continued

1972	The Professional Standards Review Organization (PSRO) legislation mandated the implementation of a system of utilization and quality review for Medicare and Medicaid.	Begins to pull existing concepts on evaluation into more specific focus.
1974	PSRO Manual identified three areas:	1. Utilization Review 2. Medical Care Evaluation —Defined as short-term, in-depth studies that assess the quality and/or nature of the utilization of medical care 3. Profile Monitoring
1977	PSRO Program manual further refines concepts. Three goals are reaffirmed and the comprehensive meaning of specific area is identified.	Utilization Review —Prospective review. —Admission review —Concurrent review —Extended duration Medical Care Evaluation identified as the overall process including: —Audit —Appraisal —Peer review —Quality assurance —Assessment in very specific form Development and Analysis of Profiles for Patterns of Care is Moving into Focus.

At this point, Medical Care Evaluation (MCE) emerges as the officially acceptable term. A variety of methodologies that mix and match the terms identified in this schematic can be used to accomplish the intent of the MCEs. The essential characteristics of MCEs are listed in the body of the chapter. Any method that includes these essential characteristics is acceptable, regardless of its local title.

JCAH and PSRO have requirements for the number of MCEs a hospital must complete. Both call for between 4 and 12 studies per year. Utilization review requirements under Medicare and Medicaid require committees in hospitals and skilled nursing facilities to have at least one such study in progress at all times.

were designed to integrate a strong planning component into health care delivery by creating a recognized body to assist providers and act as service coordinators. In 1966 the Comprehensive Health Planning and Public Health Service Amendments were enacted (PL 89-749).[3] Both programs focused on coordinated planning of health resources through established bodies. Unfortunately, no specific enforcement component was included. Willing rather than enforced cooperation was sought so as not to antagonize the powerful medical lobby. However, the assumption that medical and health care professionals would voluntarily direct their efforts into stronger coordinating efforts via additional federal dollars and agencies proved invalid.

Medicare/Medicaid, passed in 1966 (PL 89-97),[4] introduced fiscal intermediaries as middlemen between individual providers and the federal government. One of the primary procedures introduced in this legislation was utilization review. This was the spearhead of medical audit. The Medicare/Medicaid legislation of 1966 was a clear indication that the peer review concept had not been effective. Medicare opened the door to federal intervention but maintained a careful courtesy with medical professionals. It provided for delegate roles. If a hospital had an existing committee structure and program, it could incorporate the required UR elements as part of its existing committee's internal review process. This was a new dimension.

While appraisal of health care had been carried on by medical staff committees, such as infection control and tissue committees (as identified elsewhere in the text), UR targeted a specific process aimed at cost control. To more effectively utilize hospital and nursing home services would hopefully contain costs. While UR was often carried on through established hospital committees, final decisions on service reimbursement were actually made at the fiscal intermediary level. For health record professionals the major impact of this legislation was identifying the patient record as the *documented evidence* that individual health care services had been provided. Until this time, the record was used in the peer review process established within the framework of the medical staff bylaws identified in Chapter 6. The patient record was reviewed and assessed by medical staff committees and may or may not have resulted in material to be fed back into the system with the specific goal of educating the providers. This federal legislation initiated the educational element requirement. This element alerted health care providers that measurements would be applied and services would be directly affected by results of UR of health care providers' and facilities' services. UR targeted major functions for those supplying patient information. A written plan spelling out intent and process for review within the organization was required. Specific provisions for transfer of patient information among health care providers to facilitate better utilization of services as well as better patient care was initiated. Along with requirements for transferring patient information came the actual definition of the content of information to be transferred. Health record managers now had federal standards specifying the content of the records. (For instance, Medicare/Medicaid standards indicate what the record must contain and how it must be organized.) A unit medical record was mandated. This required medical record managers to provide a system for maintaining a unit record for each patient.[5]

However, utilization review goals and peer review activities remained dependent upon individual organizations and hence were only as effective as the people and systems in those organizations made them.

Table 10-1 illustrates the contrast and variety of interpretation related to the Medical Care Evaluation concept.

In 1970, Senator Bennett of Utah introduced a proposal for peer review modeled after existing physician-sponsored models. While unsuccessful in 1970, the amendment was reintroduced and passed in 1972 as part of additional amendments to the Social Security Act. The Professional Standards Review Organization (PL 92-603),[6] known as PSRO, was designed to overcome the deficiencies in the existing program for UR by changing the organizational structure of the process. The law removed primary responsibility for review from the health care facilities and placed it with the local organizations of physicians and other health care providers. The primary responsibility of PSROs is to ensure that care paid for under Medicare, Medicaid, and the Maternal and Child Health (Titles XVIII, XIX, and V,

---

Table 10-1 Medical Care Evaluation

Medical audit	Reviews carried out using hospital medical records of patients discharged (retrospective review)
	Reviews carried out using skilled nursing facility medical records of patients in the facility (concurrent review)
Quality assessment	Major focus directed to outcomes of care
Peer review	Some attention given to process of care
Medical care appraisal	Some applications in ambulatory care evolving
Medical care evaluation studies	Major focus directed to process and structure of care

respectively) programs is medically necessary, consistent with professionally recognized standards of care, and provided in the least costly setting possible. Hospitals, skilled nursing facilities, and home-based health services are all viable options).

COMPONENTS OF MEDICAL CARE EVALUATION

Quality Assurance—The Goal

A major objective of the program is quality assurance. Quality assurance is directed to assure the quality of health services provided patients in health care facilities throughout the country. It consists of the following major components.

- Ongoing MCEs to identify problems of quality or the administration of health care services through application of the scientific method utilizing objective criteria, study, and the correction of problems through education and appropriate remedial action. This is directed to medical audit.
- Ongoing programs to assure the appropriate use of hospital services. This is directed to UR.
- Periodic analysis of the performance of the health care delivery system, including review, comparative, and trend analysis of aggregate patterns of activities and experiences of patients, providers, and institutions. This is directed to pattern analysis of the results of medical audit and UR.

The responsibility of this review system rests with the PSROs with input from a variety of programs. These include state-administered review programs, UR under Medicare and Medicaid, and quality assurance through the joint commission. The legislative map was laid out, resulting in major impact. In 1973, only 9 percent of all hospitals did medical audit; in 1977 that number jumped to about 85 percent.[7]

Quality assurance is certainly described and explained in many ways. Perhaps the best approach is to consider it an umbrella under which medical and health services are reviewed, evaluated, and revised, to the benefit of the patient. Let's look at some definitions and descriptions.

- The primary goal of a quality assurance system should be to make health care more effective in bettering the health status and satisfaction of a population, within the resources that society and individuals have chosen to spend for that care.

- Quality assurance can be defined as activities performed to determine the extent to which a practice meets certain standards and, if necessary, to initiate changes in a practice so that it will meet the needed level of standards.
- Patient care audit is an objective, systematic evaluation of the quality of patient care based on two principles:
  1. It is neither necessary nor efficient to examine every aspect of the patient care process.
  2. The results of careful comparison of actual practice against certain predetermined, objective, measurable criteria accurately reflect the quality of patient care.
- Quality assurance in medical services can be viewed as a multidimensional process that requires, at minimum, accurate measures of the technical competence of the provider and provides mechanisms to improve substandard practices, once uncovered.
- The hospital shall demonstrate that the quality of care provided to all of its patients is consistently optimal by continuously evaluating it through reliable, valid measures. Where the quality of care is shown to be less than optimal, improvement in quality should be striven for.

The Role of Patient Care Evaluation

While forms and formats for patient care evaluation are still emerging, the role it is taking as a function of patient information systems is not disputed. Hospitals may establish patient care appraisal departments or UR and medical audit departments separate from or as subsystems of the medical record department. Review of the medical charts of patients has been carried out for a number of years. Previously, this review was often funneled into infection committees, tissue committees, and medical record committees that took a close look at particular aspects of care for hospitalized patients. Today's patient care evaluation process actively seeks development of more objective methods of evaluation and is vitally concerned with directing evaluation toward education of health professionals. It is also directed at changing services provided by a given institution. Within the patient information system, evaluation of care through audit programs is clearly considered within the domain of health information systems managers. Effective organization of the program will depend on the knowledge and skill of these resource persons.

The data manager can incorporate medical audit activities into general functions of the patient data processing system that we refer to as the medical record department. The record cannot be separated from the patient. Care is dependent on, drawn from, and directed by the record. The administration and direction of MCE should interface with the medical record systems in hospitals and other health agencies through clearly defined organizational ties to the medical record administrator. This can be accomplished under the medical record administrator's direct supervision or as a cooperative or mutual effort to provide quality appraisal for the organization.

In 1975 AMRA adopted a PSRO position paper[8] that clearly promoted an active leadership role in cooperatively meeting the goals of the PSRO program (see Exhibit 10-2). The areas in which HIS managers must demonstrate competency, described earlier in this chapter, incorporate and build on this philosophy. Because health information managers in all settings work with health care evaluation, imaginative adaptations and individual program designs will be required. This position paper reflected AMRA's commitment to work with other organizations and with government for the success of programs designed to improve patient care.

Exhibit 10-2 PSRO Position Paper

The American Medical Record Association (AMRA) believes that Professional Standards Review Organizations (PSROs) afford our members a unique opportunity to actively participate in efforts to improve patient care.

Varied and significant amounts of data are required by PSROs to carry out their functions. Administratively, many PSRO functions may be appropriately assigned to the medical record department since medical care review and quality assurance programs rely on information abstracted and tabulated from medical records.

AMRA's professionally and technically educated members are involved in data collection and processing functions; abstracting and coding techniques; research and statistical methods; medical record review; and the preparation and evaluation of data displays. Specifically, AMRA members can aid planners, health care administrators, and medical staffs to:

- Develop effective procedures to carry out prospective, concurrent, and retrospective patient care reviews;
- Develop and institute methods to provide statistical profiles to evaluate the quality of care and service;
- Develop and implement controls on patient care evaluation programs to ensure privacy for individual patients and physicians;
- Evaluate the feasibility and cost effectiveness of utilizing health care data services to assist the health care facility in meeting its patient care appraisal program objectives.

A major requirement in creating an effective patient care evaluation program is understanding the legislation. We have looked at the legislation and identified how the resulting requirements will affect medical and health record managers. It is critical that we understand that legislation exists at four broad levels: (1) federal, (2) state, (3) county, and (4) city.

It is not unusual to find laws at each of these levels that regulate the same activities, but laws at one level may contrast or even conflict with those at other levels. Consequently, health information managers must carefully examine the legislation at *each* level. The fundamental principle to be followed is: **The most restrictive or comprehensive requirement determines the action.**

For instance, federal requirements may call for a general evaluation program that may be delegated to committees in health organizations. However, state law may prohibit delegation. For instance, Washington State law prohibits delegation of UR for Medicaid patients to individual skilled nursing facilities. The law calls for such review to be carried out through state agencies. Effective management of the program must meet both federal and state requirements. Health record professionals assist in development of UR plans that indicate how individual facilities meet federal demands while working through the review structure required by the state. Selecting the most restrictive or comprehensive regulation is the first step. Identifying conflicting requirements and communicating them to all agencies for cooperative interpretation is the second step. Information managers can incorporate individual variations in health record department objectives, policies, and procedures to assist surveyors in accurately evaluating programs. Reviews will include licensing, accrediting, and certification for federal programs. Facilitating this process is a positive strategy.

Methods—The Selection of Means

While legislation and voluntary accreditation standards identify the goal, the choice of means to achieve it rests with individual organizations. The remainder of this chapter is devoted to four things:

- First: The specific steps involved in carrying out UR, medical audit, and patterns of care identification that will satisfy the intent of the legislation.
- Second: Examples for implementing a medical care evaluation program with a health facility.
- Third: Identification of current resources for ongoing use by health care professionals to monitor up-to-date analysis and revisions in quality assurance activities.
- Fourth: The impact of computer technology on UR and medical audit programs.

Figure 10-2 Admission Screening

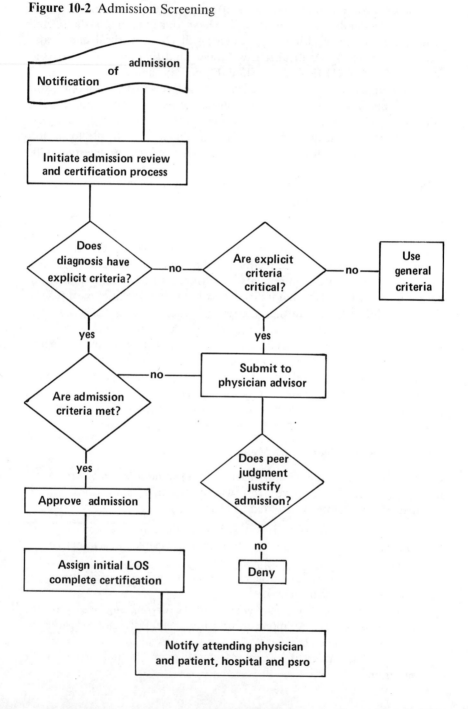

A Step-by-Step Look at UR

UR is essentially designed to provide concurrent review cases. The purpose of this is to prevent retroactive denials or overutilization of the various services within a hospital or skilled nursing facility. By establishing a program of concurrent review, beginning from the point of admission, the UR program can control cost and avoid retroactive denial. Concurrent review deals with length of stay, certification, and recertification concepts. It also investigates the rationale for extended stay duration. Active UR programs employ a UR coordinator, a review physician (most often referred to as a physician advisor), and a UR committee. These work together to accomplish the goals. The PSRO program manual explains the hospital review system as an integrated three-part major review mechanism, as noted in the preceding section[9]:

1. Concurrent admission certification in continued care review;
2. Medical care evaluation studies; and
3. Analysis of hospital, practitioner, and patient profiles.

This review system is to be implemented gradually within designated geographic areas, taking into account area size, providers, and facilities involved. Full responsibility for assuring the quality, necessity, and appropriateness of services under the Medicare/Medicaid and Maternal and Child Health programs is assumed by PSROs when they are formally established. They are to determine the necessity of hospital admission, the appropriateness of the hospital stay, and the effectiveness of discharge planning. Concurrent admission certification and continued stay review remove the need for retrospective claims review. Figure 10-2 illustrates how the UR process that deals with admissions, certification, and length of stay operates.

Utilization review monitors the units of service received by each patient in each individual transaction against normative profile data. It is carried out concurrently with the process of care so that it can affect that care during the time it is being given. It is concerned with the professions' collective responsibility to use health resources wisely.

The utilization review process is carried out in two sequential phases. The first is initiated with hospitalization and the second with discharge planning. Let's examine these in a task sequence.

Attending Physician

1. Admits patient, documents reason for admission in the medical record
2. Updates progress notes and certification as required
3. Initiates discharge planning
4. In the case of denial, discusses case with reviewing physician
5. If denial is made, determines whether to appeal the decision
6. Appeals to the appropriate party if so desired

Review Coordinator/ UR Coordinator

1. Identifies patient card at time of admission
2. Screens medical record and classifies the admission
3. Certifies those admissions that meet criteria
4. Refers questioned admits to physician review
5. Logs all denied admissions by physician and diagnosis
6. Sends admission denial letters
7. Assigns appropriate LOS
8. Reassigns LOS per significant change in the patient's condition
9. Notifies attending physician of review date
10. Assesses the 50 percentile certification note
11. Prepares review forms for the review of questioned cases
12. Receives completed review forms and processes
13. Sends continued stay denial letters
14. Coordinates activities and relays information back to the review team

When the discharge planning phase is initiated, a corresponding plan for patient information should also begin.

Discharge Planning Coordinator

1. Processes attending physician's referral for discharge planning
2. Refers request to the appropriate facility or community service, such as a skilled nursing facility

Coder/Medical Record Service Personnel

1. Codes all diagnoses, procedures, and complications for each record
2. Identifies primary codes and complication codes
3. Completes PAS or other

3. Records pertinent information in the medical record
4. Forwards the referral form to the appropriate agency upon discharge
5. Secures coordinated patient information for availability upon direct transfers

abstract forms for the discharge patient, including appropriate satisfaction of uniform hospital discharge data set

It's important to understand how the components of the overall utilization review process interact. The following tasks listed for the review physician and the review committee show the steps at which this interaction can take place.

Review Physician

1. Provides review consultation in cases of questioned admission
2. Documents pertinent information on the review form
3. Consults with the attending physician where denials are involved
4. Informs attending physician of the review decision

Review Committee

1. Reviews medical records of targeted cases on denial and appeal
2. Documents pertinent information on the review form
3. Notifies the attending physician of committee decisions
4. Provides guidance to the review program as implemented in the hospital

Medical Care Evaluation and Medical Care—The Ends

The PSRO manual goes on to explain MCE studies, which are established:

- To improve quality through an organized, systematic process
- To identify deficiencies in the quality of health care and in the organization and administration of its delivery
- To correct such deficiencies through education and administrative change
- To provide periodic follow up reassessment to assure that the improvements identified have actually been maintained

MCE studies provide the resources to determine the effectiveness of concurrent review and identify areas where concurrent review should be instituted, intensified, or dropped. They also validate criteria, norms, and standards or help provide evidence in the handling of this process by individual institutions.

> *The medical care evaluation activity is usually carried out in the medical audit program in the facility. The audit cycle (see Figure 10-3) assesses provider performance by studying criterion-referenced patterns of care. Audit is conducted on a retrospective basis so that the outcome can form the basis for the evaluation. It examines the way each practitioner fulfills the obligation to the patient.*

MEDICAL AUDIT

Medical audit may be thought of as an evaluation system similar to the management function of "controlling." The manager sets standards against which to measure performance; this process identifies problems for which corrective action is taken. Performance is then remeasured, if necessary, after an appropriate time period.

Let's look at what the JCAH considers the essential characteristics of an acceptable audit. The JCAH views patient care evaluation (audit) as an accountability mechanism by which the hospital, through its professional staff and using its own professionally directed evaluation procedure, can demonstrate that the quality of patient care it provides is consistently optimal. Furthermore, the use of such an accountability mechanism should contribute to the improvement of patient care. The essential characteristics of an acceptable patient care evaluation procedure follow:

1. Valid criteria that permit objective review of the *quality* of care provided to all patients are established.
   Valid criteria are
   - stated in *measurable* rather than descriptive terms, precise enough to permit accurate evaluation;
   - statements of *optimal achievable* care;
   - measures of *quality*, which are
     - validations of diagnoses;
     - justifications for admission, surgery, and/or special hazardous procedures;
     - statements of expected patient outcomes;
     - processes of care or patient management, under appropriate circumstances.

Figure 10-3 Medical Audit Cycle

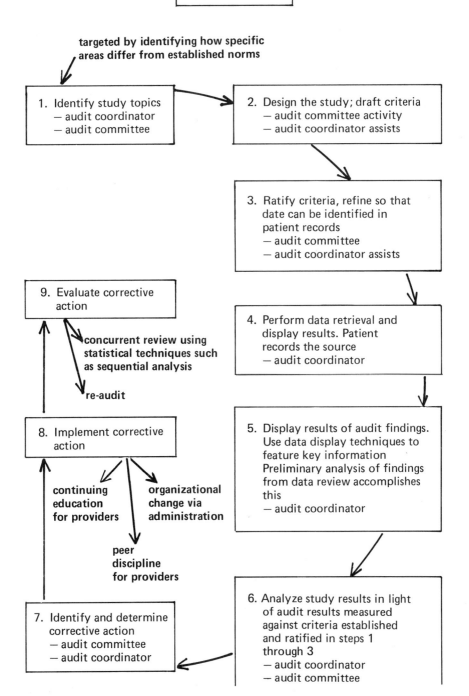

2. *Measurement* of actual practice against the criteria to produce *reliable* data.
   - *Measurement* requires comparison of actual practice to the criteria.
   - *Reliable data* requires
     - a well-defined objective method for measurement;
     - inclusion of all or a representative sample of patients and practitioners.

3. *Results* of measurement are *analyzed* by peers.
   Analysis requires
   - *identification* of conformance to and variations from the criteria;
   - explicit justification for all clinically acceptable variations;
   - identification of *problems* (not clinically acceptable variations) in the provision of patient care;
   - *attribution* of the problems to their source.

4. *Action* is taken to correct the *problems* identified.
   Action must be
   - *specific* to the *problems* identified;
   - *effective* in accomplishing change.

5. Action is *followed up*.
   Follow-up must be
   - *immediate* if problems are life-threatening;
   - *documented* to show improvement in patient care.

6. The results of patient care evaluation, that is, general findings and specific recommendations, are *reported*.
   Reported means
   - acknowledged by executive committee, chief of the medical staff, chief executive officer, and governing body (for medical studies);
   - acknowledged by chief executive officer, governing body, and chief of medical staff (for nursing service and other health care professionals' studies).

Numerical Medical Audit Requirements

Only medical or combined medical and nursing audits are acceptable for meeting the numerical requirements; however, medical audits completed in conjunction with other services will be acceptable.

Hospital Admissions for the Calendar Year Immediately Preceding Survey	Audit Studies Required at Time of Survey
Fewer than 2,500	4
2,500 to 4,999	6
5,000 to 9,999	8
10,000 to 19,999	10
20,000 and over	12

How to Do Outcome Audit

Most medical care evaluation studies or audits are outcome oriented. This means that attention is focused on the status of the patient at discharge from the hospital or from his course of primary care. Audit studies are designed by committees made up of physicians and other health care deliverers. A topic is chosen and a decision is made about how many cases to study and within what time frame. The topic can be a condition or diagnosis, a procedure, or a known or suspected problem. The committee sets criteria that it feels will effectively measure how well care has been provided.

Audit criteria generally take three forms: (1) justification for the diagnosis or procedure; (2) measurable outcome elements; and (3) nonspecific indicators, such as length of stay in the hospital or any complications of care. Each criterion is further broken down into three parts: (1) an element; (2) a standard; and (3) an exception. The audit committee determines which elements of care are of sufficient importance to warrant review of the medical record if they are not met. The screening standard is set at 100 percent (element must be found) or 0 percent (element should not be found). These standards are not intended to be standards of medical practice but rather are used as screening standards to sort out the charts that the committee wishes to review. They can add exceptions to each element if desired. These indicate justifiable nonconformance to the criterion.

The committee next defines specific instructions and definitions to help assure accurate data retrieval. Data retrieval is generally done by a nonphysician, such as a medical record practitioner or a nurse. Charts are screened by comparing data in them against the criteria and noting any variations (see Exhibit 10-3).

When the screening process is completed, variations are noted and those records are brought to the committee for review. The audit committee then determines if there was clinical justification for each variation. Unjustified variations are termed deficiencies, and these are further analyzed for attribution. This is an attempt to determine whether problems exist.

Exhibit 10-3

Example _____   A screening criterion

Element	Screening Standard 100%/0%	Exceptions	Instructions and Definitions for Data Retrieval
1. Antibiotic appropriate to culture and sensitivity (C&S)	100%	1.A. Culture taken and patient started on antibiotic pending results of C&S	1.A. See C&S report. Check to see that patient was changed to appropriate antibiotic within 24 hours of taking culture.

Problem-solving techniques are then brought into play. The data summary sheet can be used as a tool to organize an approach. For each problem to solve, ask five basic questions:

1. WHAT happened?
2. WHERE did it happen?
3. WHO is responsible?
4. WHY did it happen?
5. WHAT is the best way to correct it?

For each deficiency, the chart reproduced as Exhibit 10-4 shows what must be considered.

The audit committee's goal is to select the appropriate action to solve the problem. Appropriate feedback is given, and often ongoing monitoring is needed until the committee is assured that the problem has been solved (see Exhibit 10-5).

The audit committee reports its findings to the executive committee of the medical staff after discussing the study with the section(s) involved. Reports may be given to hospital administration, and a summary is sent to the governing board, which is ultimately responsible for the quality of care delivered in the institution.

Medical Record Professionals and Health Care Evaluation

Of individuals trained in allied health fields, perhaps none is as uniquely prepared to assist in the health care evaluation process as the medical record professionals. Because of training in, and understanding of, medical terminology, anatomy and physiology, disease processes, and diagnostic and therapeutic procedures, as well as medical record content and systems, they

Exhibit 10-4

Question	Consider	Decide			
WHAT	Problems and causes	• Nonperformance • Poor Performance • Wrong Performance			
WHERE	Patterns	• Random • Group *both by criterion and across criterion* • Individual			
WHO	Attribution	• Institution/Management • Staff			
WHY	Type	Knowledge	Environment	Feedback	Other
WHAT TO DO	Action	Teach	Restructure	Tell	Specific to problem

Exhibit 10-5

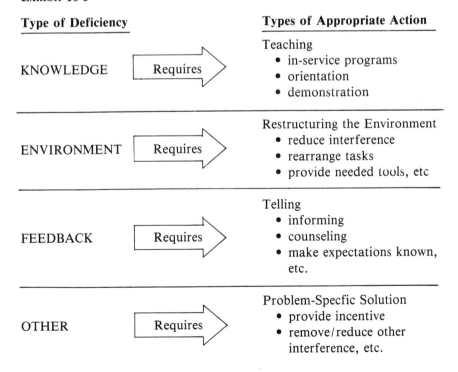

Type of Deficiency		Types of Appropriate Action
KNOWLEDGE	Requires	Teaching • in-service programs • orientation • demonstration
ENVIRONMENT	Requires	Restructuring the Environment • reduce interference • rearrange tasks • provide needed tools, etc
FEEDBACK	Requires	Telling • informing • counseling • make expectations known, etc.
OTHER	Requires	Problem-Specfic Solution • provide incentive • remove/reduce other interference, etc.

are qualified to perform the detailed analytic function required of a health data analyst. The RRA with management training is particularly qualified to coordinate all aspects of health care review. The ART, by virtue of training, is particularly qualified to analyze medical records against the screening criteria and display this data for audit committees.

In some institutions the RRA coordinates all aspects of health care review, including patient care audit; ongoing monitors of care such as morbidity/mortality, blood transfusion, antibiotics, and tissue; and the utilization review (UR). These reviews of care may be done concurrently with the patient's hospitalization, but usually are done retrospectively after the patient is discharged. The RRA's role as a coordinator may include some of the following elements:

Job Description for Director of Health Care Review

1. Manages HCR department; supervises data technicians and UR nurse.
2. Coordinates development of health care review systems and assures that the feedback loop is completed.
3. Coordinates development of health care evaluation studies; solicits topics, helps design screening criteria, facilitates with small group process techniques.
4. Provides technical assistance for data retrieval and display, concurrent monitoring of care, preadmission screening, etc.
5. Presents health care data to the review committees and assists in the analytic process.
6. Maintains procedures that comply with federal, state, institutional and accrediting agency policies and regulations.

MEDICAL CARE EVALUATION DEFINITIONS

You now have a conceptual model of medical audit. Let's move on to review particular terms and concepts and see how they will fit into this model.

Federal and Legislative Terms

A knowledge of useful terms and related concepts that deal with patient care evaluation is an essential resource. You will need these to understand this chapter and other related areas in the text. Many terms have been introduced in legislation. Others identify principles, particular agencies, and interpretive data commonly used. Exhibit 10-1 provides a description of the evolution of this concept. Let's look first at agencies and legislation.

Bureau of Quality Assurance (BQA). This division reports to the Health Care Financing Administration and is responsible for the administration of the Professional Standards Review Organization (PSRO).

Office of Professional Standards Review (OPSR). This division reports to the assistant secretary of the Department of Health, Education, and Welfare (DHEW), and is responsible for staff activities for PSRO.

Fiscal intermediary. An organization acting in an intermediate role for dispersing funds from the federal government. Blue Cross, for example, acts as a fiscal intermediary in the Medicare program.

Title V. A federal health program for maternal and child health and crippled children's services.

Title XIX, Medicaid. A federal program designed to meet the health needs for persons who receive aid through the program for families with dependent children or who have only marginal income.

Title XVIII, Medicare. A federal health insurance program for people 65 years of age and older, and some people under 65 years who are disabled.

Memorandum of understanding. A signed statement outlining the responsibilities for each party involved. Memoranda of understanding are between hospitals and PSROs and between fiscal intermediaries and PSROs.

Nonphysician health care providers. Those health professionals who do not hold a doctor of medicine or osteopathy degree but are qualified by education or licensure to practice a profession and are involved in direct patient care services.

Health care practitioners (other than physicians) are defined as those health professionals who (a) do not hold a doctor of medicine or doctor of osteopathy degree, (b) meet all applicable state or federal requirements for practice of their profession, and (c) are actively involved in the delivery of patient care or services that may be paid for, directly or indirectly, under Titles V, XVIII, and/or XIX of the Social Security Act.

Utilization Review References

These terms are likely to be found in UR plans and procedures for the health facility. One can see how the information networks from admissions, the UR coordinator on the nursing care units, medical record personnel, and medical staff committees unite in this process. The application of systems analysis techniques to the information flow in the facility, whether for manual or computer design, is a useful tool.

Utilization review. Evaluation of the necessity, appropriateness, and efficiency of use of medical services, procedures, and facilities. In a hospital this includes review of appropriateness of admissions, services ordered and provided, length of stay, and discharge practices on both a concurrent and a retrospective basis. This can be done by a UR review committee, PSRO peer review, or public agency.

Prospective review. A strategy for conducting the review process prior to the receipt of care. The purpose is to review the patient's condition and assure that the planned admission and the level of care are appropriate.

Admission certification. A set of medical elements used to determine justification for hospital admission.

Length of stay (LOS). The length of inpatients' stay in a hospital or other health facility. It is one measure of use of health facilities reported as an average number of bed days in a facility per admission or discharge. It is calculated as follows: Total number of days in the facility for all discharges and deaths occurring during a period divided by the number of discharges and deaths during the same period. In a concurrent review the LOS may be assigned to patient on admission. The average LOS varies and is measured for people with various ages and diagnoses. The LOS is a major criterion for continued stay review.

Preadmission certification. Admission that necessitates certification prior to a patient's occupying a bed in the hospital.

Length of stay certification (also called Recertification). A statement in writing by the attending physician assuring that continued hospitalization is medically necessary. It must include diagnosis, complications, plan for care, and anticipated LOS. It is what justifies additional LOS beyond the norm.

Level of care criteria. Criteria used to determine the appropriate level of care—hospital, skilled nursing facility, intermediate care—for a given patient based on the types of service that can be provided only at that level.

Percentile. A value on a scale of 100 that indicates the percent of a distribution that is equal to or less than that value. For instance, 50th percentile for a group of hospitalized patients may be 5 days. This means that 50 percent of the patients stayed 5 days or less.

Review. Examination of a medical record by a physician to determine if continued hospitalization is medically necessary.

Review coordinator. A person responsible for the smooth functioning of the review program and the communication of information between patient, attending physician, hospital, and PSRO.

Concurrent review. A form of medical care review that occurs during the patient's hospitalization. It consists of an assessment of the patient's need for a hospital level of care or a skilled nursing facility level of care. It may include an assessment of the quality of care being provided.

Continued stay review. The review carried on during a patient's hospitalization to determine the medical necessity and appropriateness of continuation of that patient's stay at that level of care.

are professionally developed expressions of the range of acceptable variation from a norm or criterion. The standard in our preceding example might require urinalysis in 100 percent of cases and a urine culture for previously untreated cases only.

Norms. Numerical or statistical measures used as a summary representation of a whole group of data. Averages are often used as norms.

Parameters. Factors that vary from one application to the next but are considered to be constants for a given application. Each health problem has a unique set of parameters. That is, plans, tests, and treatments that are individually adapted to that problem.

Elements. Specific services, tests, and/or parameters of care. Elements are identified when an audit committee sets criteria. Elements are grouped together and considered the identifiable parts that make up a criterion. For instance, a reviewer may look at three individual elements to see if a particular criterion was met.

Exception. Identified case to which specified standards do not apply. For instance, complications (that occur after the diagnosed admitting problem) that warrant an extension of the patient's stay in the hospital.

Screen. To compare documentation recorded in the medical record against preestablished criteria.

Screening. A process in which norms, criteria, and standards are used to analyze large numbers of cases to select cases that do not meet these norms, criteria, and standards for study in greater depth.

Variation. Not in agreement with the norm or standard. It may either surpass the norm or fall short of it.

Variation justification. Refers to an acceptable reason why a given finding or element is not in agreement with the norm or standard.

Variation analysis. Refers to analysis of a variation to determine whether it surpasses the norm (acceptable care) or falls short of the norm (unacceptable care).

Critical management. Describes the minimal preventive and responsive procedures that must be documented in the record to convince the audit committee that everything necessary was done to prevent the complication or that the complication was promptly recognized and appropriately treated.

Deficiency. A nonjustifiable variation from expected standards.

Monitor. To watch, observe, and check, especially to track a particular item of information.

Quality assurance mechanism. Retrospective review program by the organized medical staff. It assesses the quality of care as compared to locally or internally developed standards and verifies that the standards or exceptions are met, that deficiencies are corrected, and that the original problem is reassessed on a planned program basis.

Concurrent review. A strategy for conducting a review process concurrent with the patient's receiving medical services or commencing shortly after the patient is admitted to the hospital.

Intervention. Peer review criteria that are applied during the process of medical care of an individual patient. It may directly influence the action of the physician caring for that patient.

Delegation of review. Method of performing peer review whereby the health care facility assumes responsibility for performing actual review functions. The responsibility of actually reviewing patients in the facility is delegated to hospitals.

Denial. To deny approval for continued payment by the fiscal intermediary. In Medicare a patient may be disallowed benefits if the length of stay exceeds the norm or standard without appropriate justification.

Retroactive denial. To deny approval for payment based on retrospective review of the case. When this occurs, an appeals process is usually initiated in which further documentation from the patient's record is submitted and an additional review requested.

Figure 10-4 illustrates the sequence for audit data coordination and reporting to PSROs. The table reproduced as Exhibit 10-7 is an example of a 12-month projection for audit studies.

Profile Analysis—A Major Element

Profile analysis provides a mechanism to judge the effectiveness of a PSRO or a hospital's review program by comparing similar data over time. The concurrent review component frequently identifies potential problems within health administration and delivery. These can then be future topics for more detailed medical care evaluation studies.

Profile analysis is performed in many ways. The best way to understand it is to examine examples. Exhibits 10-8, 10-9, 10-10, and 10-11 all illustrate this activity. Drawn from the *Masters Manual* advanced audit program, they illustrate how audits are projected and how the results can be summarized for profile analysis.

Another graphic that may help differentiate between these three primary goals inherent in the medical care evaluation program is shown as Exhibit 10-12.[10] It addresses a comparative view of hospital medical care evaluation as identified by the JCAH.

Through studies and analysis of profiles, PSROs can determine areas of practice that would benefit most from ongoing intensive review. This way priority areas will emerge. The PSRO projection is comprehensive. The PSRO review system will be maintained and operated cooperatively by all the hospitals in the area and the PSRO. Once the PSRO review system is

Figure 10-4 Flow Chart for Audit Data Coordination and Reporting to
PSROs

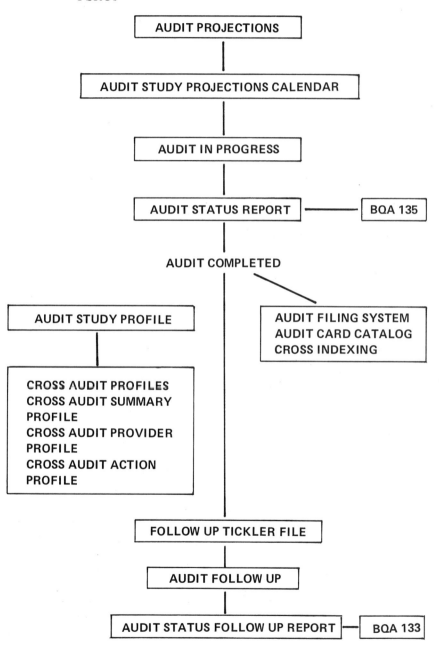

Exhibit 10-7 An Audit Study Projections Calendar for 12 Months—July 1, 1975—July 1, 1976

AUDIT STUDY PROJECTIONS CALENDAR   YEAR: 7/1/75–7/1/76

COMMITTEE	NO. TO BE COMP	AUDIT TOPICS	METH SELECT	ORIG RPT	IF RPT. DATE ORIG	EXPECT START DATE	EXPECT DATE COMPL
Medical audit committee	2	Gastroenteritis in infants	PN	Orig.		7/1/75	10/1/75
		Acute myocardial infarction	PN	Rpt.	9/1/74	10/1/75	1/1/76
Surgical audit committee	2	Surgery for urinary bladder tumors	PN	Orig.		8/1/75	12/1/75
		Cesarean section	PN	Orig.		4/1/76	7/1/76
Multidisciplinary audit committee	6	Surgery for fractured hip	PN	Orig.		9/1/75	12/1/75
		Cerebrovascular accident	OA	Rpt.	2/1/74	11/1/75	2/1/76
		Mastectomy for cancer	PN	Orig.		1/1/76	3/1/76
		Diabetic ketoacidosis	OA	Rpt.	11/73	3/1/76	6/1/76
		Alcoholism	CR	Orig.		4/1/76	7/1/76
		Hysterectomy for fibroids	PA	Orig.		5/1/76	7/1/76
Nursing audit committee	2	Congestive heart failure	PA	Orig.		8/1/75	12/1/75
		Urinary tract infection	OA	Orig.		4/1/76	7/1/76
Social service audit committee	1	Discharge planning	CR	Orig.		10/1/75	1/1/76

LEGEND: PN = Perceived need   OA = Other audit   CR = Concurrent review

Exhibit 10-8 An Audit Study Profile

An audit study profile displaying the "study data" and "audit type and participating departments and disciplines" columns completed for an audit of cerebrovascular accidents.

Reprinted with permission.

AUDIT STUDY PROFILE

STUDY DATA		AUDIT TYPE & PARTICIPATING DEPTS, DISC.		PROVIDERS* WITHOUT DEFICIENCIES	
				PROVIDER	No. REC.
AUDIT STUDY TOPIC:		PHYSICIANS ONLY	___	physician 18	2
Cerebrovascular Accident		MULTIDISCIPLINARY (PHYSICIANS AND OTHER HEALTH CARE PROVIDERS)	X	physician 72	1
		NONPHYSICIANS ONLY	___	physician 75	1
AUDIT COMMITTEE:				physician 65	1
Patient Care Audit Committee		DEPARTMENTS	DISCIPLINES	physician 35	1
		Internal medicine	nurses	physician 40	2
NUMBER OF RECORDS IN STUDY:	50	Family practice	social workers		
TOTAL NUMBER OF VARIATIONS:	160	Nursing	physical therapists		
TOTAL NUMBER OF DEFICIENCIES:	124	Social service	occupational therapists		
		Physical medicine			
DATE STARTED:	2/3/77				
DATE COMPLETED:	5/26/77				
ESTIMATED RESTUDY DATE:	2/78				

*INDIVIDUAL PROVIDERS, UNITS, ADMINISTRATION, DEPARTMENTS, SERVICES

Exhibit 10-9

An audit study profile in the audit of cerebrovascular accidents displaying the causes of and the action taken to correct deficiencies for each provider by criteria class and type.

AUDIT STUDY PROFILE   (CONTINUED)

Reprinted with permission.

DEFICIENCY ATTRIBUTION, CAUSES, AND ACTIONS

PROVIDER	No. REC.	CRITERIA CLASS AND TYPE	No. DEF.	CAUSES	ACTION
Physician 6	3	Outcome--Discharge Status	1	Documentation	Individual feedback
		Outcome--Follow-up	1	Documentation	Individual feedback
Physician 10	5	Outcome--Discharge Status	1	Documentation	Individual feedback
Physician 104	10	Outcome--Discharge Status	1	Documentation	Individual feedback
		Indicator--Length of Stay	1	Over-utilization	Individual feedback
		Indicator--Critical Process	1	Knew, did not do	Individual feedback
Physician 95	12	Outcome--Follow-up	1	Documentation	Individual feedback
Physician 150	6	Indicator--Length of Stay	1	Knew, did not do	Group feedback (memo)
Physician 25	4	Indicator--Length of Stay	1	Knew, did not do	Group feedback
Physician 30	2	Indicator--Length of Stay	1	Knew, did not do	Group feedback
Unit 2W	20	Outcome--patient knowledge	15	Documentation	Group feedback
		Indicator--Critical Mgmt.	2	Knew, did not do	Group feedback
Unit 2E	15	Outcome--patient knowledge	12	Documentation	Group feedback
Unit 3W	15	Outcome--patient knowledge	8	Documentation	Group feedback
		Indicator--Critical Process	1	Lack knowledge or skill	Individual feedback
		Indicator--Critical Mgmt.	1	Knew, did not do	Individual feedback
Nursing Administration	50	Indicator--Critical Mgmt.	6	Inadequate policy, procedure	Change procedure
Physical Medicine	30	Outcome--Discharge Status	15	Documentation	Group feedback
		Follow-up	10	Documentation	Group feedback
Social Service	35	Outcome--Discharge Status	25	Documentation	Group feedback
		Indicator--Critical Clue	20	Documentation	Group feedback
				Invalid Criterion (justification--procedure)	Change criterion for reaudit

NUMBER OF GROUP EDUCATIONAL PROGRAMS CONDUCTED TO CORRECT DEFICIENCIES _____   NUMBER OF GROUP FEEDBACKS USED TO CORRECT DEFICIENCIES _____

4

Exhibit 10-10 Completed Cross-Audit Summary Profile for 12-Month Audit Period

CROSS-AUDIT SUMMARY PROFILE

Reprinted with permission.

AUDITS COMPLETED BETWEEN 7/1/75 AND 7/1/76   TOTAL NUMBER OF AUDITS COMPLETED 13

AUDIT TYPES AND STUDY TOPICS

NUMBER PHYSICIAN ONLY 4
AUDIT STUDY TOPICS AND ID. NUMBERS:

Surgery for urinary bladder tumors	#11
Gastroenteritis in Infants	#15
Acute myocardial infection	#19
Caesarean section	#23

NUMBER MULTIDISCIPLINARY (PHYSICIANS AND OTHER HEALTH CARE PROVIDERS) 6
AUDIT STUDY TOPICS AND ID. NUMBERS:

Surgery for fractured hip	#12
Cerebrovascular accident	#13
Mastectomy for cancer	#14
Diabetic ketoacidosis	#17
Alcoholism	#21
Hysterectomy for fibroids	#22

NUMBER NONPHYSICIAN ONLY 3
AUDIT STUDY TOPICS AND ID. NUMBERS:

Congestive heart failure	#16
Discharge planning	#18
Urinary tract infections	#20

NUMBER OF RECORDS AND AUDITS PER PROVIDER

PROVIDER	No. REC	No. AUD	PROVIDER	No. REC	No. AUD	PROVIDER	No. REC	No. AUD	PROVIDER	No. REC	No. AUD

Exhibit 10-11 Completed Cross-Audit Provider Profile for One Physician Audited During a 12-Month Audit Period

CROSS-AUDIT PROVIDER PROFILE*

Reprinted with permission.

PROVIDER	AUDITS COMPLETED BETWEEN ___ AND ___				NUMBER OF AUDITS					TOTAL NUMBER OF RECORDS AUDITED ___		TOTAL DEFICIENCIES ATTRIBUTED TO THE PROVIDER ___	
CRIT. CLASS AND TYPE DEF. CAUSE	DOC	KNOWL. SKILL	KNEW, DIDN'T DO	LACK EQUIP	LACK PERS	POLICY, PROC.	M.R. FORMS	OVER-UTIL	ENVIRON-MENTAL	OTHER	TOTAL		
JUSTIFICATION Diagnosis,Problem													
Surgery													
Procedure													
Admission													
OUTCOME Discharge Status													
Pt. Knowledge													
Follow-up Plan													
Mortality													
INDICATOR Length of Time													
Critical Process													
Critical Clue													
Comp/Crit. Mgt.													
TOTAL													

FOR ONE PROFILE FOR EACH PROVIDER AUDITED DURING PERIOD

Exhibit 10-12

	Utilization Review	Patient Care Audit	Profile Analysis
Purpose	Assessment of admissions and LOS to ensure necessity and appropriate levels of care	Ensure and document that health services provided are of optimal achievable quality	Assist in identification of problems and assessment of the impact of review procedures
Focus	Individual patient transactions and assessment of patient need	Groups of similar patient transactions and assessment of patterns provider performance	Institutions and practitioners both individual and collectively and assessment of program performance
Criteria	Established or adapted by UR Committee, 3d party carrier, or PSRO	Generally established by hospital's audit committee(s)	Established by the PSRO and/or designated hospitals
	Directed to appropriateness of admissions and length of stay	Directed to validation of diagnosis and justification of admission and special procedures, the assessment of outcomes, and other discrete indicators of care	Directed to comparisons of patterns of care by similar providers and gauging impact of review procedures

Exhibit 10-12 Continued

	Utilization Review	Patient Care Audit	Profile Analysis
Timing	Concurrent	Retrospective	Retrospective
Data source	Active record, provider input	Completed record	Statistical reports
Action orientation	Certification or denial of admissions or extensions of stay	Identifies problems and directs corrective action, documents quality of services	Revision of procedures of review

established, the responsibilities currently held by Medicare contractors and the Medicaid state agencies with respect to determination of medical necessity and quality will be relinquished to the PSRO. Medicare and Medicaid through their fiscal agents will continue to retain responsibility for determination of eligibility, definition of coverage, and determination of the appropriateness of charges. The PSROs, however, will assume full responsibility for all decisions having to do with quality, appropriateness, and necessity of services. When a PSRO is carrying out its review responsibility, retroactive review will not have the potential to lead to denial of payment.

Individual Facilities Program Control

Regardless of the power of control implied in the foregoing summary, the courts have leaned toward delegating the medical care review process to individual hospitals and have instructed the PSROs to do so if at all possible. The delegation process indicates that a given hospital review committee that demonstrates a capacity for effective review can have UR and medical audit procedures delegated to the committee.

The preceding tasks defined by individuals and specific groups/committees are drawn from the six stages developed by the Health Care Evaluation Program sponsored through the Foundation for Health Care Evaluation, Minneapolis, Minnesota.[11] This health care evaluation program was established by local physicians who were concerned with providing quality health care to all patients at a reasonable cost. It is an area adaptation of the PSRO regulations and offers readers a model program designed for further modification within their own individual applications. It meets the requirements for PSRO legislation and the requirements for Title XVIII, Title XIX, and Title V. It is intended, however, to target a comprehensive review for all patients so that quality health care can be obtained. This is an example of a delegated program.

Let's look now at the process of delegation. How does a health information manager establish a program that includes the kind of task definitions, sequencing, and resource allocations we have just examined? With a clear understanding of the legislation and a model program structure in mind, let's see how this is to be accomplished in accordance with PSRO regulation.

1. The PSRO notifies the hospital of provisions contained in the legislation regarding delegation.
2. After examining the written communication, a hospital seeking delegation must provide the PSRO with a letter of intent indicating the review activities that it hopes will qualify for delegated status.

3. The PSRO must assess the hospital's capabilities for carrying on this process.
4. Within 90 days of the date of the preliminary letter of intent, the hospital must prepare and forward to the PSRO a formal review plan that conforms to requirements specified by the PSRO.
5. Following review of the hospital's formal plan and considering the findings of the PSRO's initial assessment of the hospital's capabilities, delegated status determination will be made and communicated to the hospital. This will be carried out through a written memorandum of agreement that specifies the terms of relationship between the hospital and the PSRO. This includes conditions that might lead to reassessment or reconsideration of the review activity as a result of PSRO monitoring.
6. When approved, the terms of the memorandum of agreement and the hospital's formal review plan can be implemented.
7. The PSRO will maintain responsibility and monitor the review activities that the hospital has assumed.

The PSROs will maintain responsibility in four ways:

1. They will evaluate the UR plan and UR committee structure in a given hospital.
2. They will target statistical information that must be collected and analyzed to evaluate the time limits and performance of the hospital's UR committee, as far as current review is concerned.
3. The PSROs will conduct on-site visits to witness and evaluate the review process and to be sure that the statistical data that have been collected accurately reflect activities.
4. The PSRO will evaluate medical care evaluation studies. This will include:
   a. The number of studies completed to date
   b. The number of studies in progress
   c. Description of the studies in terms of the following characteristics
   - topic
   - parameters in criteria
   - aggregate results
   - action taken or recommended on results
   - date of results or reaudit, if applicable

Medical Record Practitioner Role

In April 1977, Jane Rogers, RRA, outlined the role of practioners in PSRO *Perspective of Medical Record News.*

Increased activity in the MCE study function and involvement of health care practitioners other than physicians mandate a new management, coordination, and leadership role for the medical record practitioner. Increased demands on the medical record and medical record department require greater emphasis on planning, coordination, and education activities of the total MCE function. What can and should the medical record profession do to meet this challenge?

1. Accept the role of Medical Care Evaluation Coordinator in the health facility.
2. Review PSRO documents with health facility administration, the medical staff, and audit chairman.
3. Meet with each health care practitioner other than physician discipline in the hospital to review:
   - requirements for peer review
   - peer review activity and criteria developed by each discipline
   - statistical and data sources available from the medical record department (medical records, code books, indices, hospital statistics and reports)
   - hospital peer review activities in process and MCE methodologies used
4. Coordinate a plan for incorporating nonphysician practitioners into the present MCE study process. Place emphasis on efficiency, economy, and effectiveness of methodology.
5. Review criteria, norms, standards, methodologies, and professional journal articles prepared by allied health professionals (physical therapy, occupational therapy, podiatry, etc.).
6. Contact the local PSRO and review the proposed policies for nonphysician peer review.
7. Local and state medical record associations:
   a. Organize and become members of PSRO Advisory Groups.
   b. Invite local allied health groups to present continuing education programs on peer review in their discipline.

Coordination of the MCE study function is essential to the efficiency, economy, and effectiveness of peer review. Medical record practitioners have the background, experience, and education in audit methodology and management to provide effective leadership for the entire peer review team. We must accept this challenge.

IDENTIFYING AND APPLYING EXISTING RESOURCES

We have looked at legislation, a model structure, and the need for an active medical record professional in establishing an effective MCE system and have reviewed key terms and concepts. We'll pause now to note that using existing resources must be an integral part of an MCE program. Program developers need to explore existing models. These programs, like discharge abstract systems, must be carefully weighed against the individual facilities requirements.

We have drawn on the *Masters Manual* by Care Communications, Inc., for many of our examples in this chapter. The Masters program has all necessary elements for meeting accrediting and certification requirements. Along with the Masters program, there are other models designed to provide specific programs for health facilities. The Quality Assurance Program (QAP) for medical care in hospitals was developed by the AHA for use by hospital administrators and medical staffs in the development of a hospital program to assure the quality of care given in the hospital. It is another example of a currently available model resource. The Computerized Audit and Record Evaluation System (CARE) is a system developed to specifications for Kings County Hospital Center in Brooklyn, New York. It is an example of a tailored system designed for a particular application. Health facilities may design their own individual programs. In many states the PSRO has designed MCE programs for use in nondelegated hospitals.

Potential audit coordinators need to investigate all such resources before making a decision for their particular application. They also need to establish and maintain a library for reference in working with audit systems. Criteria banks, data retrieval procedures, and data display techniques are all helpful tools. The list in Exhibit 10-13 is a directory to current publications that will keep audit coordinators informed about up-to-date analysis and revisions of quality assurance expectations.

Reading over this list of resources, the reader can readily determine that there is a wide range of sources and regulating bodies that profoundly affect patient care appraisal systems. An interesting factor is that the JCAH is still recognized as an authority in the field of standardization of health care. That recognition is reflected in the Medicare legislation itself. Section 1861 of the Medicare law designates JCAH accreditation as one of the requirements for eligibility for reimbursement, so that to even participate in the federal programs, hospitals must first meet the criteria established by the JCAH.

COMPUTER TECHNOLOGY—A USEFUL TOOL

The impact of computer technology has been felt at all levels of medical care evaluation. Several UR computer systems now exist and more are being developed. Medical audit, while not as fully developed, is also employing this technology. Pattern analysis is most amenable to established software packages that perform statistical analysis in a data base management mode.

Exhibit 10-13 Current Resources about Up-to-Date Analysis and Revision of Quality Assurance Expectations

- Guidelines and intermediary letters from the Bureau of Health Insurance of the Social Security Administration
- Regulations in the *Federal Register*
- Interpretation of guidelines made by Medicare intermediaries
- Guidelines in the PSRO program manual
- Interpretation of the PSRO manual by local PSROs
- Technical Assistance Documents (TADs) identified as numbered transmittals by the PSRO
- Guidelines and regulations written by state agencies for the Medicaid program
- Interpretations of these guidelines and regulations as well as the Medicare guidelines and regulations by the state licensing bureaus
- Recommendations by the JCAH
- Recommendations by state medical associations and hospital associations
- Recommendations by the AMA and the AHA
- Recommendations by abstracting services, such as the Professional Activities Study Medical Audit Program (PAS/MAP)
- Recommendations by medical care foundations for starting prepaid health plans or health maintenance organizations

Health record professionals working with MCE must develop an understanding of these applications as well as of the skills necessary to provide leadership and direction in computer systems planning. Chapter 9 outlined the particular skills required by patient data managers in developing computer applications generally. These will be critical here. Recalling that objectives setting and output design are among the first tasks involved in planning such a system, let's look briefly at how these two components translate into planning a computerized utilization review program. Objectives of such a program might be to:

- Collect all data necessary to meet PSRO federal reporting requirements
- Facilitate data use for patient review and facility management
- Provide production reports that monitor facility utilization of resources that can be used for evaluating overall effectiveness of the UR plan
- Include methods for updating and refining file resources within the system, including changes in LOS norms and updating criteria and standards

- Provide for timely, planned updates to the system to review current operations and plan new applications
- Incorporate an interface with existing computer applications inside and outside the facility
- Develop specific plans for interface with planned computer applications inside and outside the facility
- Save costs that would be incurred by maintaining the existing system
- Provide methods for direct transfer of data to the PSRO through magnetic tape as feasible
- Provide daily screen displays or printouts that can be used both as output documents for review assistance and as a basis for data feedback into the system

These are some of the objectives that might be used in planning this application. Let's look at potential outputs. Remember that output descriptions are drawn from the established objectives and are the performance specifications of the system. An on-line, interactive computerized utilization review system could produce the following outputs:

- An automatically generated patient discharge abstract form for all discharged patients
- An automatically generated BQA Form 121, Concurrent Review Summary
- An automatically generated BQA Form 131, MCE Study Abstracts
- An automatically generated BQA Form 133, Restudy Report
- An automatically generated BQA Form 135, MCE Study Status Report
- Other specified forms judged by the health facility to be cost-beneficial byproducts of the system
- Automatic transmission of data to PSRO

As identified in Chapter 9, individual facilities have many options in developing computerized URs. They may use existing resources when available, through purchase of UR packages. They may build a system to their own specifications, such as the CARE system described in preceding sections. They can consider acquisition of minicomputers or microprocessors for the application, or they can participate in a Time Share System. Many computer resources are directing efforts to employ teleprocessing to create networks so that participating health facilities may work from CRT terminals on site and transmit data for processing and manipulation over phone lines to a host computer in a central location. Systems analysis should pinpoint the most appropriate decision in each case.

When we turn to medical audit systems for implementing effective medical care evaluation systems, the computer is used essentially as a support and screening aid component of the system. This area is not as well developed as the utilization review components, but still reveals imaginative applications when investigated. Figure 10-5 on the following page is a schematic showing screening sequence in a medical audit application.[12] As you review it, consider some sample objectives of such a system.

- To assure the quality of care for all patients in the facility
- To assure effective provider decisions based on comprehensive access to patient care information
- To target system breakdowns in the structure and/or process of the health care delivery system
- To maximize computer technology in screening aids and exception reporting methods to expedite and monitor the MCE process
- To assure a comprehensive continuing education program for providers based on analysis and evaluation of existing health care services.

Looking at the schematic, can you think of some output descriptions like the ones identified in the utilization review application?

- Can you see how this system might be interfaced with the UR system we just described?
- Are there functional operations within a hospital that might already maintain some of the data elements needed to construct this type of application?
- What are some specific questions you would like to ask about this type of application?

Again, using the process identified in Chapter 9, analytical, top-down viewing will be a critical resource to medical record professionals.

Pattern analysis is fraught with technologic possibilities. Excellent statistical analysis software packages are available. Many of these are options of Time Sharing Programs. Others may be purchased and used on individual microprocessors within a health facility. As MCE programs build up data resources through the reviewing activities, a gradual data base will be developed. Computer technology is the only way that appropriate statistical analysis can unveil patterns of care and accomplish it on a cost-effective and comprehensive basis. PSROs and health facilities need to explore the options. Data analysis and manipulation can be done in batch-run operations or in on-line mode. This potential underscores the major philosophy of this text. Health information is collected, processed, stored, and retrieved for *use* by providers for individual care and by planners and

Figure 10-5 An Operational Model of Systematic Peer Review

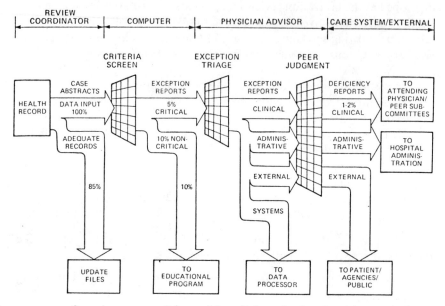

An operational model of systematic peer review

Screening sequence. Schema of flow of information from its origin in medical record, preparation of a case abstract for input into the data system (computer processing), reporting of an exception (deviation) from preset criteria, rendering of a judgment by a physician advisor that a true care deficiency has occurred, ranking of these deficiencies as to type and origin, and referral of these deficiencies from level 1 to level 2 peer groups. Progressively fewer cases are passed through the screens, as there are data sinks at each step.

Source: Ertel, P.Y., and Aldridge, M.G., Medical Peer Review, The C.V. Mosby Company, 1977. Reprinted with permission.

---

evaluators for collective care. This is a key example of emerging potential in the analysis of patient and health data for the express purpose of using it to plan and put into practice the best, most effective health care system possible.

NOTES

1. P.L. 79-725, Hill-Burton Law, 1946.

2. P.L. 89-237, Regional Medical Programs, 1965.

3. P.L. 89-749, Comprehensive Health Planning and Public Health Service Amendment, 1966.

4. P.L. 89-97, Medicare/Medicaid Amendments to the Social Security Act, 1965.

5. U.S. Department of Health, Education and Welfare, *Standards for Certification for Participation in Title XVIII for Hospitals* (Washington, D.C., 1965), p. 22.

6. P.L. 92-603, Professional Standard Review, 1972.

7. Leslie Fox, Gerry Stearns, and Walter Imbiorski, *The Masters Manual* (Chicago, Ill.: Care Communications, Inc. 1977), p. 4.

8. AMRA, "PSRO Position Paper," *Medical Record News* 46, no. 6 (December 1975), p. 29.

9. U.S. Department of Health, Education and Welfare, Office of Professional Standards Review, *PSRO Program Manual* (Rockville, Md., 1974).

10. Comparative Aspects of Medical Care Evaluation, Joint Commission on Accreditation of Hospitals, "Quality Review Seminar on Medical Audit," (JCAH), p. 9.

11. Sharon Van Sell Davidson, ed., *PSRO Utilization and Audit in Patient Care* (St. Louis, Mo.: C.V. Mosby Co., 1976), p. 95.

12. Paul Y. Ertel and Gordon C. Black, "An Operational Model of Systematic Peer Review," *Medical Peer Review* (St. Louis, Mo.: C.V. Mosby, 1977), p. 205.

REFERENCES

Ainsworth, Thomas H., Jr. *Quality Assurance in Long Term Care*. Germantown, Md.: Aspen Systems Corp., 1977.

Davidson, Sharon Van Sell, ed. *PSRO Utilization and Audit in Patient Care*. St. Louis, Mo.: C.V. Mosby Co., 1976.

Ertel, Paul Y. and Aldridge, M. Gene., ed. *Medical Peer Review Theory and Practice*. St. Louis, Mo.: C.V. Mosby, 1977.

Greene, Richard. *Assuring Quality in Medical Care*. Cambridge, Mass.: Ballinger Publishing Co., 1976.

Glossary

Abortion—the expulsion or extraction of all (complete) or any part (incomplete) of the placenta or membranes without an identifiable fetus, with a live born infant or a stillborn infant weighing less than 500 gm, or after an estimated length of gestation of less than 20 completed weeks (139 days) calculated from the first day of the last normal menstrual period.

Abiscissa side—the horizontal side of a graph, used for values.

Accession number—the number given each order as it occurs.

Accreditation—a process of evaluation of the physical, medical, and administrative as well as social and rehabilitative services provided by a health care facility.

ACS—American College of Surgeons.

Active medical staff—physicians and dentists who are responsible for the greatest amount of medical practice within the hospital and who perform all significant staff, organizational, and administrative functions.

Adjunct diagnostic or therapeutic unit (ancillary unit)—an organized unit of a hospital, other than an operating room, delivery room, or medical care unit, with facilities and personnel to aid physicians in the diagnosis and treatment of patients through the performance of diagnostic or therapeutic procedures.

Administrator—an individual who works at the direction of the Board of Trustees to carry out the specific functional activity of the organization.

Admission certification—a set of medical elements that are used to determine justification for hospital admission.

Agencies, associations, societies—extensions of the individuals who deliver or participate in the delivery of health care; organized groups.

AHA—American Hospital Association.

665

AHR—Association for Health Records; a multidisciplinary forum for the exchange of information among all persons in the field of medical and health information.

AMRA—American Medical Record Association.

Aperture card—punch card with film attached.

ART—Accredited Record Technician; an individual who has achieved a specified educational level and successfully completed a national qualifying examination.

Associate medical staff—physicians or dentists who are new to the staff and are being considered for advancement to the medical staff.

Audit measurement—comparison of actual practice to preestablished criteria.

Audit trial report — a report of an audit or check on the accuracy of a computer application. These reports can be computer generated as a part of a data security program.

Auxiliary computer storage—supplements to the main storage which are usually of higher capacity and lower speed or longer access time. Because central memory is limited and expensive relative to the size of programs and the data sets requiring processing, most computers have devices, usually disks, attached to them which store large amounts of data (millions or billions of characters). Data are then transferred in blocks between auxiliary storage and central memory as the data in central memory are exhausted. Transfer of data between auxiliary storage and central memory is slower than the rate at which data may be moved between the CPU and memory. Secondary storage can also include magnetic tape, magnetic drum, and card readers.

Average daily inpatient census — the average number of inpatients present each day for a given period of time.

Average length of stay — the average length of hospitalization of inpatients discharged during the period under consideration.

Bar charts — the depiction of relationships among elements. The rectangle is the essential representation of the area of the bar.

Batch processing method — the processing of the data that has been accumulated in advance such that each accumulation of data or batch thus formed is processed during the computer run. An in-house computer system could use batch processing to prepare a discharge analysis of services each month.

Board of Directors of AMRA — a ten member board elected by the active membership of the American Medical Record Association.

Board of trustees — governing body; the highest level of organization administration, it bears full legal and moral responsiblity for professional services provided by the facility.

Bureau of Quality Assurance (BQA) — agency which reports to the Health Services Administration and is responsible for the administration of the Professional Standards Review Organization (PSRO).

Business records as evidence — a record of an act, condition, or event which, insofar as it is relevant, shall be competent evidence if the custodian or other qualified witness testifies to its identity and the mode of its preparation, if it was made in the regular course of business at time near the time of the act, condition, or event, and if in the opinion of the court the source of information, method, and time of preparation were such as to justify its admission. This refers to admitting the medical record to the court as evidence and the testimony by the medical record administrator or a designee that this is in fact a record kept in the regular course of business.

CARE — Computerized Audit and Record Evaluation System.

Cathode Ray Tube Terminals (CRTs) — common instruments for transmitting data to a computer retrieving data from the computer and displaying them in a visual manner so that anyone can read them. Cathode ray terminals may have typewriter keyboards for communication and display data on a TV-like screen.

Census — the number of inpatients present in a health care facility at any one time.

Central Processing Unit (CPU) — the part of a computer system that contains the circuits which control the interpretation and execution of instructions, including the arithmetic, logic, and control functions.

Centralized filing system — a system in which all information is filed in one central location.

Charge-out devices — simple cardboard ledgers in a file that a user or a clerk fills out, noting date and destination of chart.

Chart analysis — careful review of the entire record; identification of specific areas that are incomplete.

Chart-out guide — a file ledger that records the date and name of the person removing the record and the reason for removing it.

Clinic — a physical site that provides office space for several physicians who are organized to serve patients through their cooperative efforts.

Clinical algorithm — application of algorithms which are procedures consisting of a finite number of steps for solving a problem in medicine. Algorithms may contain a number of branch points where the next step depends on the outcome of the preceding step.

Cluster sampling — a sampling procedure that selects population elements in groups or clusters. Medical record administrators may use sampling when ascertaining particular growth patterns of cards in a master patient index file, for example.

CMT — current medical terminology; a dictionary of preferred terms in medicine.

Coding — a numerical assignment that provides an organized approach to data retrieval. Codes are symbolic abbreviations that allow information to be categorized into succinct forms for ease of storage and use.

COM — computer output microfilm system; the process of translating computer-generated information into a miniature image on film.

Complication — a detrimental condition arising after the beginning of hospital observation and treatment and modifying the course of the patient's illness or the medical care required.

Computer conversion plan — a formal plan for converting to a new computer system.

Computer interactive processing (mode, conversational) — an operation of data processing systems such that the user, at an input-output terminal, carries on a conversation with the system. Since a prompt response is obtained from the system as each unit of input is entered, a sequence of runs can take place between the user and the system typical of a conversation.

Computer primary or main storage (also referred to as main memory) — a device in a computer in which the binary bit representations of program instructions and data are stored. The memory device is very closely linked with the CPU so that individual program instructions and data elements may be obtained from memory very rapidly.

Computer program — a set of instructions stored in the computer which directs it to perform a specific process.

Computer system design and resource allocation phase — the process of formulating a plan which describes the specifications determined in the study phase. It includes allocation of staff time, determination of required software, identification of required documentation for computer operations programs and user applications, and determination of required hardware functions.

Computer system development and conversion planning phase — time period or phase in which the actual computer programs are written, hardware purchased, and conversion plan formally prepared for a specific computer application.

Computer system operation phase — the phase in which the computer system becomes operational and its performance is reviewed and measured against original objectives.

Computer system study phase — a fundamental examination of an operation that needs to be improved or evaluated. It includes problem identification and can include all the steps of a feasibility analysis. It may be used synonymously with feasibility analysis.

Computer user manual — a procedure manual for computer applications usually prepared in the computer system design process as part of the documentation of the system.

Computerized word processing system — a system, based on microprocessor technology, in which medical stenographers type dictation directly into computer terminals. Errors can be easily corrected by inserting items or lines where appropriate. This information, once it is proofread, is then printed out on an impact printer.

Concurrent review — a form of medical care review that occurs during the patient's hospitalization. It consists of a review of the patient's need for a hospital or skilled nursing facility's level of care and may include an assessment of the quality of care being provided.

Confidential information — a statement made to a lawyer, physician, or clergyman in confidence with the implicit understanding that it should remain a secret.

Confidentiality — status accorded to data or information which is sensitive for some reason and therefore must be protected against theft or improper use and disseminated only to individuals or organizations authorized to have it.

Consent — concurrence of wills; voluntary yielding of one's will to the proposition of another; acquiescence or compliance.

Consulting medical staff — staff members who provide consulting services to other members of the staff on an on-call or regularly scheduled basis.

Contestant — one contesting a decision.

Continued stay review — the review carried on during a patient's hospitalization to determine the medical necessity and appropriateness of continuation of care at that level.

Control selection — a technique of sampling developed to increase the likelihood (over that of random sampling) of choosing a preferred combination of sampling units while maintaining probability methods.

Controlled-decentralized system — a system in which all forms, requisitions, filing procedures, methods, and processes are standardized so that records in the various areas are maintained identically.

Courtesy medical staff — physicians or dentists who have privileges to admit patients only occasionally.

CPT — current procedural terminology; a coding method for diagnostic and therapeutic procedures in surgery, medicine, and the specialties.

Criteria — predetermined elements against which aspects of the quality of medical service may be measured; for instance, two criteria for care of a urinary tract infection might be a urinalysis and urine culture.

Critical management — the minimal preventive and responsive procedures concerning a complication that must be documented in the record to convince the audit committee that everything necessary was done to prevent the complication or that the complication was promptly recognized and appropriately treated.

Daily inpatient census — the number of inpatients present at the census-taking time each day, plus any inpatients who were both admitted and discharged after the census-taking time the previous day.

Data Collection Network (DCN) — a computer-coordinated system that collects, stores, and disseminates information from a computer center. The information is collected initially from several health care institutions or agencies, which also have access to a central computer or group of linked computers.

Data entries — all the items of information that are entered into a health record.

Data entry — inputting information into a computer for processing.

Data security — the policies and procedures established by an organization to protect its information from unauthorized or accidental modification, destruction, and disclosure.

Data Security Administrator — a specially trained medical record administrator who is proficient in information science, medical information handling, and data security systems maintenance and supervision. The person must be trained and/or certified by a recognized authority verifying the individual's level of expertise.

Debug — to detect, identify the source, and fix errors in a computer program.

Decentralized filing system — a system in which files are usually located close to the source of their active use.

Defendant — a person required to make answer in an action or suit; a person to whom an action is brought. In malpractice this could be the physician and the hospital.

Deficiency — a nonjustifiable variation from expected standards.

Delegation of review — method of performing peer review whereby the PSRO delegates to the health care facility responsibility for performing actual review functions.

Denial — disapproval of continued payment by the fiscal intermediary. In Medicare a patient may be disallowed benefits if the length of stay exceeds the norm or standard without appropriate justification.

Denominator — number that represents a large group of related conditions, individuals, or events counted; the part of the fraction below the line.

Deposition — the written testimony of a sworn witness in response to interrogation, testimony taken on oath in writing outside of the courtroom to be used as evidence.

Descriptive statistics — numerically described events, services, patients, charges, and other agency activity to demonstrate and quantify the operations of the agency.

Direct patient data — facts that the patient actually states or displays to another person.

Discharge analysis — the tabulation of data on discharged hospital patients to reflect the professional services provided in the hospital.

Discharge transfer — the disposition of an inpatient to another health care institution at the time of discharge.

Disease and operation index — a numerical index of patient problems, diagnoses, and procedures by individual categories.

Dividers — heavy-weight fabric forms of pressboard, used to designate alphabetical breaks in the folders or highlight numerical divisions within the filing system.

DSM — Diagnostic and Statistical Manual of Mental Disorders.

ECF — extended care facility. This term preceded SNF (Skilled Nursing Facility) to designate nursing homes which had been certified to care for Medicare patients.

Elements — specific services, tests, and/or parameters of care which are grouped together and considered the identifiable parts that make up a criterion. For instance, a reviewer may look at three individual elements to see if a particular criterion was met.

Emergency — any condition which could result in serious permanent harm to a patient or aggravation of injury or disease, or in which the life of a patient is in immediate danger and any delay in administering treatment could add to that danger.

Evidence (primary) — that evidence that suffices for the proof of a particular fact until contradicted or overcome by other evidence.

Exception — identified case to which specified standards do not apply. For instance, complications may warrant an extension of the patient's stay in the hospital.

Executive committee of the medical staff — group of staff members empowered to act for the staff in intervals between medical staff meetings.

Expert witness — a person testifying to facts within his or her own knowledge who may give opinions upon assumed facts.

Family numbering — a system in which the family is assigned one number and the individual family members are assigned subnumbers.

Feasibility analysis — the process that examines, identifies, and ranks alternative solutions to a problem. It evaluates the probable soundness of such elements as hardware, software, cost analysis, and staffing against performance specifications required in a given application.

Federal Register — a publication that makes regulations and legal notices issued by federal agencies available to the public.

File folders — solid, two-sided binders of Kraft, manila, pressboard, or patented composition used to store paper records.

Fiscal intermediary — an organization acting in an intermediate role for dispersing funds from the federal government. Blue Cross, for example, acts as a fiscal intermediary in the Medicare program.

Focused review — a review of target areas or cases identified through analysis of the data system as questionable in effective utilization of resources. This allows a utilization review program to bypass repetitive activities on well-defined topic areas that have exhibited consistent effective utilization of services.

Format — the arrangement of a form, or an organization of forms in a permanent file folder, which directs the type of entries, the way entries are made, and the future use of those entries.

Frequency distribution — a number of predetermined classes with counts of the number of cases or observations that fall within the interval for each class.

GANTT chart — a program management chart that tracks the progress of a project against a predetermined schedule.

Glossary of hospital terms — hospital statistical terms, definitions, and formulas.

Grants — projects funded through federal appropriations approved by the U.S. Congress and provided through the direction of federal agencies and programs for ongoing and new health care programs.

Gross autopsy rate — the ratio during any given period of time of all inpatient autopsies to all inpatient deaths.

Group practice — care provided by a group of physicians who usually represent a fairly broad spectrum of medical specialties.

Hardware — the physical machinery and equipment that comprise a computer system.

Health — the state of complete physical, mental, and social well-being.

Health care — the restoration or preservation of health; the providing of relief, comfort, and healing to the sick.

Health care delivery — a set of separate, related, but essentially nonunified health care activities not all working toward a single purpose.

Health care practitioners — other than physicians, those health professionals who (a) do not hold a doctor of medicine or doctor of osteopathy degree, (b) meet all applicable state or federal requirements for practice of their profession, and (c) are actively involved in the delivery of patient care or services that may be paid for, directly or indirectly, under Titles V, XVIII, and/or XIX of the Social Security Act.

Health information — any data pertaining to the physical, mental, or social well-being of an individual or group of individuals.

Health record — documentation of direct or indirect health care services to patients/clients by providers and users of the data in any type of health-related institution.

Hearsay — statements not made under oath by someone who is not a party in interest, nor a party to the action.

HEW — Department of Health, Education and Welfare.

HMO — health maintenance organization.

Honorary staff — those individuals recognized for their noteworthy contributions to patient care, outstanding professional reputation, and/or their long service to the hospital.

Hospital autopsy rate (adjusted) — ratio of autopsies actually performed to the number of bodies of deceased persons available for autopsy.

Hospital cesarean section rate — the ratio of cesarean sections performed in a hospital to deliveries. For statistical purposes, a delivery resulting in a multiple birth is counted as one delivery.

Hospital computer system — a hospital electronic data processing and communications system which provides on-line processing with interactive responses for patient data within the hospital and its outpatient department, including ancillary services such as clinical, laboratory, x-ray, pharmacy, etc.

Hospital fetal death — a death prior to the complete expulsion or extraction from the mother, in a hospital facility, of a product of conception, irrespective of the duration of pregnancy. Death is indicated by the fact that, after such separation, the fetus does not breathe or show any other evidence of life such as beating of the heart, pulsation of the umbilical cord, or definite movement of voluntary muscles.

Hospital inpatient — a hospital patient who is provided with room, board, and continuous general nursing service in an area of the hospital where patients generally stay at least overnight.

Hospital inpatient autopsy — a postmortem examination performed in a hospital facility, by a hospital pathologist or by a physician of the medical staff to whom the responsibility has been delegated, on the body of a patient who died during inpatient hospitalization.

Hospital live birth — the complete expulsion or extraction from the mother, in a hospital facility, of a product of conception which, after such separation, breathes or shows any other evidence of life such as beating of the heart, pulsation of the umbilical cord, or definite movement of voluntary muscles, whether or not the umbilical cord has been cut or the placenta is attached; each product of such a birth is considered live born.

Hospital patient — an individual receiving, in person, hospital-based or coordinated medical services for which the hospital is responsible.

Hospital record — a written account of all the services provided the patient from the time of admission until discharge. It identifies the dates and ward or room where the patient was physically located, names of the physicians, nurses, and other health professionals who provided care, and the results of the care.

House of Delegates of the AMRA — the official legislative body of the American Medical Record Association.

ICD — international classification of diseases; a basic three-digit code with four- and five-digit categories in some areas.

ICF — intermediate care facility.

ICHPPC — international classification of health problems in primary care; a method of classification for use by physicians in general and family practice throughout the world.

IMR — institution for the mentally retarded.

In loco parentis — in the relationship of a parent.

Independent contractor — one who exercises an independent calling and is subject to the control of no one in his or her work.

Index — an organized, condensed list of data that reflects more extensive data pertaining to one subject or source of information.

Indirect patient data — information which comes from the patient but requires an interpretation before it is usable.

Individual plan of care — document established to view the patient from the aspect of each health care provider. It pulls all portions of the available information together to develop a coordinated, individual plan for use by health care providers or family in further treatment programs.

Infection committee — committee responsible for substantiation of hospital v. nonhospital acquired infections, control of infection, and coordination of all other activities regarding infection control, including the reporting, evaluating, and maintaining of records of infections among patients and personnel.

Inference statistics — an analysis of population samples, services, or treatment results which is used to make an inferred judgment or assessment on the whole. Medical research, patient care appraisal, utilization review, length of stay by selected diagnosis, projected effects of new therapy, and studies on effects of nutrition on underprivileged children are all examples of inference statistics.

Information — knowledge or intelligence; facts, data.

Information activity list — a detailed record that provides information about the usage of patient information, i.e., how often it is requested.

Inpatient admission — the formal acceptance by a hospital of a patient who is to be provided with room, board, and continuous nursing service in an area of the hospital where patients generally stay at least overnight.

Inpatient bed count — the designated number of available hospital inpatient beds, both occupied and vacant, on any given day.

Inpatient bed occupancy ratio — the proportion of inpatient beds occupied, defined as the ratio of inpatient service days to the inpatient bed count days in the period under consideration; percent occupancy; occupancy percent; percentage of occupancy, occupancy ratio.

Inpatient census — the number of inpatients present at any one time.

Inpatient discharge — the termination of a period of inpatient hospitalization through the formal release of the inpatient by the hospital.

Inpatient service day — a unit of measure denoting the services received by one inpatient in one 24-hour period.

Interim patient record — a paper record made up primarily of computer printouts in those settings where patient information is maintained on the computer until discharge or cessation of treatment.

Intervention — peer review criteria that are applied during the process of medical care of an individual patient which may directly influence the action of the attending physician during care.

JCAH — Joint Commission on Accreditation of Hospitals.

Job description — a document containing information about a position such as required education or training, experience, lines of authority and designation of supervisor, as well as a general description of the job and major job objectives.

Judicial contest — any controversy that must be decided upon evidence.

Length of stay — the number of calendar days from admission to discharge of one inpatient.

Length of stay certification (also called recertification) — a statement in writing by the attending physician assuring that continued hospitalization is medically necessary. It must include diagnosis, complications, plan for care, and anticipated length of stay. It justifies a length of stay beyond the norm.

Letter distribution classification — a list prepared by the Department of the Navy and the Social Security Administration which shows how certain letters of the alphabet expand in a filing system. The expansion of each letter is described in percentages.

Level of care — the degree of services and health care available. The degree may be extensive or minimal depending on the health care needs of an individual patient.

Level of care criteria — standards used to determine the appropriate level of care—hospital, skilled nursing facility, intermediate care—for a given patient based on the types of service that can only be provided at that level.

Liability — state or quality of being liable; that which is under obligation to pay. Hospitals, nursing homes, and health care providers can all be considered liable for services they render.

Liability insurance — insurance to cover answerable claims, such as malpractice insurance.

Line chart — a graph which depicts movement and generally aids the reader in comprehending the material.

Litigation — the act of carrying on a suit in a law court.

Longitudinal health record — a patient record that includes medical information collected over an extended time, such as a family practice record that includes all medical data on an individual from birth to the present.

Majority — that age which qualifies an individual as legally responsible for his or her own acts; 21 years of age in most states.

Malpractice — improper, careless, or ignorant treatment.

Management data — data used by those who support the development, retention, and retrieval of patient data through their professional direction; information used by providers and users as well as patients, such as policy and procedure manuals, memos, bylaws, budgets, correspondence, and individual or specialized worksheets developed for individual departmental needs.

Master patient index — a condensed listing of data that provides identification and location information regarding medical or health records.

Mean — the arithmetic average of the value of a sample.

Median — the point at which half of the values of a sample fall above and half below.

Medicaid — the federal health program designed for the recipients of categorical aid programs, i.e., the medically indigent.

Medical audit — an evaluation system in which established standards are used to measure performance. Once corrective action has been taken on problems identified through a review process, performance is remeasured after an appropriate time period.

Medical audit committee — committee responsible for evaluation of the quality of patient care provided to patients by the medical and other professional staff who are directly responsible for patient care.

Medical audit follow-up — action taken as a result of medical audit committee recommendations. Action must be immediate if problems are life-threatening and must be documented to show improvement in patient care.

Medical care appraisal programs — program components which include utilization review of services, assessment of the patient's treatment, and examination of the end result of patient care.

Medical care evaluation — a structured program to measure the quality of care given to patients. It is a global term that encompasses methods used to carry out such measurement functions as audit, appraisal, peer review, quality assurance, and assessment in various specific forms.

Medical care evaluation studies (MCEs) — a retrospective medical care review in which an in-depth assessment is made of the quality and nature of the use of identified health services.

Medical care outcome — the end result of a patient's state of illness during an episode of treatment or a period of care during chronic illness.

Medical consultation — the response by one member of the medical staff to a request for consultation by another member of the medical staff, characterized by review of the patient's history, examination of the patient, and completion of a consultation report giving recommendations and/or opinions.

Medical Record Administrator — the individual responsible for developing and directing the objectives and activities that comprise an information system to compile and distribute patient/client data.

Medical record committee — committee which sees that accurate and complete medical records are developed and retained for every patient treated.

Medical staff — qualified medical personnel responsible for the quality of all medical care provided to patients and for the ethical conduct and professional practices of individual physicians.

Medical staff bylaws — rules and regulations which define duties, qualifications, and method of selection of officers of the medical staff.

Medicare — the federal health care program designed for persons over 65 years of age.

MEDLARS — Medical Literature Analysis and Retrieval System: a computer-based system derived from journals indexed for *Index Medicus, Index to Dental Literature,* and the *International Nursing Index.*

MEDLINE — MEDLARS on-line; a shortened form of the MEDLAR system.

Memorandum of understanding — a signed statement outlining the responsibilities of each party involved. Memoranda of understanding are between hospitals and PSROs and between fiscal intermediaries and PSROs.

Microfilming — a process of photographing and reducing a given report to a miniature of the original on film.

Mode — the one value in a sample that occurs with most frequency.

Monitor — to watch, observe, and check, especially to track, a particular item of information.

Morbidity — the incidence of disease or the proportion of diseases in a given population; statistical data that represents rates or ratios of disease.

Mortality — the incidence of deaths or the proportion of deaths in a given population; statistical data that represents rates or ratios of deaths.

MRP — medical record practitioner; an individual who works with medical records but has not successfully completed a national qualifying examination.

MSIS — Multi-State Information System, an automated information system for mental patients' records.

NAMCS — National Ambulatory Care Survey.

Negligence — failure to exercise the reasonable prudent care that the circumstances justly demand.

Net autopsy rate — the ratio during any given period of time of all inpatient autopsies to all inpatient deaths minus unautopsied coroners' or medical examiners' cases.

Nominal scales — the enumeration of attribute data, i.e., survival status. The summary measure is the proportion of cases that exhibit the attribute.

Non compos mentis — of unsound mind, including all forms of mental unsoundness.

Nonphysician health care providers — those health professionals who do not hold a doctor of medicine or osteopathy degree but are qualified by education or licensure to practice a profession and are involved in direct patient care services.

Nonprobability samples — samples which at some stage of sampling permit arbitrary choice of sampling units by the sampler.

Norm — a numerical or statistical measure of usually observed performance. Norms are identified by analyzing statistical data that record particular activities and results of a defined problem, diagnosis, or treatment.

Normal distribution — the bell-shaped curve which is a method of mathematically explaining the frequency of occurrences.

Notary public — public officer whose function is to administer oaths and to attest and certify by his or her hand or official seal certain classes of documents to give them authenticity in foreign jurisdictions.

Notary subpoena — an order issued by a notary public for the medical record to be taken to an attorney's office instead of to court. Used as part of a pretrial discovery procedure, this type of subpoena is intended to expedite the trial of cases.

Number index — a chronological listing of all numbers issued with cross references to the names of the patients to which the numbers have been assigned.

Numbering system — an identifying method that utilizes assigned numbers to label each record for filing in a systematic manner for easy retention and retrieval.

Numerator — that number representing the actual number of conditions, individuals, and events counted; the part of the fraction above the line.

Numerical continuum scale — the continuous along which clinical measurements such as blood pressure, height, and weight fall.

Objectives — a determination and a description of activities, stated in measurable terms, that lead toward a unified goal. They must be formulated in such a manner that all participants in the system understand what is to be achieved. The objective should have specific activities identified to describe what is to be done between the date of establishing the plan and the target date for reaching the goal.

Office of Professional Standards Review (OPSR) — agency which reports to the Assistant Secretary of the Department of Health, Education and Welfare (DHEW) and is responsible for staff activities for PSRO.

On-line — a device that currently is an operating part of the computer system. A terminal is on-line if it is logged into the system. An idle service is on-line if it may be activated by the computer.

On-line patient records — computerized patient records stored on a storage device which permits direct, immediate access through terminals.

Ordinate axis — the vertical side of a graph, usually used to designate the frequency.

Output descriptions — a detailed explanation of what will result from a computer action in a specific application. For example, a new form, format, or other combination of documents that produces data previously unavailable, such as a printout produced in the main file room that automatically prints all chart requests in two-part labels. The labels include patient number, name, requesting party, authorization code number (which tells the staff the requestor is authorized to access the chart), date, and time of request. One label is placed on the outguide and one on the chart. Another example is an activity summary produced at the end of the day that lists the number of charts requested, distribution of request frequency, and a list of all charts not returned for that day.

Parameters — values which vary according to the circumstances of their application. Each health problem has a unique set of parameters, that is, plans, tests, and treatments that are individually adapted to that problem.

Patient care audit — an objective, systematic evaluation of the quality of patient care based on two principles: (1) it is neither necessary nor efficient to examine every aspect of the patient care process; and (2) the results of careful comparison of actual practice against certain predetermined, objective measurable criteria accurately reflect the quality of patient care.

Patient carried personal health record — the written information which people keep about their personal health care and actually are responsible for physically storing and transporting.

Patient data — information gathered during a patient encounter with a professional health care provider.

Pattern analysis — a program to evaluate the effectiveness of medical care evaluation by comparing similar data over time. It is generally directed at the comparison of data regarding particular topics or characteristics.

PEP — performance evaluation procedure for auditing and approving patient care. Originated by the Joint Commission on Accreditation of Hospitals, this procedure originally focused on patient care outcomes.

Percentile — a value on a scale of 100 that indicates the percent of a distribution that is equal to or below it. For instance, 50th percentile for a group of hospitalized patients may be five days, which means that 50 percent of the patients stayed five days or less.

Performance testing — a dry run of the particular computer application to see if the results produced match the specifications laid out in the study phase.

PERT — Program Evaluation Review Technique.

Pharmacy committee — committee responsible for development of policies and practices relating to the selection and distribution of drugs.

Pharmacy profile record system — a system which provides immediate retrieval of information necessary for the pharmacist to identify previously dispensed medication at the time a prescription is presented. One profile card may be maintained for all members of a family living at the same address and possessing the same family name.

Pie charts — graphic presentation of relationships as percentages.

Plaintiff — one who commences personal action or suit to obtain a remedy for injury to his or her rights; the complaining party in any litigation. A patient suing a physician for malpractice would be the plaintiff.

Plan (POMR) — notation in the problem oriented medical record consisting of three parts: the plan for (1) collecting further data; (2) for initial treatment; and (3) for patient education. It explains what the patient must do, the results of the patient's own activities in the management of that problem, the results of the tests, and any prognosis that is available; it educates the patient regarding changes that may have to come about in life style in order to recover fully or live comfortably with a particular problem.

Playscript procedure — a procedure written in two columns in which the source or person carrying out the step is listed in the left-hand column and the steps to be carried out are listed in the right-hand column in exact chronological sequence.

Policy — a basic guide to action that prescribes the boundaries within which activities are to take place.

POMR (Problem Oriented Medical Record) — a system of organizing data entries in a patient record by titled and numbered problems that are determined by the clinician in reviewing the patient's direct data and the data base. The data base includes medical history, physical findings, and patient life-style information. Plans for investigation, treatment, and patient education as well as progress recording are all keyed to the problem numbers and titles.

Preadmission certification — a preadmission process that provides for formal certification of necessity for hospitalization prior to a patient occupying a bed in the hospital.

Prefix with the year — a system in which a number including the year of current treatment is assigned.

Prepaid care — health program which offers the patient the opportunity to pay for health care regularly whether it is needed or not, in exchange for which no charge is made when care is provided.

Prima facie — evidence sufficient to establish the fact and, if not rebutted, conclusive of the fact.

Printout — the printed data document from a computer operation. An on-line patient admission system in a hospital may create a printout of the admission information to be used as an identification and summary sheet in the hospital patient record.

Privacy — a right. To declare information confidential is to recognize formally the patient's inherent right to privacy.

Privileged communication — any information acquired by a physician or surgeon in attending a patient which was necessary to enable him or her to prescribe or act for the patient and which cannot be revealed in a civil action without the consent of the patient.

Problem — an aspect of the patient that disturbs or endangers the patient's health and that requires further attention for diagnosis, treatment, or observation.

Process — components of the total health care activity that are evaluated to determine adequacy of care. For instance, process components might include contraindicated drugs, excessive exposure to radiation, surgical intervention without documented workup, misfiled lab work, denied admission, adjustments in the care plan to accommodate changes in a patient's condition, routine physical exams, follow-up of abnormal lab or x-ray findings, etc. Process can be performed concurrent with care, addresses all direct and indirect providers, can directly interface and depend on patient's actions, and can relate directly to administrative and fiscal controls. The process of care also refers to effective documentation of the details of the patient's history and physical examination, other diagnostic measures, and specific treatment procedures. The Problem Oriented Medical Record is particularly geared to in-depth, effective operation of process audits.

Processing cycle — *see* Batch processing method, Computer interactive processing, Real time processing.

Professional — one who renders a personal service, possesses a specialized body of knowledge, observes ethical principles, maintains high standards, and participates in continuing education.

Profile analysis — a mechanism to judge the effectiveness of a PSRO or a hospital's review program by comparing similar data over time. It is generally directed at the comparison of data regarding a particular physician or health care provider.

PROMIS program — hospital-based computerized problem oriented medical record program that uses specific computer applications to aid health providers in recalling the memory elements of the patient record via CRT terminals.

Prospective review — a procedure for conducting the review process prior to the receipt of care. The purpose is to review the patient's condition and assure that the planned admission and the level of care are appropriate.

Provisional staff — individuals who have only recently been appointed to the medical staff. All initial appointments to the medical staff, except honorary and consulting, are provisional.

PSRO — Professional Standards Review Organization.

Punch cards — 80- or 96-column cards widely used for computer input. The hole combinations punched into cards are converted with electronic pulses by the card readers and sent to the CPU for processing.

QAP — Quality Assurance Program.

Quality assurance — activities performed to determine the extent to which a phenomenon fulfills certain values and standards, and to assure changes in practice that will fulfill the highest or a predetermined level of values.

Quality assurance mechanism — retrospective review program by the organized medical staff. It assesses the quality of care as compared to locally or internally developed standards and verifies that the standards or exceptions are met, that deficiencies are corrected, and that the original problem is reassessed on a planned program basis.

Quantitative analysis — descriptive statistics; a basic means of describing and understanding the population served by the health care system. There are three basic types: (1) numbers and demographic information; (2) health status, commonly referred to as morbidity (sickness) and mortality (death) information; and (3) utilization of goods and services.

Rate — a numerical expression that describes a relationship per time interval.

Ratio — a numerical expression that describes a relationship per number of total relationships.

Real time processing — a form of interactive processing in which the computer system records each change immediately and updates all the necessary files, etc. immediately. In health information a computerized on-line appointment system could be real time; intensive core computers that monitor patient heart functions, breathing, etc. are real time systems.

Rebuttal — defeat or removal of the effect of something; testimony intended to deny or contradict.

Recommended medical audit action — specific steps determined by the medical audit committee as a result of a completed audit. It must be specific to the problems identified and effective in accomplishing change.

Record control — that part of record retention and retrieval that provides (1) procedural elements that assure a permanent location for data to be maintained, (2) defined limits on retrieval of the data by particular users, and (3) methods to communicate continually the current location of a record.

Record destruction program — a plan that includes a time schedule and facility for routinely eliminating selected records from the files.

Record linkage — the process of connecting one individual's records, even though they were developed at different times and in different places, and combining them into one file by means of a common identifier.

Recorded instruments — certified copies of any deconveyance, bond, mortgage, or other writing that has been recorded, which can be accepted as evidence.

Refutation — the act of proving the falsity or error in a statement, a proposition, or an argument.

Register — a log that records all requests for information.

Registry — a synopsized listing of data that categorizes a larger group of data.

Release — a written instrument by which some claim or interest is surrendered to another person.

Reliable data — information obtained by means of a well-defined objective method for measurement which involves all or a representative sample of patients and practitioners.

Reported — acknowledged by executive committee, chief of the medical staff, chief executive officer, and governing body (for medical studies); acknowledged by chief executive officer, governing body, and chief of medical staff (for nursing service and other health care professionals' studies).

Res ipsa loquiter — "The occurrence speaks for itself" (the proof that an accident took place).

Research Grants Index — annual publication which is a source of information on health research currently supported by the health agencies of DHEW.

Research sampling techniques — alternative methods used to select appropriate representation of a given population; to use analysis of that representation to draw conclusions on the population.

Respondeat superior principle — principle that states "Let the master answer." Two factors must exist: employee-employer relationship, that is, the person must be employed by a facility, and the employee must act within the scope of his or her employment. This doctrine says the employer is responsible for the act of his or her agent or servant. A patient who sues a nurse also sues the hospital because the nurse is employed by the hospital.

Retention/retrieval — keeping information so that it may be used in the future; planning, implementation, and control of a system that safeguards the physical and information characteristics of medical or health data for future use.

Retention/retrieval manual — a written manual that describes what is to be completed, the method to be used, and the productivity level expected.

Retroactive denial — disapproval of payment based on retrospective review of the case. When this occurs, an appeals process is usually initiated in which further documentation from the patient's record is submitted and an additional review requested.

Retrospective review — an in-depth assessment of the quality or nature of the utilization of health services performed after the patient has been discharged.

Review — examination of a medical record by a physician to determine if continued hospitalization is medically necessary.

Review coordinator — a person responsible for the smooth functioning of the review program and the communication of information among patient, attending physician, hospital, and PSRO.

RFP — request for proposal.

RFVC — reason for visit classification.

RRA — Registered Record Administrator; one who has achieved a specified educational level and has successfully completed a national qualifying examination.

Rules of exclusion — rules that evidence offered will be excluded from the record of proceedings or from being received in evidence if it is not properly qualified or not properly identified. For this reason, medical record administrators direct staff to take medical records to court and testify to their identity as medical records from the institution in which they originated.

Satellite record system — a system in which the majority of records are filed in one major location but some records needed in other areas may be moved and may be kept in those areas for a certain period of time, being returned to the central file room only for permanent filing.

SCM — Society for Computer Medicine; an association which promotes the use of computers in medicine.

Screen — to compare documentation recorded in the medical record against preestablished criteria.

Screening — a process in which norms, criteria, and standards are used to analyze large numbers of cases in order to select cases not meeting these norms, criteria, and standards for study in greater depth.

Serial numbering — a system of numbering in which the patient is assigned a new number each time treatment is received.

Serial unit numbering — a system in which patients are assigned a new number each time they enter the system. All previous records are brought forward and reassigned the new number.

Service or care unit — a group of patients who have related diagnoses and/or kinds of treatment; a group of inpatient beds designated for a single specialty of the medical staff.

Shared Computer Systems — a commercial program that collects, processes, and reports statistics on patient services and needs assessments, based on analysis of abstracts of hospital discharges. Studies comparing individual hospital performance with similar facilities are available to client hospitals.

Shop book rule — a rule of evidence allowing the admission in evidence of a party's account books of original entry, that is, the business record of the facility. The medical record is in this category.

Simple random sampling — method of sampling in which every unit in the population is assured an equal and independent chance of selection. A table of random numbers applied to sequential accession numbers assigned to clinic patients is an example of this.

SNF — skilled nursing facility.

SNODO — standard nomenclature of disease and operations.

SNOMED — systematized nomenclature of medicine.

SNOP — systematized nomenclature of pathology.

SOAP (POMR) — subjective objective assessment plan. S subjective; notation of items, as symptomatic complaints of the patient, that cannot necessarily be measured or strictly defined and are considered subjective. O objective; notation of items that are observable and measurable, such as laboratory findings, color of skin, results of tests, blood pressure, pulse rate, and any other activity that can be observed by one of the health care providers. A assessment; a statement of what is currently happening to the patient, the severity of the illness, any changes or conclusions to be drawn about diagnoses, prognosis, or change in the patient's statement. P plan; short-range, diagnostic, patient educational, or long-range treatment, according to the assessment.

Social Security numbering — a system of numbering in which records are identified by the individual patient's Social Security number.

Software — the programs (and associated documentation) produced to operate the computer system.

Soundex system — a phonetic filing system that uses a combination of letters and code numbers to designate names.

Source document — document on which data are originally recorded (handwritten or typed) and from which data elements are extracted for input into a computerized data system.

Source oriented record — a record that maintains all reports and data from a given department in one section and keeps them in chronological sequence within each subsection.

Standard — generally, a measure set by competent authority as the rule for measuring quantity or quality. Conformity with standards is usually a condition of licensure, accreditation, or payment of services.

Standardization — the establishment of a baseline guide as to the minimum acceptable level of performance.

State statutory law — written law that is created and enacted by the state legislature. It is also referred to as administrative code.

Statistical display — a graphic arrangement of statistical information; for example, tables, charts, graphic illustrations, and computer plots.

Statute of limitations — a law limiting the period of time during which an action must be brought; the legal requirement regarding retention time periods for various business and medical documents.

Step chart — illustration of patterns of motion often used in place of a line chart.

Straight numerical filing — a method of filing in which documents are filed according to chronological sequence of assigned number.

Stratified sampling — dividing the patient population into homogenous groups according to some characteristic such as the type of service (surgical or cardiology) or source of payment (such as Medicare) and selecting a separate sample within each of those categories.

Subpoena duces tecum — a notice compelling the attendance of a person in court and ordering them to bring the books, documents, or other evidence described in the writ. It is signed by a clerk of the court or a deputy and directs a record administrator or employee of a medical record department to bring a particular record to court.

Suit — an action or process in a court for the recovery of a right or claim.

Summons — a process (document) served on a defendant in civil court action to secure his or her appearance in the action.

Surgical operation — one or more surgical procedures performed at one time for one patient via a common approach or for a common purpose.

System — related elements that are coordinated to form a unified result, specifically people, activities, equipment, materials, plans, and controls, working together to achieve a unified objective or whole; an array of components that interact to achieve some objective through a network of procedures that are integrated and designed to carry out a major activity.

Systematic sampling — the selection of every x number of individuals from a list or card file of patients, i.e., every fifth entry on a registrar or index, or all patients admitted on a certain day or intervals of days during a month.

Systems analysis — a problem-solving method for an overall, thorough analysis of an activity to determine the most appropriate method for accomplishing it. It is directed, but not limited to, knowledge and processes required for planning and implementing computer-based systems in health and patient information handling.

Tabs — the identifying extensions of folders.

Teleprocessing — data processing through the use of a combination of data processors, or computers, and telecommunications facilities.

Temporary staff — physicians or dentists who have been granted privileges for a limited period of time by the chief medical staff officer on the recommendation of the chief of a particular department.

Terminal digit filing — a method of filing by the last digits of a number instead of by the first digits. The entire number is broken into groups of twos or threes, with the last group being filed first.

Third party payment — that type of payment utilized by those who spend a regular part of their income or work benefits on health care insurance and, in turn, receive full or partial payment for their health care.

Time sharing operation — a system in which a number of users buy time and share resources of a central computer.

Tissue committee — committee responsible for the review of surgical procedures in the facility.

Title V — a federal health program for maternal and child health and crippled children's services.

Title XIX, Medicaid — a federal program designed to meet the health needs of persons who receive aid through the program for families with dependent children or who have only marginal income.

Title XVIII, Medicare — a federal health insurance program for people 65 years of age and older, and some people under 65 years who are disabled.

Tort — an injury or wrong committed with or without force to the person or property of another. Tort claims deal with civil or federal wrongs.

Total inpatient service days — the sum of all inpatient service days for each of the days in the period under consideration.

Total length of stay — the sum of the days stay of any group of inpatients discharged during a specified period of time.

Transfer (intrahospital) — a change in medical care unit, medical staff unit, or responsible physician of an inpatient during hospitalization.

Transfer data — an abstract or summary of an individual patient care plan to accompany the patient to another care facility.

Trial court — the formal examination of the matter in issue in a case before a competent tribunal for the purpose of determining such issues; the court before which issues of fact and law are first determined.

Type of care — the facilities and personnel available for health care and, more importantly, the objective of the care.

Unit numbering — a system in which only one number is assigned to the patient's record and is retained permanently.

Unit record system — a method that compiles all information on a single patient or subject and records it in one document and file folder.

Utilization review — the evaluation of the necessity, appropriateness, and efficiency of the use of medical services, procedures, and facilities. In a hospital this includes review of the appropriateness of admissions, services ordered and provided, length of stay, and discharge practices on the concurrent and retrospective basis. This can be done by a utilization review committee, PSRO peer review, or public agency.

Utilization review committee — committee which reviews all aspects of care in order to assure high-quality patient care through the effective use of equipment, personnel, materials, and the facility as a whole.

Valid criteria — standards stated in measurable rather than descriptive terms, precise enough to permit accurate evaluation; statements of optimal achievable care; measures of quality, which are (1) validation of diagnosis, (2) justification for admission, surgery, and/or special hazardous procedures, (3) statement of expected patient outcomes, and (4) processes of care or patient management, under appropriate circumstances.

Variation — finding or element not in agreement with the norm or standard.

Variation analysis — identification of conformance to and variations from the audit criteria. It requires explicit justification for all variations that are clinically acceptable, identification of problems in the provision of patient care (variations that are not clinically acceptable), and attribution of the problems to their source.

Variation justification — an acceptable reason why a given finding or element is not in agreement with the norm or standard.

Verdict — the finding or decision of a jury on the matter submitted in trial; decision or judgment; opinion pronounced.

Waiver — the voluntary relinquishing of a known right.

Witness — one who testifies to facts within his or her own knowledge.

WONCA — World Organization of National Colleges, Academies, and Academic Associations of General Practitioners/Family Physicians.

Written authorization — a written statement to clothe with legal power; to empower.

Index

C

CPHA. *See* Commission on
Professional and Hospital Activities
CPT. *See Current Procedural
Terminology*
Criteria, defined, 644
Critical management, defined, 645
Current Medical Terminology, 466
Current Procedural Terminology, 466

D

Daily inpatient census, 129
See also Census
Data base, in problem-oriented medical
records, 181
Data collection, 65, 67
methods, 167
for research evaluation, 108, 109
Data development, 434-435
Data entries, 39-85
accuracy in, 61, 63-73
characteristics, 76
direct, 57
for documentation, 82
financial, 51-52, 53
identification, 41-51, 53
indirect, 57
locations of, 39
medical, 54, 57
need for updating, 82
as payment initiation, 82
social, 52
types, 40
updating, 82
as verification of care, 83
Data processing industry, and
confidentiality, 268-270
Data retrieval methods, 100
See also Retention and retrieval
systems
Data security
and hardware, 269-270
measures urged, 282
See also Confidentiality
Data systems, recommendations for,
279-280

Databanks in a Free Society, 265
Defendant, defined, 274
Deficiency, defined, 645
Delegation
and professional standards review
organizations, 655-656
of review, defined, 646
Denial, in medical audit, 646
Department of Health, Education and
Welfare, 158, 423
agencies of, 29
and confidentiality, 266
scope, 28
Deposition, defined, 274
Descriptive statistics, 111-151
frequency distribution, 145-146
hospital use of, 113-128
scales of measurement, 142,
144-145
Designing forms, 161-199
Development of data, 434-435
Development phase of systems analysis,
588-589
*Diagnostic and Statistical Manual of
Mental Disorders,* 468
Direct data entries, 57
Direct patient data, 57, 59
Discharge abstracting, 139
Discharge analysis, 122-126, 591
Discharge days, 127
Discharge planning, 104, 105
Discharge summaries, in problem-
oriented medical records, 185
Disease classification, 466, 467, 468
Doctor's office. *See* Physician's office
Documentation of health care, history,
2, 392
Duties. *See* Responsibilities

E

E.G. Meyer Memorial Hospital, 102
Education
and health care data, 92-93
patient, 198